Practical Management of Affective Disorders in Older People

Practical Management of Affective Disorders in Older People

A multi-professional approach

Edited by

Professor STEPHEN CURRAN
Consultant in Old Age Psychiatry
Fieldhead Hospital
Wakefield

and

Professor JOHN P WATTIS
Visiting Professor of Old Age Psychiatry
Centre for Health and Social Care Research
University of Huddersfield

Foreword by

Professor KEN WILSON
Professor of Old Age Psychiatry
University of Liverpool

Radcliffe Publishing
Oxford • New York

Radcliffe Publishing Ltd
18 Marcham Road
Abingdon
Oxon OX14 1AA
United Kingdom

www.radcliffe-oxford.com
Electronic catalogue and worldwide online ordering facility.

British Library Cataloguing in Publication Data

A catalogue record for this book is available from the British Library.

ISBN-13: 978 184619 101 5

Typeset by Pindar NZ (Egan Reid), Auckland, New Zealand
Printed and bound by TJI Digital, Padstow, Cornwall, UK

Contents

Foreword   vii
Preface   ix
About the editors   x
Contributors   xi

1   Affective disorders in the new millennium   1
    John P Wattis

2   Affective disorders in old age: detection and clinical
    features   17
    Cornelius Katona

3   Aetiology of late-life affective disorders   25
    Adrian Lloyd

4   Pharmacological management of depression in older
    people   54
    Stephen Curran, Andrew Byrne and John P Wattis

5   Pharmacological treatment of bipolar affective disorder in
    old age   80
    Naila Jawaid and Robert Baldwin

6   Electricity, magnetism and mood   94
    Susan Mary Benbow

7   Psychotherapy with older people   108
    Ian Andrew James

8   Depression in physically ill older patients   126
    Graham Mulley

9   Relationship between physical illness and affective
    disorders   144
    Richard Marriott

10 Depression in primary care   161
    Stephen Iliffe

11 The role of the nurse in the assessment, diagnosis and
    management of patients with affective disorders   173
    Richard Clibbens and Paula Rylatt

12 Occupational therapy and affective disorders   194
    Mary Duggan

13 Social services for older people with depression   205
    Jill Manthorpe

14 Carer and service user perspectives of affective disorders
    in older adults   217
    Virginia Minogue

15 Cultural aspects of affective disorders in older people   230
    Anilkumar Pillai

16 Religion/spirituality and depression in old age   242
    Rachel Dew and Harold Koenig

17 An overview of human drug development   253
    Chris Bushe

    Index   265

Foreword

This book shines a light into the dark room of depression. The editors have built a unique perspective through expert contributions from a wide range of specialists, service providers, service users and researchers. The reader is taken on an exciting and informative journey through current literature, contentious issues and the diversity of affective disorders in older people.

The first chapter gives an overview of depression and bipolar affective disorder in both a historical and contemporaneous context. The progression of subsequent chapters takes the reader deeper into diagnosis, aetiology and management. Having been provided with a strong foundation, the reader moves on to those areas that continually frustrate, puzzle and excite clinicians, researchers and service providers. Despite the paucity of research, these areas provide some of the most contentious and difficult challenges facing modern medicine. The relationships between affective disorders and physical health, cognitive integrity, psychosocial and spiritual aspects of the human condition are explored. These issues are reflected in the chapters devoted to intervention and management. Within these chapters are updates on electro-convulsive treatments and, interestingly, on the use of magnets in the treatment of depression. There is an easy-to-read but well-informed chapter on psychotherapy with useful case illustrations. The chapter relating to drug treatments is well founded in scientific evidence and also draws attention to the developing public interest in herbal and other remedies.

One of the main attractions of this book is the way in which the editors have managed to cater for an eclectic readership. In other books, this approach can be at the expense of focus and clarity. However, the complexity of affective disorders in older people and the acknowledged practice of working in multi-professional teams and crossing boundaries between secondary, primary and social care demands such an approach. The informed and useful inclusion of service users' perspectives and the innovative and interesting chapter on spirituality adds to the adventure.

There is no doubt that this book is good, fun and interesting. The editorial style makes it easy to read and the reader will come away with enthusiasm for working in this field, which is, after all, probably one of the most challenging and interesting fields you can be involved in.

Professor Ken Wilson
Professor of Old Age Psychiatry
University of Liverpool
February 2008

Preface

This is the fourth in a group of books for professionals working with the elderly. The parent book *Practical Psychiatry of Old Age* has proved popular and enduring and is now in its fourth edition. This introductory book has now been supplemented by multi-professional works which explore different areas of old age psychiatry in greater detail and from a variety of perspectives. *Practical Management of Dementia: a multi-professional approach* was the first of these. This was followed by *Practical Old Age Psychopharmacology: a multi-professional approach* and now by this volume on affective disorders.

Our aim in editing these multi-author works is not only to go into more depth than is possible in a general introductory text like *Practical Psychiatry of Old Age* but also to develop an overview from a variety of perspectives. This view is intended to provide a balanced and inclusive view about the different contributions of different disciplines, patients and carers into the practical management of the main disorders of mental health in old age.

In this volume we have invited chapters from a variety of experts on areas such as aetiology, diagnosis and psychological and pharmacological treatment. In addition, we have included chapters that adopt a more contextual approach to the management of affective disorders in areas like primary care and geriatric medicine. Other chapters look at what specific disciplines such as nursing, social work and occupational therapy have to offer. We have sought to include the user and carer viewpoint and the important and often neglected spiritual aspects of managing affective disorders. We trust, therefore, that this book will be a useful resource for all members of the multi-professional team. It will help them understand the contributions of other disciplines but most of all it will help them adopt a balanced and practical approach to the management of a very important group of disorders in old age.

Stephen Curran and John P Wattis
February 2008

About the editors

Stephen Curran works as a Consultant Old Age Psychiatrist in Wakefield and is a Visiting Professor in Old Age Psychiatry at the University of Huddersfield. He graduated in psychology in 1983 and completed his undergraduate medical training in 1986. He then worked as a Research Fellow and Lecturer in Old Age Psychiatry at the University of Leeds before moving to Wakefield in 1998. His research interests include old age psychopharmacology and drug monitoring. He is Director of the Ageing and Mental Health Research Group at the University as well as being Associate Medical Director for Education and Training.

John P Wattis is Visiting Professor of Psychiatry for Older Adults at Huddersfield. Before this appointment he was responsible for pioneering old age services in Leeds where he worked as a Consultant and Senior Lecturer for nearly 20 years. He completed his psychiatric training in Birmingham and Nottingham where he was Lecturer in the Department of Health Care of the Elderly that combined psychiatric and medical teams. He has experience of management as Medical Director of a large Community and Mental Health Trust. He is a former Chairman of the Faculty for Psychiatry of Old Age and the Higher Training Committee for General and Old Age Psychiatry at the Royal College of Psychiatrists. He has published research on the development of old age psychiatry services, alcohol abuse in old age, the prevalence of mental illness in geriatric medical patients, educational issues in old age psychiatry and outcomes of psychiatric care for older people. He has written or edited a number of books and contributed numerous chapters in the area of old age psychiatry and has been Director of Research and Development in three NHS Trusts. Prior to his retirement from his last NHS post in Huddersfield he trained as a life and executive coach. He now divides his time between his academic work in old age psychiatry, management support and coaching, mostly in the NHS setting, and extended weekends.

Contributors

Professor Robert Baldwin
Consultant Old Age Psychiatrist and Honorary Professor
Manchester Royal Infirmary
Manchester

Professor Susan Mary Benbow
Consultant Psychiatrist (Old Age Psychiatry)
Wolverhampton City PCT;
Professor of Mental Health and Ageing
Centre for Ageing and Mental Health
Staffordshire University

Dr Andrew Byrne
Specialist Registrar in Old Age Psychiatry
Calder Unit
Fieldhead Hospital
Wakefield

Dr Chris Bushe
Clinical Research Physician
Eli Lilly and Company Ltd
Basingstoke

Richard Clibbens
Nurse Consultant for Older People's Mental Health
Calder Unit
Fieldhead Hospital
Wakefield

Dr Rachel Dew
Research Fellow
Center for Ageing and Human Development
Duke University Medical Center
Durham, NC

Mary Duggan
Senior Portfolio Manager
Fieldhead Hospital
Wakefield

Professor Stephen Iliffe
Professor of Primary Care for Older People
Centre for Ageing Population Studies
Department of Primary Care and Population Studies
University College London

Dr Ian Andrew James
Clinical Psychologist and Head of Challenging Behaviour Service
Newcastle Centre for the Health of the Elderly
Newcastle General Hospital;
Research Tutor
Newcastle University

Dr Naila Jawaid
Consultant Psychiatrist in Old Age
Avenue Clinic
Nuneaton

Professor Cornelius Katona
Dean
Kent Institute of Medicine and Health Sciences
University of Kent;
Honorary Consultant Psychiatrist
Kent and Medway NHS and Social Care Partnership Trust

Professor Harold Koenig
Professor of Psychiatry and Behavioural Sciences and Associate Professor of
    Medicine
Duke University Medical Center
VA Medical Center
Durham, NC

Dr Adrian Lloyd
Consultant and Honorary Senior Clinical Lecturer
School of Neurology, Neurobiology and Psychiatry
University of Newcastle
Royal Victoria Infirmary
Newcastle upon Tyne

Professor Jill Manthorpe
Professor of Social Work and Director
Social Care Workforce Research Unit
King's College London

Dr Richard Marriott
Consultant Old Age Psychiatrist with a Special Interest in General Hospital
    Liaison Psychiatry
Calder Unit
Fieldhead Hospital
Wakefield

Dr Virginia Minogue
Head of West Yorkshire Mental Health Research and Development Consortium
Leeds

Professor Graham Mulley
Professor of Elderly Medicine
St James's University Hospital
Leeds

Dr Anilkumar Pillai
Consultant in Old Age Psychiatry
St Luke's Hospital
Huddersfield

Paula Rylatt
Specialist Practitioner in Psychosocial Interventions for Older People
South West Yorkshire Mental Health NHS Trust
Community Mental Health Team
Castleford, Normanton and District Hospital
Castleford

CHAPTER 1

Affective disorders in the new millennium

JOHN P WATTIS

Introduction

While concepts of depressed mood or melancholia have been with us for many centuries, it is only in the last 50 years or so that our understanding of the biochemistry and physiology of depression (and mania) have advanced significantly. 'Evidence-based' psychological and psychopharmacological treatments are also relatively recent, though the roots of psychodynamic therapy go back a little further. The whole evidence-based approach to healthcare[1] has resulted in a more standardised approach to treatment, exemplified in the National Institute for Clinical Excellence (NICE) guidance on the management of depression.[2] The social, political and economic contexts of psychiatric practice are changing rapidly. In the Western world the nuclear family has largely replaced the extended family and capitalism is now the dominant economic system worldwide. People in the richer countries have access to a wide range of treatments for mental disorder though these may be constrained in different ways depending on how healthcare is funded. Improvements in communication and the phenomenon of 'globalisation' have brought different cultures, religions and world-views into contact, sometimes resulting in positive collaborations and synthesis and sometimes in conflict.

Two trends are particularly relevant to the subject of affective disorders in old age at the beginning of the new millennium. The first is the vast shift in the age structure of the population, now affecting virtually all continents and cultures. Many developed countries now have 15% or more of the population in the over-65-years age group and numbers are increasing across the world. In the UK, the proportion of the population aged 65 and over has increased from around 5%

1

in 1900 to around 16% currently. Over the period 1971–2005, the percentage of people aged 65 and over increased from 13% to 16%. Within this age group even greater increases were seen for those aged 85 and over. The proportion of those aged 65 and over who were aged 85 and over increased from 7% in mid-1971 to 12% in mid-2005. The Office of National Statistics predicts that population ageing will continue during the first half of this century, since the proportion of the population aged 65 and over will increase as the large numbers of people born after the Second World War and during the 1960s baby boom become older. The proportion of population at working ages is set to fall as the baby boomers move into retirement and are replaced by the smaller numbers of people born in each year since the 1960s.[3] Reduced infant mortality and better healthcare generally now mean that other countries are undergoing a similar demographic shift.

The second major trend is the increasing synthesis of psychological, social, physical, spiritual and pharmacological viewpoints in the understanding and management of affective disorders. Biomedical sciences are no longer seen as necessarily in opposition to the 'softer' psychosocial sciences and the false opposition between science and religion is weakening. This is reflected in the contents and multidisciplinary authorship of this volume.

Depression is an important cause of morbidity and mortality in old age. Mania is much less common but can have a devastating impact when it does occur. In this introductory chapter we will first consider depression in some detail. Then we will consider mania and hypomania more briefly. In this overview, there will inevitably be some overlap with the contents of the chapters that follow and we will point to these as appropriate.

Depression

In this section we will consider the following.
- Clinical features.
- The classification of depression.
- Epidemiology, including:
  - associations with physical illness and disability/handicap
  - exercise
  - gender differences
  - detection and measurement of outcome.

Clinical features

Severe depression changes life completely. It affects behaviour, relationships, emotions, motivation, thinking, sleep and other somatic functions. The person who could mix well socially suddenly becomes isolated and reclusive. Everything is too much trouble. Personal appearance is neglected and the capacity for enjoyment is reduced. Appetite is often diminished, food is not enjoyed and weight is lost (though sometimes 'comfort eating' leads to weight gain). Often sleep is disrupted and waking early in the morning may be compounded by diurnal variation of mood with mood generally (but not always) worse first thing. Severe depression reduces motivation and slows mind and body. It distorts thinking and even memories, resulting in preoccupation with negative themes such as poor physical health, guilt, self-reproach and unworthiness. Agitation sometimes complicates depression and may paralyse the patient's capacity to make decisions or manifest itself in constant seeking for comfort and reassurance. Weepiness is more common in women than men but is often reported indirectly by friends, relatives and carers since the patient may feel she has to conceal her true feelings from strangers. Suicide risk is high, especially in men. Depression in older men differs in a number of respects from depression in older women (this is discussed in more detail in a later section).

Classification and definitions

The major international system for classifying diseases, *The International Classification of Diseases*, 10th edition (ICD-10),[4] groups all mood disorders together under seven main categories as follows:

F30   **Manic episode**
F31   **Bipolar affective disorder (includes recurrent mania)**
F32   **Depressive episode**
F33   **Recurrent depressive disorder**
F34   **Persistent mood disorder**
F38   **Other mood disorder**
F39   **Unspecified mood disorder.**

Each category is subdivided according to severity (mild, moderate or severe) and the presence or absence of psychotic symptoms. There are also coding provisions to record the presence or absence of somatic symptoms (anhedonia, mood worse in the morning and early morning waking). This generates around 30 different categories for depression, though in practice some are more common than others.

Unfortunately, the need for consistency in diagnosis can generate very complicated rules. For example, a diagnosis of *mild* depressive episode rests on the following:

1   The syndrome must be present for at least *two weeks*, there must be no history of mania/hypomania and the depression must not be attributable to organic disease or psychoactive substances (the difficulty of this will become evident when we examine associations with physical illness in more detail).
2   At least *two* of the following three symptoms must be present:
   a   Depressed mood to a degree that is definitely abnormal for the individual, present for most of the day and for almost every day, and largely uninfluenced by circumstances
   b   Loss of interest or pleasure in activities that are normally pleasurable
   c   Decreased energy or increased fatiguability.

3   Additional symptoms from the following list to give a total of at least four:
   a   Loss of confidence or self-esteem
   b   Unreasonable self-reproach or excessive and inappropriate guilt
   c   Recurrent thoughts of death or suicide; suicidal behaviour
   d   Complaints or evidence of diminished ability to think or concentrate, such as indecisiveness or vacillation
   e   Change in psychomotor activity with agitation or retardation (either subjective or objective)
   f   Sleep disturbance
   g   Change in appetite/weight.

To be classified as moderate, at least *two symptoms* from list 2 above and additional symptoms from section 3, to a total of six, must be present. To meet the criteria for severe depression: all three symptoms from section 2 must be present and at least *five* from section 3 (at least *eight symptoms from 2 and 3 in total*).

Depressive episodes (F32), whether or not occurring in the context of *recurrent depressive disorder* (F33) or *bipolar disorders* (F31), and *manic or hypomanic episodes* (F30) are our main concern in this volume. However, *dysthymia (F34.1)* is also important. It describes people whose outlook is persistently depressed but whose depression is not sufficiently severe or acute in onset to be described as a depressive episode. Anxiety symptoms are often prominent. The relationship between dysthymia and depressive disorder is not exclusive. Dysthymia may follow or complicate a depressive episode and it is not always clear that they are different conditions either in terms of causation or treatment.

Epidemiologists and others who research into the relationships between depression and other conditions in old age often resort to less complicated definitions. The main diagnostic classifications (and the rating scales developed from them) have largely been developed in relation to younger adult patients and may not always be applicable to older adults.[5] In addition epidemiologists have to employ case-finding instruments which may be *mapped* on to diagnostic systems but may employ variable definitions of 'caseness'. *Pervasive depression* has been used as a term to define a level of caseness that defines depression of a type and severity likely to warrant medical or psychological intervention. Depression in epidemiological studies is diagnosed using instruments such as the Geriatric Mental State (GMS) Examination[6] or the Short-CARE[7] schedule. Sometimes self-assessment measures such as the Geriatric Depression Scale (GDS),[8] the Brief Assessment Schedule for Depression in the Elderly-Cards (BASDEC)[9] or the Hospital Anxiety and Depression (HAD) scale[10,11,12] are used. The correspondence between the categories produced by these latter scales and the more rigorous categories of the ICD-10[4] and the American Diagnostic and Statistical Manual (DSM-IV)[13] is at times sketchy. However, even the simplest self-assessment scales like the HAD measure something that can properly be described as depression and that responds to treatment.

Epidemiology

In this section we consider the prevalence of depression in old age and its associations with other diagnoses, disabilities, handicaps and social factors. Depression is associated with increased mortality.[14,15] Depressive disorder is essentially treatable but under-diagnosed and under-treated in many different settings[14,16–19] and its higher prevalence in particular groups makes people in those groups ideal candidates for early detection and intervention.

When we are considering prevalence, we need to distinguish carefully between overall prevalence and the prevalence of depression in subgroups which, for one reason or another, are at higher risk of developing or continuing to suffer from depressed mood. For example, a large-scale epidemiological study using the GMS[20] showed that having *ever* been a heavy drinker (for a period of at least two years) increased the relative risk of depression in old age fourfold. Depression is more common among elderly acute medical inpatients,[21] among disabled isolated elders[22] and in residential settings.[23] It contributes to morbidity, mortality and increased usage of non-psychiatric medical services.[24] These associations are often complicated and difficult to tease out. Overall, *pervasive depression* probably affects around 12% or 13% at any one time (past month 'point' prevalence),[25] but only about 2–3% of older people have a depression that would meet the categoric criteria for severe *depressive episode*. There has long been conflict of opinion about whether depression is more or less common with increasing age. One study showed that prevalence of depression increased over the age of 80 years but that this was mostly associated with chronic health problems and functional impairment rather than a direct effect of ageing.[26]

We will now briefly examine the prevalence of depression in different settings, in different ethnic groups and cultures, and in different sexes. We will also consider the effect of depression upon mortality, and its association with different illnesses, social factors, disability and handicap. Some of these issues will be addressed at greater length in later chapters of the book.

Depression in different settings

In residential homes[23] and hospitals[21] depression is two or three times more common than in the community. One Italian study showed a very high prevalence of 20% 'major' depression, 4% dysthymic disorders and 13% 'atypical' depression in a geriatric day hospital where there was no distinct old age psychiatry service,[27] emphasising the interaction between patterns of service and apparent prevalence. A UK study, using the GMS, of people in receipt of Home Care services found the prevalence of depression to be 26%, half of it severe, and often not recognised.[28] A follow-up study of older medical inpatients showed that, when physical illness was controlled for, those who were depressed before discharge saw physicians more frequently, were more often hospitalised and more often needed nursing home care than controls without depression.[29]

Depression, culture and ethnicity

There have been few studies of the symptomatology, prevalence or outcome of depression by race. One relatively large-scale study suggested there is at least little difference in symptomatology between African-Americans and non-African-Americans.[30] A European study using the same case-finding methods in a number of different countries found a wide variation in prevalence from 9% in Iceland to 24% in Munich. The difference was even marked between two UK cities, London (17%) and Liverpool (10%).[31] Explanations for these differences are only speculative at present but the issue of depression and culture is addressed at greater length in Chapter 15.

Depression and mortality

Overall, point prevalence of depressed mood (mostly DSM-III dysthymia) did not predict short-term mortality among the elderly in the community when other factors such as high age, gender, smoking, disability, somatic illnesses and number of medications taken was controlled for.[32] However, depression persisting over five years was associated with increased mortality.[33] Also, given the associations between hypertension, heart disease and cancer and depression discussed later, there remains a question as to how logical it is to control for physical illness which is itself associated with disability and depression. Another, hospital study, reported later,[34] showed an association between depressed mood (measured dimensionally using the HAD) and increased mortality.

Depression and physical illness

One carefully controlled large-scale (n=1286) study with a four year follow-up showed that older people who reported depressive symptoms were at higher risk of subsequent physical decline in simple tests of motor function (odds ratio 1.55; 95% CI 1.02–2.34).[35] For medical inpatients (n=454), high depression scores on the HAD were associated with mortality at 22 months (multivariate odds ratio 1.9; 95% CI 1.2–3.1, p<0.01).[34] Another study of outcome for depressed patients in hospital with physical disability showed that, on average 47 weeks after discharge, depression and disability varied together,[36] furnishing further evidence of the strong links between depression and disability in old people that will be explored further later. An interesting ethnic difference emerged in this study in that black people tended to have a better outcome for mood regardless of whether or not physical disability improved.

Moving to more specific associations, cardiovascular disease, cancer, stroke, hypertension and diabetes are all associated with depression.[37] In a Finnish community study, coronary heart disease, physical disability, and widowhood or divorce were associated with self-reported depression in men. In women the association was between a history of clinical depression, physical disability and the use of angiotensin-converting enzyme inhibitors and depression.[38] A prospective hospital-based study in the USA of people having elective cardiac catheterisation for coronary artery disease showed that at the time of catheterisation self-reported physical function differed by the number of arteries stenosed, and by observer-rated baseline anxiety and depression quartiles. Deterioration in physical function at one year was associated with baseline anxiety or depression but not with baseline artery status. Surgical or medical treatment seemed to neutralise the effect of coronary stenosis on physical function at one year but not the negative effect of baseline anxiety or depression.[39] The association between depression and heart disease is strong and depression may precede as well as follow heart disease.[40]

Another large-scale study (n=4825) showed that, after controlling for other known risk factors, depressed mood persisting over six years increased the hazard ratio for developing cancer to 1.88 (95% CI =1.13–3.14). This risk was consistent across most kinds of cancer and was not confined to cigarette smokers.[41]

A thorough evaluation of 277 patients from three to four months after an ischaemic stroke[42] found DSM-III-R major depression in 26% and minor depression in a further 14%. Major depression with no explanatory factor apart from stroke was present in 18%. Analysis showed that dependency in daily life was associated with an increased risk of depression (odds ratio [OR] 1.8; 95% CI 1.1–3.1) with an even greater association with major depression (OR 2.0; 95% CI 1.6–5.5). Previous episodes of depression were also associated with a markedly increased risk of post-stroke depression. A survey of stroke and hip fracture survivors living in private households[43] found high levels (41%) of HAD depression or anxiety and of severe or very severe disability (57%). Not surprisingly, there was a strong association between severe disability and anxiety (p<0.0005 OR not given) and severe disability and depression (p<0.0001). These authors also looked at the impact of social contact and found that there was a strong association between social contact and lower prevalence of anxiety (p<0.01) or depression (p<0.0001). The association with stroke is not only that of depression as a post-stroke phenomenon but also as a possible risk factor for stroke.[44] Caregivers also may become anxious or depressed following a stroke in the person they look after. Survivors of stroke and their relatives were asked at six months to complete the General Health Questionnaire (GHQ – a measure of emotional distress) and the HAD. Over half the carers were in the abnormal range on the GHQ. Caregivers were more likely to be depressed if the patients were severely dependent or emotionally distressed themselves (p<0.01, OR not quoted).[45]

Depression is common, though notoriously difficult to diagnose, in Parkinson's disease (PD). Symptoms such as cognitive slowing (bradyphrenia) are hard to distinguish from psychomotor retardation. One study found major depression in 16.5% and dysthymia and other forms of depression in 25.7% of patients with PD. Low abilities in activities of daily living correlated with the diagnosis of depressive disorder and with high scores on the Hamilton Depression Rating Scale (an observer rating scale commonly used in trials of antidepressants).[46]

Depression and dementia

A review of depression in dementia estimated 17–30% of patients have depressive symptoms. Depression-related behavioural problems in patients with Alzheimer's dementia were distressing to caregivers. This was reflected by a prevalence of over 75% of depressed mood in those caring for patients with both dementia and depression.[47] A study of over 1000 older people in a district of Stockholm, Sweden found a surprisingly high prevalence of dementia (28% by DSM-III-R criteria). More importantly for present purposes, it found the prevalence of major depression at around 12% was around three times higher than in the non-demented. Increased disability was associated with major depression in both demented and non-demented subjects.[48] A French incidence study in which 397 older people with subclinical cognitive impairment were followed up over three years found 11% developing dementia without depression and 5% dementia with depression. Those with dementia plus depression showed significantly greater decrements at three years in dressing, washing, use of the telephone and continence.[49]

Depression, impairment, disability, handicap and social factors

Conditions such as depression produce impairments of function that result in a loss of ability (disability). The social response (or lack of response) to this can produce handicap. Depression is very common in selected groups of old people with a variety of disabling illnesses (and in those caring for them). Depression is often associated with increased disability and the direction of causality may be both ways. There are also hints in the studies cited above of a protective effect against depression through social contacts. This takes us back to the now classic study by Murphy on the social origins of depression in old age.[50] She found an association between severe life events, major social difficulties, poor physical health and the onset of depression. Working class subjects had a higher incidence of depression and this was associated with both poorer health and greater social difficulties. Lack of a confiding relationship (associated with lifelong personality traits) increased vulnerability to depression. A more recent large-scale study failed to support some of these findings but it clearly demonstrated a link between declining health, increasing disability and the onset of depression.[51] Further clarification of the relationship between impairment, disability, handicap, depression and social factors was provided by the 'Gospel Oak' series of studies in London. The prevalence of 'pervasive' depression in this relatively deprived area was 17%. Impairment, disability and particularly handicap were strongly associated with depression. The adjusted odds ratio for depression in the most handicapped quartile compared to the least was 24.2 (95% CI 8.8–66.6). Adjusting for handicap abolished or weakened most of the associations between depression and social support, income, older age, female gender and living alone.[52] When the overarching effect of handicap was put aside there was a moderate association between depression and the number of life events experienced over the previous year. Personal illness, bereavement and theft were reported as the most salient events. There was a stronger relationship between the number of social support deficits and depression. Social support deficits also related to age, handicap, loneliness and the use of home care services. Loneliness was itself associated with depression (OR 12.4 (7.6–20)).[53] A follow-up study a year later found that the one-year onset rate for pervasive depression was 12% and the maintenance rate for those initially depressed 63%. There was a high mortality rate among depressed people. Disablement, especially handicap, was the strongest predictor of onset of depression. Lack of contact with friends was a risk factor for onset of depression. For men marriage was protective, but for women it was a risk factor. Maintenance of existing depression was predicted by low levels of social support and social participation rather than by disablement.[54] Intervention studies are needed to see how far enhanced social support and opportunities for participation can contribute to reducing duration of depression.

Exercise and depression

The image of inactive, isolated, depressed old people, evoked by the studies above, contrasts with emerging research on the benefits of exercise in treating mild to moderate depression. In the UK, evidence-based NICE guidance on the management of depression[2] recommends that GPs should prescribe exercise as a first line treatment for mild to moderate depression. There is evidence that exercise improves the outcome for older adults with poorly responsive depressive symptoms[55] and the Mental Health Foundation has issued a report and run a campaign to make GPs aware of the 'exercise option' in treating mild to moderate depression in all age groups.[56] A systematic review of the effects of exercise on depressive symptoms in old people[57] points in the same direction but cautions that more research is needed. Given the beneficial effects of exercise on cardiovascular disease, diabetes and hypertension, the known association between these disorders and depression and the incidental social benefits of engaging in an exercise programme, there seems little doubt that exercise programmes should be recommended for the treatment and perhaps for the prevention of mild to moderate depression in old age. They may also prove to have a secondary preventative effect in people who have recovered from a major depression.

Gender differences in depression

Depression is less common in older men in the community than in older women. Robust epidemiological studies have shown that the overall prevalence of depression in the over sixty-fives is around 12% (14% for women and 8% for men).[31] In selected groups, however, depression may be more common in men than women. For example, a community study in Perth showed that four months after stroke there was no significant difference between the rates of depression in men and women but at 12-month follow-up over three-quarters of the men remained depressed whereas most of the women had recovered.[58] Unfortunately, the study did not examine incident cases of depression over the study period. A population-based study of older people with coronary heart disease also showed a relatively higher prevalence in men (29%) compared with women (20%).[38]

The presentation of depression may also be different. In focus groups conducted in the USA by the National Institute of Mental Health to assess depression awareness,[59] men described their own symptoms of depression without realising that they were depressed. Many were unaware that 'physical' symptoms, such as headaches, digestive disorders, and chronic pain, could be associated with depression. In addition, they feared that contact with mental health services or being labelled with a diagnosis of mental illness would cost them the respect of their family and friends, or their standing in the community.

The interplay between physical symptoms and physical disease is complicated. As we have seen above, men with major cardiovascular disease may be more likely to be depressed than women with the same problems. At the same time, they may be less likely to acknowledge depressed mood, manifesting it by preoccupation with physical symptoms and health anxiety.

Some think that the relatively low prevalence of depression in older men (only two-thirds that in older women) is an artefact because depression is less likely to be recognised in older men. However, recent research[60] suggested that the genetic basis of severe (early onset) depression in men and women may be different. Certainly, depressed older men often describe their symptoms differently.

The profile of older people who deliberately self-harm more closely approximates to the profile of those who kill themselves than to the profile of younger people who deliberately self-harm.[61] This implies that older people who self-harm are more often 'failed' suicides than people who are making a 'cry for help'. At all ages, men are more likely to kill themselves than women. One study showed that contact with mental health services is lower for males under 65 and for both sexes over 65 years.[62] General Practice contact rates were higher but still lower for men than women with one study finding a higher GP consultation rate in older people (though not necessarily for overt depression).[63]

Detecting depression and measuring outcome

In this section we will not be concerned with diagnostic interview schedules such as the GMS,[6] Short-CARE[7] and others which are largely used in epidemiological research or in-depth observer rater scales such as the Montgomery Asberg Scale[64] and similar scales used mostly to rate outcomes in drug trials. We will consider the importance of a high 'index of suspicion' for the diagnosis of depression in older people, particularly those in 'high risk' groups and look at short scales that can be used effectively, especially in high risk populations, to enhance the diagnosis of depression and for the systematic evaluation of outcome in routine clinical practice with depressed old people.

'Screening' for depression in older people

Screening is generally more effective in high risk populations. The geriatric depression scale (GDS) is most widely used for this purpose. It has been validated in a variety of settings, cultures and languages[65] and a number of short forms have been developed.[66–68] The BASDEC[9,69] is a simple card-sort test which has been validated in an inpatient geriatric population. It has a potential advantage in that the questions are repeated in different languages on the reverse of the card but it has not been validated across cultures or different languages. The EBAS-DEP[70] is a related scale. As even five questions from the GDS appear reasonably sensitive and specific at least in a setting with a high prevalence (46%) of depression,[68] it may be that the value of these scales is as much in prompting clinicians always to ask about depression as in their intrinsic psychometric properties. Certainly, one study has shown that systematising the information already gathered when patients are admitted to acute geriatric inpatient care can potentially result in higher detection rates.[71]

Measuring outcome for depression in old people

Patient self-report is the most obvious way to measure outcome. When a variety of different interviewers are involved, a self-rating scale such as the GDS has obvious advantages in ensuring that the same factors are being considered. The Hospital Anxiety and Depression Scale, which does not work well as a screening instrument in geriatric inpatients,[72] does, however, correlate well with more sophisticated measures of severity[11,12] and appears to function well as an outcome measure in depressed elderly psychiatric inpatients.[73]

Mania and hypomania

Research into mania/hypomania specifically in old age is relatively limited.

ICD-10[4] defines *hypomania* as a disorder characterised by persistent mild elevation of mood, increased energy and activity and usually marked feelings of well-being and both physical and mental efficiency. Increased sociability, talkativeness and other features are present but *not to the extent* that they lead to severe disruption or social rejection. Especially in older subjects, irritability (and sometimes suspiciousness) may take the place of the usual euphoria. *Manic* patients show a more severe degree of the same symptoms with excitability, loss of attention and concentration and pressure of speech and activity of a degree that significantly interferes with normal function. In *mania with psychotic symptoms* delusions, hallucinations or complete incoherence complicate the picture. Sometimes these states may be hard to distinguish from some forms of *excited delirium* and it is therefore important for the health professional to consider the possibility of underlying physical disorder. Single episodes of mania are rare. By convention, repeated episodes of mania or hypomania along with the more usual pattern of depressive episodes interspersed with mania/hypomania are classified as 'bipolar' disorders. The relationship between mania and depression was recognised by Kraepelin[74] when he developed the concept of manic-depressive illness. He and other more recent authors[75] emphasised the occurrence of mixed states where some depressive and some manic symptoms coexisted and early accounts suggested these were more common in old age, though systematic analyses have shown no significant differences in clinical features between older and younger patients with bipolar disorder.[76] One-year prevalence of mania in the over sixty-fives is only 0.1%, but they are over-represented in specialised old age psychiatry inpatient units, accounting for up to 12% of admissions.[77]

Though mania and hypomania often show themselves at an early age in bipolar disorder, some patients with recurrent depressive disorder develop mania or hypomania for the first time in late life. There is some evidence that this may be due to the precipitation of these conditions by organic brain damage (up to 40%) which does not necessarily presage dementia.[76,78,79]

Treatment of depression and mania in old age is affected by different susceptibilities to the side-effects of treatment and sometimes by changes in the metabolism or renal clearance of drugs, especially lithium (see later).

Conclusions

In this chapter we have reviewed the basic facts about the definition, impact, diagnostic classification and associations of affective disorders in old age. We have emphasised how the changing age structure of the population makes management of affective disorders in old age a key priority. The association of depression with mortality and morbidity leads to the conclusion that the detection and treatment of depression in late life is very worthwhile and simple, brief self-rating scales can assist both in detection and in measuring the outcomes of intervention. Depression is particularly prevalent in certain settings and in association with particular conditions and it is in these settings that screening is likely to be most effective.

Mania or hypomania may be part of a lifelong bipolar disorder or may arise for the first time in late life. Onset may be associated with non-dementing organic brain damage and possible precipitation by medical conditions or treatment. A distinction should be made between mania and excited delirium where the treatment of the underlying medical condition is vital.

We have tried to support the trend towards synthesising different areas of knowledge and practice to promote a holistic approach to the management of these disorders. Their understanding and management includes medical, psychological, physical, social, occupational and spiritual perspectives. The structure of this book aims to provide some depth in understanding of detection and diagnosis, aetiology, psychological and physical treatment and some breadth by considering the perspectives of psychiatry, primary care and geriatric medicine, social work, nursing and therapy professions. In addition we have asked contributors to look specifically at the often neglected cultural and spiritual dimensions and have asked another contributor to look at drug developments and future treatments.

KEY POINTS

▶ Increasing numbers of old people and the high prevalence of affective disorders (especially depression with its associated morbidity and mortality) make this a vital area of practical concern.

▶ The association with chronic physical illness, disability and social deprivation means that primary care practitioners, social workers and clinicians in geriatric medicine need to be alive to the possibility of depressive illness and its management.

▶ While mania and hypomania are less common than depressive disorder in old age they are potentially very destructive and hard to manage when they occur.

▶ Close cooperation with specialist old age psychiatry services is necessary for the effective management of more severe depressive disorder and probably in virtually all cases of mania and hypomania.

▶ Good management of these disorders is inevitably multifaceted, taking into account physical, psychological, pharmacological and social perspectives. It demands a team approach.

REFERENCES

1 Sackett DL, Tugwell P, Guyatt, G. *Clinical Epidemiology: a basic science for clinical medicine.* 2nd ed. Philadelphia: Lippincott-Raven; 1991.

2 National Institute for Clinical Excellence. *Depression: management of depression in primary and secondary care* (CG023); 2004. Available from: http://www.nice.org.uk/CG023NICEguideline

3 Office of National Statistics. http://www.statistics.gov.uk/CCI/nugget.asp?ID=949&Pos=&ColRank=1&Rank=326 (accessed 2006).

4 World Health Organization. *The ICD-10 Classification of Mental and Behavioural Disorders: clinical descriptions and diagnostic guidelines.* Geneva: World Health Organization; 1992.

5 Weiss IK, Nagel CL, Aronson MK. Applicability of depression scales to the old person. *J Am Geriatr Soc.* 1986; **34**: 215–18.

6 Copeland JRM, Kelleher MJ, Kellet JM, *et al.* A semi-structured clinical interview for the assessment and diagnosis of mental state in the elderly: the Geriatric Mental Status schedule. *Psychol Med.* 1976; **6**: 439-49.

7 Gurland B, Golden RR, Teresi JA, *et al.* The SHORT-CARE: an efficient instrument for the assessment of depression, dementia and disability. *J Gerontol.* 1984; **39**: 166–9.

8 Herrmann N, Mittmann N, Silver IL, *et al.* A validation study of the Geriatric Depression Scale short form. *Int J Geriatr Psychiatr.* 1996; **11**: 457–60.

9 Adshead F, Day Cody D, Pitt B. BASDEC: a novel screening instrument for depression in elderly medical inpatients. *BMJ.* 1992; **305**: 397.

10 Zigmond A, Snaith P. The hospital anxiety and depression scale (HAD). *Acta Psychiatr Scand.* 1983; **67**: 361–70.

11 Kenn C, Wood H, Kucyj M, *et al.* Validation of the Hospital Anxiety and Depression Rating Scale (HADS) in an elderly psychiatric population. *Int J Geriatr Psychiatr.* 1987; **2**: 189–93.

12 Wattis J, Burn WK, McKenzie FR, *et al.* Correlation between Hospital Anxiety Depression (HAD) scale and other measures of anxiety and depression in geriatric patients. *Int J Geriatr Psychiatr.* 1994; **9**: 61–3.

13 American Psychiatric Association. *Diagnostic and Statistical Manual of Mental Disorders: (DSM-IV).* 4th ed. Washington, DC: APA; 1994.

14 Murphy E, Smith R, Lindesay J, *et al.* Increased mortality rates in late life depression. *Br J Psychiatr.* 1988; **152**: 347–53.

15 Pulska T, Pahkala K, Laippala P, *et al.* Follow up study of longstanding depression as predictor of mortality in elderly people living in the community. *BMJ.* 1999; **318**: 432–3.

16 Green BH, Copeland JRM, Dewey ME, *et al.* Factors associated with recovery and recurrence of depression in older people: a prospective study. *Int J Geriatr Psychiatr.* 1994; **9**: 789–95.

17 Koenig HG, Meador KG, Cohen HJ, *et al.* Detection and treatment of major depression in older medically ill hospitalised patients. *Int J Psychiatr and Med.* 1988; **18**: 17–31.

18 Baldwin B. Late life depression: undertreated? *BMJ.* 1988; **296**: 519.

19 Snowdon J, Burgess E, Vaughan R, *et al.* Use of antidepressants, and the prevalence of depression and cognitive impairment in Sydney nursing homes. *Int J Geriatr Psychiatr.* 1996; **11**: 599–606.

20 Saunders PA, Copeland JRM, Dewey ME, *et al.* Heavy drinking as a risk factor for depression and dementia in elderly men: findings from the Liverpool longitudinal community study. *Br J Psychiatr.* 1991; **159**: 213–16.

21 Burn WK, Davies KN, McKenzie FR, *et al.* The prevalence of psychiatric illness in acute geriatric admissions. *Int J Geriatr Psychiatr.* 1993; **8**: 171–4.

22 Prince MJ, Harwood RH, Blizard RA, *et al.* Impairment, disability and handicap as risk factors for depression in old age: the Gospel Oak Project V. *Psychol Med.* 1997; **27**: 311–21.

23 Mann A, Graham N, Ashby D. Psychiatric illness in residential homes for the elderly: a survey in one London borough. *Age Ageing.* 1984; **13**: 257–65.

24 Beekman AT, Deeg DJ, Braam AW, *et al.* Consequences of major and minor depression in later life: a study of disability, well-being and service utilisation. *Psychol Med.* 1997; **27**: 1397–409.

25 Gurland BJ. The comparative frequency of depression in various age groups. *J Gerontol.* 1976; **31**: 283–92.

26 Roberts RE, Kaplan GA, Shema SJ, *et al.* Does growing old increase the risk for depression? *Am J Psychiatr.* 1997; **154**: 1384–90.

27 Turrina C, Siciliani O, Dewey ME, *et al.* Psychiatric disorders among elderly patients attending a geriatric day hospital: prevalence according to clinical diagnosis (DSMIIIR) and AGECAT. *Int J Geriatr Psychiatr.* 1992; **7**: 499–504.

28 Banerjee S. Prevalence and recognition rates of psychiatric disorder in the elderly clients of a community care service. *Int J Geriatr Psychiatr.* 1993; **8**: 125–31.

29 Koenig HG, Kuchibhatla M. Use of health services by medically ill depressed elderly patients after hospital discharge. *Am J Geriatr Psychiatr.* 1999; **7**: 48–56.

30 Blazer DG, Landerman LR, Hays JC, *et al.* Symptoms of depression among community-dwelling elderly African-American and white older adults. *Psychol Med.* 1998; **28**: 1311–20.

31 Copeland JRM, Beekman AT, Dewey ME, *et al.* Depression in Europe: geographical distribution among older people. *Br J Psychiatr.* 1999; **174**: 312–21.

32 Pulska T, Pahkala K, Laippala P, *et al.* Six-year survival of depressed elderly Finns: a community study. *Int J Geriatr Psychiatr.* 1997; **12**: 942–50.

33 Pulska T, Pahkala K, Laippala P, *et al.* Follow up study of long-standing depression as a predictor of mortality in elderly people living in the community. *BMJ.* 1999; **318**: 432–3.

34 Herrmann C, Brand-Driehorst S, Kaminsky B, *et al.* Diagnostic groups and depressed mood as predictors of 22-month mortality in medical inpatients. *Psychosom Med.* 1998; **60**: 570–7.

35 Penninx BW, Guralnik JM, Ferrucci L, *et al.* Depressive symptoms and physical decline in community-dwelling older persons. *JAMA.* 1998; **279**: 1720–6.

36 Koenig HG, George LK. Depression and physical disability outcomes in depressed medically ill hospitalised older adults. *Am J Geriatr Psychiatr.* 1998; **6**: 230–47.

37 Dinan TG. The physical consequences of depressive illness. *BMJ.* 1999; **318**: 826.

38 Ahto M, Isoaho R, Puolijoki H, *et al.* Coronary heart disease and depression in the elderly: a population based study. *J Fam Pract.* 1997; **14**: 436–45.

39 Sullivan MD, LaCroix AZ, Baum C, *et al.* Functional status in coronary artery disease: a one year prospective follow up of the role of anxiety and depression. *Am J Med.* 1997; **103**: 348–56.

40 Ferketich A, Scwartzbaum J, Frid D, *et al.* Depression as an antecedent to heart disease among women and men in the NHANES I Study. *Arch Intern Med.* 2000; **160**: 1261–8.

41 Penninx BW, Guralnick JM, Pahor M, *et al.* Chronically depressed mood and cancer risk in older persons. *J Nat Cancer Inst.* 1998; **90**: 1888–93.

42 Pohjasvara T, Leppavuori A, Siira I, *et al.* Frequency and clinical determinants of poststroke depression. *Stroke.* 1998; **29**: 2311–17.

43 Bond J, Gregson B, Smith M, *et al.* Outcomes following acute hospital care for stroke or hip fracture: how useful is an assessment of anxiety or depression for older people? *Int J Geriatr Psychiatr.* 1998; **13**: 601–10.

44 Williams LS. Depression and stroke: cause or consequence? *Semin Neurol.* 2005; **25**: 396–409.

45 Dennis M, O'Rourke S, Lewis S, *et al.* A quantitative study of the emotional outcome of people caring for stroke survivors. *Stroke.* 1998; **29**: 1867–72.

46 Liu CY, Wang SJ, Fuh JL, *et al.* The correlation of depression with functional activity in Parkinson's disease. *Neurol.* 1997; **244**: 493–8.

47 Teri L. Behavior and caregiver burden: behavioral problems in patients with Alzheimer disease and its association with caregiver distress. *Alzheimer Dis Assoc Disord.* 1997; **11**(Suppl. 4): S35–8.

48 Forsell Y, Winblad B. Major depression in a population of demented and nondemented older people: prevalence and correlates. *J Am Geriatr Soc.* 1998; **46**: 27–30.

49 Ritchie K, Touchon J, Ledesert B. Progressive disability in senile dementia is accelerated in the presence of depression. *Int J Geriatr Psychiatr.* 1998; **13**: 459–61.

50 Murphy E. The social origins of depression in old age. *Br J Psychiatr.* 1982; **141**: 135–42.

51 Kennedy GJ, Kelman HR, Thomas C. The emergence of depressive symptoms in late life: the importance of declining health and increasing disability. *J Commun Health.* 1990; **15**: 93–104.

52 Prince MJ, Harwood RH, Blizard RA, *et al.* Impairment, disability and handicap as risk factors for depression in old age: the Gospel Oak Project V. *Psychol Med.* 1997; **27**: 311–21.

53 Prince MJ, Harwood RH, Blizard RA, *et al.* Social support deficits, loneliness and life events as risk factors for depression in old age. The Gospel Oak Project VI. *Psychol Med.* 1997; **27**: 323–32.

54 Prince MJ, Harwood RH, Blizard RA, *et al.* A prospective population-based study of the effects of disablement and social milieu on the onset and maintenance of late-life depression: the Gospel Oak Project VII. *Psychol Med.* 1998; **28**: 337–50.

55 Mather AS, Rodriguez C, Guthrie MF, *et al.* Effects of exercise on depressive symptoms in older adults with poorly responsive depressive disorder. *Br J Psychiatr.* 2002; **180**: 411–15.

56 The Mental Health Foundation. *Up and Running: the role of exercise therapy in mild to moderate depression in primary care.* London: MHF; 2005.

57 Sjosten N, Kevela SL. The effects of physical exercise on depressive symptoms among the aged: a systematic review. *Int J Geriatr Psychiatr.* 2006; **21**: 410–18.

58 Burvill PW, Johnson KA, Jamrozik KD, *et al.* Prevalence of depression after stroke: the Perth community stroke study. *Br J Psychiatr.* 1995; **166**: 320–7.

59 National Institute of Mental Health. http://menanddepression.nimh.nih.gov/clientfiles/menanddep.pdf (last accessed October 2006).

60 New Scientist News. http://www.newscientist.com/article.ns?id=dn2104 (last accessed October 2006).

61 Nowers M. Deliberate self-harm in the elderly: a survey in one London borough. *Int J Geriatr Psychiatr.* 1993; **8**: 609–14.

62 Evans J. The health service contacts of 87 suicides. *Psych Bull.* 1994; **18**: 548–50.

63 Vassilas CA, Morgan HG. General practitioners' contact with victims of suicide. *BMJ.* 1993; **307**: 300–1.

64 Montgomery S, Asberg M, Jornestedt L, *et al.* Reliability of the CPRS between the disciplines of psychiatry, general practice, nursing and psychology in depressed patients. *Acta Psychiatr Scand.* 1978; **271** (suppl.): S29–32.

65 Montorio I, Izal M. The Geriatric Depression Scale: a review of its development and utility. *Int Psychogeriatr.* 1996; **8**: 103–12.

66 Lesher EL, Berryhill JS. Validation of the Geriatric Depression Scale – Short Form amongst inpatients. *J Clin Psych.* 1994; **50**: 256–60.

67 Shah A, Herbert R, Lewis S, *et al.* Screening for depression among acutely ill geriatric inpatients with a short Geriatric Depression Scale. *Age Ageing.* 1997; **26**: 217–21.

68 Hoyl MT, Alessi CA, Harker JO, *et al.* Development and testing of a five-item version of the Geriatric Depression Scale. *J Am Geriatr Soc.* 1999; **47**: 873–8.

69 Loke B, Nicklason F, Burvill P. Screening for depression: clinical validation of geriatricians' diagnosis, the Brief Assessment Schedule Depression Cards and the 5-item version of the Symptom Check List among non-demented geriatric inpatients. *Int J Geriatr Psychiatr.* 1996; **11**: 461–5.

70 Allen N, Ames D, Ashby D, *et al.* A brief sensitive screening instrument for depression in late life. *Age Ageing.* 1994; **23**: 213–8.

71 Hammond MF, O'Keeffe ST, Barer DH. Development and validation of a brief observer-rated screening scale for depression in elderly medical patients. *Age Ageing.* 2000; **29**: 511–15.

72 Davies KN, Burn WK, McKenzie FR, *et al.* Evaluation of the Hospital Anxiety and Depression scale as a screening instrument in geriatric medical inpatients. *Int J Geriatr Psychiatr.* 1993; **8**: 165–9.

73 Wattis JP, Butler A, Martin C, *et al.* Outcome of admission to an acute psychiatric facility for older people: a pluralistic evaluation. *Int J Geriatr Psychiatr.* 1994; **9**: 835–40.

74 Kraeplin E. *Manic Depressive Insanity and Paranoia.* Edinburgh: Livingston; 1921 (reprinted New York: Ages Company Publishers; 1976).

75 Clothier J, Swann AC, Freeman T. Dysphoric mania. *J Clin Psychopharm.* 1992; **12**(Suppl.), S13–16.

76 Broadhead J, Jacoby R. Mania in old age: a first prospective study. *Int J Geriatr Psychiatr.* 1990; **5**: 212–22.

77 Shulman K. Mania. In: Butler R, Pitt B, editors. *Seminars in Old Age Psychiatry.* London: Gaskell; 1998.

78 Shulman K, Post F. Bipolar affective disorder in old age. *Br J Psychiatr.* 1980; **136**: 26–32.

79 Shulman K, Tohen M, Satlin A, *et al.* Mania compared with unipolar depression in old age. *Am J Psychiat.* 1992; **149**: 341–5.

CHAPTER 2

Affective disorders in old age: detection and clinical features

CORNELIUS KATONA

Introduction

The syndromes included within this chapter include major depression, bipolar disorder and dysthymia which between them affect about 6% of the population aged 65 and over, and the 'subsyndromal' but still significantly disabling depressions which may affect as many as a further 14%.[1]

Affective disorders are therefore clearly very common; they are also all too often not identified or not treated. Recognition of their clinical features (and how these features differ from those of the affective disorders occurring earlier in life) is crucial for all members of primary care teams as well as those working in mental health and general hospital settings. In view of the greater prevalence of depression in residential and nursing home residents, staff working in such settings should also be aware of how depression may present.

Clinical features of depression in old age

The clinical features of depression identified with the standard classificatory systems such as *The International Classification of Diseases* (ICD-10; 2) (*see* Chapter 1) and the *Diagnostic and Statistical Manual of Mental Disorders* (DSM-IV-TR;[3]) may still be used for older people but are more problematic in this group. For major depressive disorder, for example, DSM-IV-TR requires the presence for at least two weeks of at least five features from the list shown in Table 2.1, with one of them having to be depressed mood or diminished interest. The syndrome should lead to significant distress or functional impairment and 'not be a direct effect of a medical condition or bereavement'.

TABLE 2.1 Summary of DSM-IV-TR core depressive symptoms and signs

- Depressed mood
- Diminished interest
- Loss of pleasure in all/almost all activities
- Weight loss or gain (at least 5% of premorbid body weight)
- Insomnia or hypersomnia
- Psychomotor agitation or retardation
- Reduced ability to concentrate
- Recurrent thoughts of death or suicide

Five (including depressed mood or diminished interest or pleasure) required for major depressive episode. Two or more required for minor depressive disorder (same minimum duration). Sad mood on most days and two other symptoms for at least two years required for dysthymia.

The most obvious problem is the high prevalence of medical conditions (which are almost inevitable in the very old) and in particular the strong associations between depression and neurological conditions such as stroke.[4] This has led Alexopoulos[4] to propose that a number of specific 'geriatric depression syndromes' should be recognised in future classificatory systems, including 'depression due to a general medical condition' and (in view of the many potentially depression-inducing medications older people take) 'substance-induced depression'. There is also a much higher likelihood of recent bereavement in older people, in which context it may be difficult to distinguish between typical grief (whose expression may vary widely depending on cultural norms), atypical grief and frank depression. Severity, persistence and disproportionate functional incapacity following bereavement are all pointers towards true depressive illness.

Several studies have suggested that the pattern of symptoms may differ between older and younger patients. The classic paper by Brown *et al.*[5] on 'involutional melancholia' compared depressed patients with a first onset of illness after the age of 50, with younger depressed patients and with a group of older patients who had had previous episodes of depression when aged less than 50. Regardless of age of initial onset, older patients had more somatic complaints, sleep disturbance (particularly initial insomnia) and agitation, but were less likely to express feelings of guilt. More recently a more specific association has been reported between depression and painful symptoms in older people, strongest for neck and back pain.[6] Prince *et al.*[7] identified two symptom clusters in older depressed patients. The first, 'affective suffering' (depression, tearfulness and the wish to die), was associated with female gender. A second 'motivation' factor (loss of interest, poor concentration and lack of enjoyment) was more often found in very old people.

Other symptoms that may be useful pointers towards depression in older people include social withdrawal and increased dependency.[8] Persistent sleep disturbance has been found to be significantly associated with depression in community-residing elderly people and may predict subsequent depression.[9,10] Although reduced depth and duration of sleep are commonly found as part of the ageing process, relatively abrupt changes in sleep pattern should be seen as useful indicators of underlying or forthcoming depression. Among very elderly people living in long-term care facilities, loss of interest in previously enjoyed activities and increased irritability may indicate depression.[11] Patterns of care utilisation may also be markers for depression in old age. Older people with depression consult their general practitioners more frequently.[12] Iliffe *et al.*[13] examined the interrelationship between depression, physical disability and contact with services in 239 primary care patients aged over 75 years. Home care use was associated with depression, even after adjustment was made for functional impairment.

Subsyndromal depression

Depression-like symptoms are also often found in older subjects whose 'core' symptoms are insufficient in number to fulfil criteria for major depression, minor depression or dysthymia. Kessler *et al.*[14] compared older people with minor depression, those with major depression but only five or six 'core' symptoms and those with major depression and seven or more 'core' symptoms. They showed that minor and major depression had very similar clinical characteristics in terms of number of episodes, average length of first episode, degree of functional impairment, comorbidity and family psychiatric history. The incidence of non-major depression is particularly high in people aged over 80. Such 'subsyndromal' depression 'is associated with significant functional and psychosocial disability'[15] and 'a significantly increased risk remains of developing a major depression, having an accident or experiencing a serious illness'.[1]

Screening for depression in older people

In the light of these differences in symptom pattern, screening instruments specific for the elderly may be particularly useful in identifying older people with disabling depression, in primary care, general hospital and institutional settings. Watson and Pigmore[16] have recently reviewed the performance of a range of depression-screening instruments for older adults in primary care. Probably the most widely used instrument is the Geriatric Depression Rating Scale (GDS)[17] which Watson and Pigmore reported as having a sensitivity range of 79–100% with specificity 67–80%. The GDS has been shown to be sensitive and specific in both hospital and primary care settings.[18,19] It exists in 30 and 15 item versions and is designed for self-completion. It thus has the advantage of not requiring any rater training.

The use of such rating scales is perhaps particularly appropriate in older people with one or more specific risk factors for depression (summarised in Table 2.2). Residential and nursing home care staff and nursing staff on medical wards are ideally placed to carry out such screening. Other health and social care professionals in close contact with older people, such as podiatrists and home care staff, also have excellent opportunities to screen for depression in the vulnerable older people they see. It must, however, be borne in mind that screening is no substitute for diagnosis and that the workload resultant from further assessment of patients with 'false positive' screening results may be considerable. The GDS has also recently been shown to be a useful indicator of improvement or deterioration in depressive symptoms, even in people aged over 85.[20] An interview-based rating scale specifically designed to be sensitive to change is also available but not as yet in wide use.[21]

TABLE 2.2 Risk factors indicating high risk of depression in old age[1,4]

- Medical illness
- Residential or nursing care
- Recent bereavement
- Neck/back pain
- Social isolation
- Caregiving for spouse with dementia

Depression and suicide

The risk of suicide must always be borne in mind when assessing depressed patients. The link between depression and suicide is stronger in old age than earlier in life since other mental health problems associated with suicide, such as schizophrenia, personality disorders and drug and alcohol abuse, are less often involved. Particular indicators of suicidal risk include severity of depression, disruption of social ties (e.g. by bereavement), prominent feelings of hopelessness, and previous suicidal attempts. These features of the history and mental state should be elicited carefully at initial assessment, and the mental state features monitored closely during treatment.

Depression and anxiety

The diagnosis of depression in old age may be obscured by the presence and indeed prominence of anxiety symptoms. Anxiety disorders have a similar overall prevalence in older people to that of depression, with considerable diagnostic overlap.[22] This study found that both phobic disorders and generalised anxiety commonly coexisted with depression; only phobic disorder was also frequently 'stand-alone'. Panic disorder is rare in older people.

Depression and cognitive impairment

Cognitive impairment is also frequently found in association with depression in older people. It may hinder diagnosis but may also be informative as an indicator of aetiology and of prognosis. Particularly prominent cognitive dysfunction in the context of (often less obvious) depression, reversible with successful antidepressant treatment, is sometimes referred to as 'depressive pseudodementia'. The long-term prognosis of such initially reversible cognitive impairment, however, is poor. Alexopoulos et al.[23] reported an almost fivefold increase in risk of subsequent dementia in people whose original depressive presentation included prominent cognitive dysfunction. Prior depressive episodes have been shown to be associated with increased risk of Alzheimer's disease (AD) in twins discordant for AD.[24] Kessing et al.[25] suggest that the risk of subsequent dementia increases with the number of previous depressive episodes. Vascular risk factors may contribute to the development both of depression in old age and to dementia.[26] People whose first episode of depression occurs in old age may be particularly vulnerable to cognitive deterioration and associated neurodegenerative change.[27] Alexopoulos's group[28] have proposed a link between late first onset, vascular disease, poor response to antidepressants, neuroimaging abnormalities and a symptom pattern characterised by the relative absence of agitation and of guilt feelings, but relatively marked loss of insight and of functional abilities. More recently, Alexopoulos[4] has proposed that two distinct patterns of brain dysfunction may increase vulnerability to depression. In 'vascular depression', which occurs in people with a history of stroke and/or other evidence of vascular brain damage, verbal fluency and object naming tend to be particularly impaired. The depressive syndrome in these patients is characterised by apathy, retardation and poor insight. Alexopoulos[4] identifies a separate syndrome of 'depression-executive dysfunction syndrome', also characterised by retardation and poor insight but in addition by reduced interest and motivation and disproportionate impairment of daily living skills. This suggests that it is therefore particularly important to assess cognitive function (especially executive and other frontal lobe functions) in older people with apparent depression. Where the diagnosis is in doubt, and where there has been a poor response to treatment, full neuropsychological testing (as well as neuroimaging) may be very informative.

Depressive symptoms are also common in people with established dementia. As long ago as 1989, Wragg and Jeste[29] reviewed several studies of the phenomenology and prevalence of depressive symptoms and depressive illness in patients with established AD. They found that depressed mood was recorded in a median of 41%, and depressive disorder (including dysthymia) in a median of 19% of the subjects studied. Somewhat higher rates of depressive diagnosis (ranging from 22% to 54%) have been reported in a more recent review[30] which also found that depression in AD was usually mild and had a characteristic symptom pattern involving indecisiveness, poor concentration and sleep disturbance. Overt complaints of depressed mood were rare. The detection of depression in subjects with coexistent dementia remains difficult. Information from relatives (or from nursing or care staff) may be crucial in detecting significant depression in people with AD. As with depression in general, rating scales may be helpful. The GDS has limited validity in the presence of dementia but may be helpful where cognitive impairment is relatively mild. The Cornell Scale[31] is the most widely used scale in this context; it incorporates information from both patient and carer interviews.

Bipolar disorders

There is little evidence that older people with bipolar disorder present differently to those with unipolar depression when the episode in question is purely depressive. Apparent cognitive impairment or subjective confusion may occur but (as discussed below) this is also frequently the case in unipolar depression. The presentation of bipolar disorder may, however, be particularly confusing in the case of older people with bipolar disorder during manic or mixed episodes. Manic episodes represent a substantial minority (between 5 and 19%) of episodes of affective disorder of sufficient severity to warrant inpatient hospital care.[32] Some studies also suggest that the new incidence of bipolar disorder may actually rise in the eighth and ninth decades in men.[33] Survival into old age may also reveal bipolarity in people who have previously had multiple episodes of apparently unipolar depression. It is therefore important to be familiar with the clinical presentation of such patients and how best to assess them.

Some manic patients present with elation, over-activity, pressure of speech, rapid but intelligible flight of ideas and disinhibition, much as is the case earlier in life. Often, however, the picture is more mixed with rapid fluctuation in mood between sadness and elation. Delusions, where present, tend to have persecutory rather than grandiose content. Frailty, comorbid physical illness, medication effects and ill-fitting dentures (all of which may make rapid speech hard to understand) as well as prominent subjective confusion can contribute to a presentation in which apparent confusion dominates the clinical picture. The differential diagnosis is thus of delirium (acute organic confusional state), dementia and agitated depression. Excluding possible causes of delirium such as acute infections, drug toxicity, and recent myocardial infarction or stroke is vital, though it must be borne in mind that 'true' manic episodes in older people are often triggered by acute physical illness, particularly stroke. Neuropsychological testing may be helpful in preventing the (potentially disastrous) misidentification of mania as dementia, but such testing is usually not practical until the acute manic episode has begun to respond to treatment. Neuroimaging may also be helpful, though it should be borne in mind that both atrophy and subcortical hyperintensities have been reported in older people with mania in the absence of clinical evidence of dementia.[34]

KEY POINTS

▶ Depression in older people is often triggered by bereavement or by medical conditions.

▶ Social withdrawal and increased dependency may indicate underlying depression.

▶ Subsyndromal depression is associated with substantial disability.
▶ Vascular risk factors are particularly important in late first-onset depression.
▶ Mania in old age may mimic delirium or dementia.

REFERENCES

1 VanItallie TB. Subsyndromal depression in the elderly: underdiagnosed and undertreated. *Metabolism.* 2005; **54**(Suppl. 1): S39–44.

2 World Health Organization. *International Classification of Disease.* Geneva: World Health Organization; 1992.

3 American Psychiatric Association. *Diagnostic and Statistical Manual of Mental Disorders (DSM-IV-TR).* 4th ed. Washington, DC: American Psychiatric Association; 2000.

4 Alexopoulos GS. Depression in the elderly. *Lancet.* 2005; **365**: 1961–70.

5 Brown RP, Sweeney J, Loustsch E, *et al.* Involutional melancholia revisited. *Am J Psychiatr.* 1984; **141**: 24–8.

6 Carrington Reid M, Williams CS, Concato J, *et al.* Depressive symptoms as a risk factor for disabling back pain in community-dwelling older persons. *J Am Geriatr Soc.* 2003; **51**: 1710–17.

7 Prince MJ, Reischies F, Beekman ATF, *et al.* Development of the EURO-D Scale: a European Union initiative to compare symptoms of depression in 14 European centres. *Br J Psychiatr.* 1999; **174**: 339–45.

8 Reynolds CF. Depression: making the diagnosis and using SSRIs in the older patient. *Geriatr.* 1996; **1**: 28–34.

9 Livingston G, Blizard B, Mann A. Does sleep disturbance predict depression in elderly people? A study in inner London. *Br J Gen Pract.* 1993; **43**: 445–8.

10 Newman AB, Enright PL, Manolio TA, *et al.* Sleep disturbances, psychosocial correlates and cardiovascular disease in 5201 older adults: the Cardiovascular Health Study. *J Am Geriatr Soc.* 1997; **45**: 1–7.

11 Burrows AB, Satlin A, Salzman C, *et al.* Depression in a long-term care facility: clinical features and discordance between nursing assessment and patient interviews. *J Am Geriatr Soc.* 1994; **43**: 1118–22.

12 Livingston G, Thomas A, Graham N, *et al.* The Gospel Oak Project: the use of health and social services by dependent elderly people in the community. *Health Trends.* 1990; **22**: 70–3.

13 Iliffe S, Tai SS, Haines A, *et al.* Assessment of elderly people in general practice. 4. Depression, functional ability and contact with services. *Br J Gen Pract.* 1993; **43**: 371–4.

14 Kessler RC, Shanyang Z, Blazer DG, *et al.* Prevalence, correlates and cause of minor depression and major depression in the national comorbidity survey. *J Affect Disord.* 1997; **45**: 19–30.

15 Copeland JRM, Davidson IA, Dewey ME *et al.* Alzheimer's disease, other dementias, depression and pseudo-dementia: prevalence, incidence and three-year outcome in Liverpool. *Br J Psychiatr.* 1992; **161**: 230–9.

16 Watson LC, Pigmore MP. Screening accuracy for late-life depression in primary care: a systematic review. *J Fam Pract.* 2003; **52**: 956–64.

17 Yesavage JA, Brink TL, Rose TL, *et al.* Development and validation of geriatric depression screening scale: a preliminary report. *J Psychiatr Res.* 1983; **17**: 37–49.

18 D'Ath P, Katona P, Mullan M, *et al.* Screening, detection and management of depression in elderly primary care attenders. 1. The acceptability and performance of the 15-item Geriatric Depression Scale (GDS-15) and the development of short versions. *J Fam Pract.* 1994; **11**: 260–6.

19 Ramsay R, Wright P, Katz A, *et al.* Psychiatric morbidity and bed-occupancy in geriatric in-patients. *Int J Geriatr Psychiatr.* 1991: **6**: 861–6.

20 Vinckers DJ, Gusselkoo J, Stek ML, *et al.* The 15-item Geriatric Depression Scale (GDS-15) detects changes in depressive symptoms after a major negative life event: the Leiden 85-Plus study. *Int J Geriatr Psychiatr.* 2004; **107**: 54–60.

21 Ravindran AV, Welburn K, Copeland JRM. Semi-structured depression scale sensitive to change with treatment for use in the elderly. *Br J Psychiatr.* 1994; **164**: 522–7.

22 Livingston G, Watkin V, Milne B, *et al.* The natural history of depression and the anxiety disorders in older people: the Islington community study. *J Affect Disord.* 1997; **46**: 255–62.

23 Alexopoulos GS, Meyers BS, Young RC, *et al.* The course of geriatric depression with 'reversible dementia': a controlled study. *Am J Psychiatr.* 1993; **150**: 1693–9.

24 Wetherell JL, Gatz M, Johansson B, *et al.* History of depression and other psychiatric illness as risk factors for Alzheimer's disease in a twin sample. *Alzheimer Dis Assoc Disord.* 1999; **13**: 47–52.

25 Kessing LV, Andersen PK. Does the risk of developing dementia increase with the number of episodes in patients with depressive disorder and in patients with bipolar disorder? *J Neurol Neurosurg Psychiatr.* 2004; **75**(12): 1662–6.

26 Cervilla JA, Prince M, Joels S, *et al.* Does depression predict cognitive outcome 9 to 12 years later? Evidence from a prospective study of elderly hypertensives. *Psychol Med.* 2000; **30**(5): 1017–23.

27 van Ojen R, Hooijer C, Jonker C, *et al.* Late-life depressive disorder in the community, early onset and the decrease of vulnerability with increasing age. *J Affect Disord.* 1995; **33**: 159–66.

28 Alexopoulos GS, Meyers BS, Young RC, *et al.* Vascular depression hypothesis. *Arch Gen Psychiatr.* 1997; **54**: 915–22.

29 Wragg RE, Jeste DV. Overview of depression and psychosis in Alzheimer's disease. *Am J Psychiatr.* 1989; **146**: 577–87.

30 Zubenko GS, Zubenko WN, McPherson S, *et al.* A collaborative study of the emergence and clinical features of the major depressive syndrome of Alzheimer's disease. *Am J Psychiatr.* 2003; **160**(5): 857–66.

31 Alexopoulous GS, Abrams RC, Young RC, *et al.* Cornell Scale for depression in dementia. *Biol Psychiatr.* 1988; **23**: 271–84.

32 McDonald WM, Nemeroff CB. The diagnosis and treatment of mania in the elderly. *Bull Menninger Clin.* 1996; **60**: 174–96.

33 Sibisi CDT. Sex differences in the age of onset of bipolar affective illness. *Br J Psychiatr.* 1990; **156**: 842–5.

34 McDonald WM, Krishnan KRR, Doraiswamy PM, *et al.* The occurrence of subcortical hyperintensities in elderly subjects with mania. *J Psychiatr Res.* 1991; **40**: 211–20.

CHAPTER 3

Aetiology of late-life affective disorders

ADRIAN LLOYD

Introduction

Affective disorders in late life may begin prior to and then persist into old age or may have their very first onset later in life. Initial aetiological factors in early-onset illnesses are, by definition, those described in standard texts on psychiatry of working-age adults. This chapter will not revisit these in detail but will focus on factors that are of increasing importance in old age. It must be recognised throughout that factors evolving in later life may precipitate new episodes of illness or add to pre-existing maintaining factors that slow recovery in both early-onset and late-onset disorders.

The distinction between early- and late-onset illness varies between studies from around 45 to around 65 years. For the current discussion the definition of late-onset will be taken as 60 or above unless otherwise stated. Bipolar affective disorder and unipolar depression are considered separately as their aetiologies may differ.

A number of age-related processes may be important in late-onset affective disorders, including reduced neurotransmitter levels (e.g. 5-Hydroxytryptamine (5-HT) and noradrenalin (NA)),[1,2] increasing vascular burden,[3] early degenerative processes,[4-6] increasing vulnerability to oxidative stress[7] and disordered neuroendocrine function, particularly of the hypothalamo-pituitary-adrenal (HPA) axis.[8] These biological factors occur within a changing psychosocial milieu as individuals age and there may be important interplay between them.

Bipolar disorder

Compared with the extensive literature on bipolar disorder in younger individuals and on unipolar depression at all ages, data regarding bipolar affective disorder in the elderly are relatively scant and are generally cross-sectional and retrospective.[9,10] The research cut-off between early- and late-onset bipolar disorder is often in the fourth or fifth decade, not fitting particularly well with the generally accepted distinction between working age and elderly populations. Onset of mania peaks first prior to age 30 in all subjects, then again in the late forties in females and in the eighties or nineties in males.[10] The validity of using an age of onset distinction at all in bipolar illness has been questioned.[11,12]

Most patients experiencing mania for the first time in late life have had depressive episodes (i.e. onset of affective illness) earlier in life or have illness that is secondary to other neurological insults.[13] Family history of affective disorder is increased in relatives of bipolar patients of any age-of-onset, but is more prevalent in relatives of those with early-onset illness:[10,14–17] e.g. positive family history in 58% of early-onset versus 36% of late-onset patients.[18] Lower socioeconomic status in subjects with early-onset bipolar disorder is probably due to the cumulative disruptive effect of greater illness duration.[19]

Krauthammer and Klerman,[20] supported by subsequent authors,[15,21,22] introduced the concept of mania secondary to physical illness: the proportion of elderly patients where mania is temporally related to physical problems ranging from 8% to 12%.[14] Reviewing the literature, Shulman et al.[23] conclude that late-onset mania is not generally precipitated by the dementias (except possibly dementia with Lewy bodies) and note a relative lack of true manic symptoms other than the disinhibition that can also occur in frontal lobe syndromes. Case reports record a wide range of neurological disorders associated with mania, most commonly cerebrovascular disease.[24] Other disorders range from trauma through cerebral tumours to AIDS and neuroendocrine disturbances. A predominance of right-sided pathology and lesions involving the orbito-frontal areas, temporal lobe and the basal ganglia emerges.[9,23,24]

Pre-existing neurological disease is more common in manic syndromes of late-onset than early-onset (in up to 25% with onset after age 50). Also neurological disorders appear to be more commonly associated with late-onset mania than with late-onset unipolar depression (e.g. 36% versus 8%). Again, however, most studies are retrospective and cross-sectional and examine patients with manic symptoms rather than a rigorous diagnosis of bipolar disorder.[10,15,25] A study examining clearly defined bipolar disorder supported the stronger relationship of organic conditions with late-onset (2.8%) compared with early-onset mania (1.2%) but the absolute proportions are small and contrast with the much higher rates described with more broadly defined manic symptoms.[19]

Neuroimaging defines a range of structural and functional abnormalities in the prefrontal cortex (especially anterior cingulate, orbito-frontal and ventral areas), amygdala, and striatum. There is also an association with increased MRI hyperintensities. These data are reviewed at length elsewhere.[26–32] Interesting findings in bipolar disorder that contrast with unipolar depression (see later) include some evidence for amygdala enlargement and little evidence for hippocampal change.[33–40] Paucity of data makes it difficult to draw conclusions about the effect of age-of-onset of bipolar disorder on structural changes beyond middle age and independently of generalised ageing effects.

Elevation in mood can occur secondary to medication use – this is summarised along with the findings for depression in Table 3.1.

Unipolar depression

While the point prevalence of major depressive episodes in later life (approximately 1–3%) remains similar to that for the disorder overall (1.5–4.9%) with a constant female:male ratio of 2:1, the prevalence of depressive symptoms below the threshold for a depressive episode is strikingly high at 10–15%.[41,42] Also, the cumulative percentage of individuals with depression in any given birth cohort rises with age.[43] This raises an important question: is the aetiology of depression the same throughout life or do alternative or additional factors come into play with increasing age? Lesser importance of family history in late-onset depression has been recognised for over 40 years.[44]

Organic conditions associated with late-onset depression
The dementias

Unipolar depression is associated with Alzheimer's disease (AD), vascular dementia and dementia with Lewy bodies (DLB)[42,45–48] While many psychiatric disorders (including schizophrenia and neuroses) are predictive of dementia, the strongest relationship is with affective disorders.[45] Up to 63% of patients with Alzheimer's disease will have depressive symptoms and up to 25% a depressive episode,[45,49–52] figures strikingly higher than in the general population. Additionally, cell loss in aminergic nuclei is greater in depressed sufferers of AD than in those without depression.[53] Depression in dementia appears unlikely to be due simply to the psychological impact of suffering a degenerative disorder, as its relationship with specific dementias varies in terms of persistence, suggesting that the underlying pathology may modify the course of depression (persistence of depression at six months: vascular dementia 50%, DLB 42%, AD 11%).[45] Retrospective analysis of patients with dementia and longitudinal follow-up of depressed elderly subjects both indicate depression to be a risk factor for future cognitive decline.[4,6,54–61] Depression presenting with cognitive impairment as a temporary clinical feature carries a two- to five-fold increased risk of future dementia than that without cognitive features,[62–67] although a small number of studies have not found this relationship[68–69] and it is apparent in psychiatric patients rather than in community samples.[70–72]

Family history, Apolipoprotein E and other genetic markers

Family history of affective illness is perhaps twice as common in early-onset than in late-onset depression, indicating a greater genetic aetiological component to early-onset illness.[73–78] In view of the well-recognised relationship between the Apolipoprotein E-ε4 (APOE-ε4) genotype and Alzheimer's disease and the above relationships between depression and dementia, APOE-ε4 status has been investigated in depression. Most studies have failed to establish any link between depression and APOE-ε4.[71,79–90] Only indirect associations with medial temporal lobe structural change, cognitive impairment or greater risk of progression to dementia in depressed cohorts[91–93] are described. APOE-ε4 has been found to have an association with white matter (and thus by extrapolation possibly vascular) change.[94–95] These associations add little to the possible demographic links between degenerative and affective disorders.

Other candidate genetic markers include the methylene tetrahydrofolate reductase gene mutation C677T: homo- or heterozygosity for this mutation and clinical vascular risk factors have been reported as higher in late-onset depression. Also worthy of mention, though rare, is the link of depression with CADASIL (cerebral autosomal dominant arteriopathy with subcortical infarcts and leukoencephalopathy) in which depression is often an early presenting feature.[10]

Vascular disease and vascular risk factors

A significant body of evidence links cardiovascular and cerebrovascular disease with depression.[24,96–100] This includes coronary heart disease,[42,101–103] 20–25% of patients with serious heart disease having depression. Depression is also an independent risk factor for ischaemic heart disease.[98] Stroke and risk factors for cerebrovascular disease are similarly closely related to depressive illness,[77,100,104–108] 25–50% suffering depression, with lesion location relating to onset of depression soon after stroke but not one year later.[10] Lesion laterality and relationship to depression has contradictory evidence (e.g. right-sided;[109] no significant effect of laterality[110]), although more studies suggest a relationship to left-sided insults and give a reasonable weight of findings implicating frontal lobe lesions in particular.[26,111–117] As with cardiovascular disease, the direction of cause and effect is uncertain as depression increases the risk of cerebrovascular disease two- or three-fold and there is evidence for a dose-response relationship between severity of depression and subsequent risk of vascular disease.[3,118] Depression may have a predictive effect comparable to that of left-ventricular function on outcome following myocardial infarction and may increase the rate of cardiac death more than three-fold. Also, treatment of depression improves cardiovascular outcome.[119–122]

Increased rates of depression have been reported associated with lower high-density lipoprotein cholesterol (but normal total cholesterol) and previous cerebrovascular disease,[123] reduced total cholesterol[124] and both elevated and lowered total cholesterol in the same study.[118] Kim *et al.*[118] have speculated that two separate mechanisms may be operating: low cholesterol being associated with general frailty or possibly lowered serotonin levels, and elevated cholesterol being associated with vascular disease; both factors having importance in the aetiology of depression. This issue is open to further clarification as other contradictory findings also exist (e.g. no association with lowered cholesterol;[123,125] controlling for confounding factors removes associations of low cholesterol with depression;[126] treating hypercholesterolaemia with statins does not increase depression).[127]

Whilst some population-based studies[128–130] do not find an association between vascular risk and depression, the weight of evidence increasingly supports the existence of this relationship.[3,131] Also, pathologically defined vascular disease, particularly of the cerebral vessels, has been shown to be increased in depressed subjects compared to matched, psychiatrically healthy controls,[132] as has the presence of inflammatory markers involved in the genesis of vascular pathology.[133–134]

Possible explanations for these relationships are not entirely clear but include:[98,100,135–136] atherosclerosis leading to both cardiac disease and vascular brain pathology; increased platelet reactivity in depression; HPA-axis activation in depression with consequent adverse effects on lipid metabolism, blood pressure and vascular intimal healing; increased immune activation; abnormal adrenal medullary function; sympathetic dysregulation and hypotensive episodes. Biogenic amines implicated in affective disorders also fulfil autonomic functions. These relationships need not be mutually exclusive and such processes may even potentiate one another.

Glucocorticoids and the hypothalamo-pituitary-adrenal (HPA) axis

Cortisol secretion can increase with increasing age[137–140] and old age may be a time of reduced adaptability to stress.[141] Glucocorticoid secretion is known to be disordered in affective illnesses, particularly in the elderly, up to half of patients with late-life depression having elevated cortisol.[137,142–149] The 'Glucocorticoid Cascade Hypothesis'[150] draws these concepts together: the hippocampus down-regulates the HPA axis and hippocampal neurones are vulnerable to damage from elevated cortisol. Hypercortisolaemia in affective illness may (via neuronal damage/loss) reduce glucocorticoid receptor sites, attenuating the hippocampal response to raised cortisol and hence up-regulating the lower components of the HPA axis. This may perpetuate or further increase hypercortisolaemia in a feed-forward cascade. An additional factor may exacerbate this effect in the elderly: Dehydroepiandrosterone (DHEA)[151] is an endogenous antiglucocorticoid that may limit hypercortisolaemic damage. From a maximum between puberty and around age 30 DHEA secretion declines into old age, potentially amplifying cortisol-related neurotoxicity. As well as its direct effect on neurones, elevated cortisol may render nerve cells vulnerable to damage from other mechanisms such as the action of excitatory amino acids.[152–155] Further evidence implicating the HPA axis and hippocampal integrity in depression comes from the observation in Cushing's syndrome of (reversible) low mood[156–161] and hippocampal volume reduction.[162,163]

Links between HPA function and monoamines involved in the control of mood[164-170] include, in particular, altered 5-HT turnover in the hippocampus. Not only may cortisol be elevated in depression but abnormalities are reported at higher levels in the HPA axis: namely elevated ACTH at the circadian nadir[171] and some evidence for altered corticotropin releasing factor (CRF) function.[147,172,173] Interestingly, successful antidepressant or ECT treatment can lead to normalisation of HPA function in patients with treatment-responsive, but not treatment-resistant, depression.[166,173-180]

Other important associations

Up to one quarter of patients with cancer have depression.[42] In Parkinson's disease,[44,181-185] the prevalence of depression (50% in clinical research samples and 10% in community samples) is in excess of that expected in the general population – even in those with similarly disabling conditions – and is likely to be directly related to degenerative processes affecting not only the substantia nigra but, variably, also the ventral tegmental area, hypothalamus, locus coeruleus and dorsal raphe nuclei; implicating dopamine, serotonin and noradrenalin systems.

Limbic and fronto-subcortical circuitry in affective disorders

An anatomical framework is helpful in understanding the common end result (mood disorder) of a wide variety of changes in different brain areas (discussed below) and in tying in the diverse biological associations reviewed above with the presentation of depressive illness. Two major sets of connections require consideration: 1) the interconnection of limbic structures and 2) the circuits that give reciprocal connections between the prefrontal cortex and deeper brain nuclei.

Limbic connections

The main connections between limbic structures are summarised in Figure 3.1. There are many further connections between these structures and other subcortical nuclei and also areas of frontal and temporal cortex. The most important circuit within these connections is as follows: hippocampus→fornix→mamillary bodies→thalamus→cingulate gyrus→hippocampus – the reverberating circuit of Papez.

Fronto-subcortical circuits

Fronto-subcortical circuits or, perhaps more accurately, *cortical-basal ganglia-thalamocortical circuits*, are well-defined.[186-191] Three pathways are of relevance in affective disorders and, with minor variations, these share the structure illustrated in Figure 3.2. Connections from each of three prefrontal cortical regions (dorsolateral, lateral orbital, anterior cingulate) project to progressively more focused subcortical structures and finish with a reciprocal connection back to the respective cortical area.

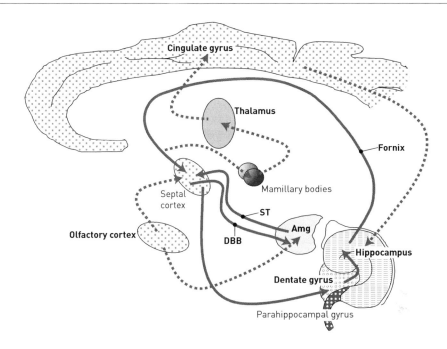

FIGURE 3.1 Limbic system connections. ST = Stria terminalis. DBB = diagonal band of Broca. Amg = amygdala.

It can be appreciated from these neural pathways that disordered function at any point – from cortical processing problems to small, discrete lesions of subcortical structures or of the fibre tracts that connect components – may have similar effects on mood.

Evidence for altered brain structure in depression

The structural brain changes associated with depression (largely defined by neuroimaging) are myriad, including reductions in frontal and temporal lobe volumes, increased ventricular volumes, basal ganglia changes and increased white matter hyperintensities on MRI. A number of reviews give a thorough overview of this topic.[26,192–197] Associations of generalised structural brain changes (e.g. indices of brain atrophy, increased burden of white matter change) with depression have been recognised for over 20 years,[68,198–201] some studies finding the relationship to be specifically with late-onset illness.[199,201–203] Basal ganglia changes are primarily of caudate volume reduction,[204] possibly more so in late-onset than in early-onset illness.[205] Structural changes that relate particularly to age of illness onset are enlarged ventricular volumes, hippocampal volume loss and white matter hyperintensities.

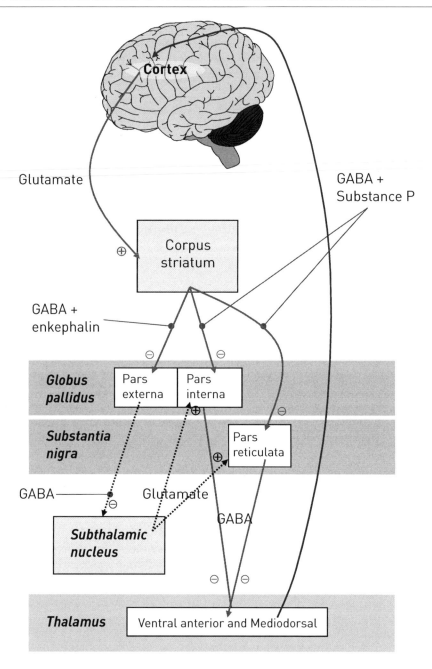

FIGURE 3.2 Affective fronto-subcortical circuit structure. GABA = gamma-aminobutyric acid. ⊕ = excitatory ⊖ = inhibitory.

Increased ventricular size/brain atrophy

In late-life depression overall findings have been equivocal,[200–201,206–209] but in late-onset illness evidence for ventricular enlargement is stronger[201,203,206,210] and associated with increased mortality.[202] Some studies report increased third ventricle volume, suggesting possible atrophy of adjacent structures – the thalamus and hypothalamus. Increased ventricle:brain ratio is reported in depression in general,[211] more so in the elderly[212] and especially in late-onset illness,[68,198,213–214] although negative findings also exist.[209,215–217] Evidence for brain volume reduction *per se* is more mixed with studies both supporting[192,199,218] and arguing against[219–222] its relationship with depression. Frontal lobe volume loss may be related to depression, perhaps particularly in severe illness[223] and later life.[204,224] Evidence for overall temporal lobe atrophy in unipolar illness is weak,[26] but medial temporal lobe volumes may be reduced in late-onset illness and be related to cognitive impairment.[205]

Hippocampal volume

Within the medial temporal lobe, evidence for hippocampal volume loss in older depressed subjects[8,154,225–234] is much stronger than that for amygdala volume change. This contrasts with bipolar disorder (mixed evidence for increased amygdala volume and little evidence for hippocampal change) and perhaps indicates some divergence in aetiology. In samples ranging in age from younger adults to the elderly an association has been shown of greater cumulative exposure to depression correlating with hippocampal volume loss, supporting the glucocorticoid cascade hypothesis.[225] In samples of elderly subjects only, however, there is evidence for greater hippocampal atrophy occurring in patients with late-onset illness,[228,233] suggesting that in late life other biological factors may modify, or have greater effects than, glucocorticoid dysregulation. Hippocampal volume reduction should also be considered in the context of the epidemiological link between Alzheimer's disease, in which hippocampal atrophy is striking, and depression: might some late-life depression represent a pre-cognitive presentation of Alzheimer's pathology, as already discussed?

MRI hyperintensities

These occur largely in the white matter (periventricular lesions (PVL) adjacent to the ventricular walls and deep white matter lesions (DWML) remote from the ventricles) and also in deep grey nuclei. Figure 3.3 illustrates their appearances. They occur in many conditions and also in normal ageing, and are associated with vascular risk factors.[106,114,135,195,212,235–248] While there are some common features to the neuropathology of PVL and DWML there are also distinctions between them. PVL are characterised by discontinuity of the ventricular ependymal lining, subependymal gliosis and myelin pallor, with increasing vascular pathology as lesions extend deeper into the white matter; DWML tend to show vascular changes and myelin pallor, fibre loss and gliosis being evident only in larger lesions.[136,249–253] The association of hyperintensities with unipolar depression is equivocal in younger adults[26] but is well defined in the elderly, independently of vascular risk factors.[26,114,136,241–243,254] Most studies examining age of onset describe more hyperintensities in late-onset than early-onset illness.[200,208,211,236,243,255–257] Depression

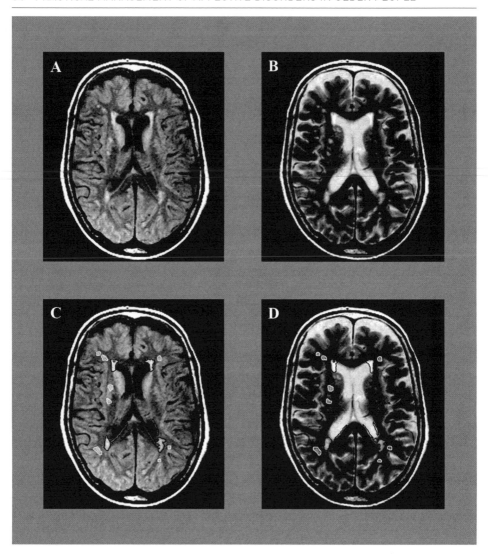

FIGURE 3.3 Axial magnetic resonance images illustrating white matter hyperintensities. Un-annotated images showing periventricular and deep white matter lesions (panels A and B) with duplicate images (panels C and D) in which lesions are outlined: black outlines = periventricular lesions, white outlines = deep white matter lesions. Panels A and C: Proton density-weighted MRI scans. Panels B and D: T2-weighted MRI scans.

is more closely associated with DWML and basal ganglia hyperintensities than with PVL[201,235,240,242,243,258,259] and possibly particularly with lesions of the frontal lobes.[241,243,258] PVL tend to be increased in patients with impaired cognition as a feature of depression and in those who later develop dementia.[259] Interestingly, subjects with dementia alone and dementia with comorbid depression have excess PVL rather than DWML.[260,261] The direction of cause/effect between depression and DWML is difficult to prove, but the association with late- rather than early-onset suggests they are more likely to be an aetiological factor in the development of depression in older individuals than to result from depression that developed earlier in life.

Functional brain imaging

Functional MRI, positron emission tomography and single photon emission tomography have demonstrated a range of activity changes in different brain regions in affective disorders, those most frequently implicated being the anterior brain structures (both cortical and subcortical) consistent with structures and connections of the affective circuits described above. There are, however, few data that allow exploration of a direct relationship between structural and functional findings and only a small proportion of studies consider elderly subjects specifically. These studies often highlight regions of the brain implicated in the genesis of depression, rather than informing on specific aetiologies in their own right, but can inform on transmitter changes – the serotonin system being particularly indicated.[262–271]

Vascular depression hypothesis

In the late mid- to late-1990s the concept evolved of a sub-type of depression in which vascular aetiology is particularly important – 'vascular depression'.[10,107,272,273] This was defined clinically as late-onset, associated with vascular risk factors, having cognitive (especially executive) impairments, more prominent vegetative and less prominent psychological depressive symptoms and possibly treatment resistance,[77,105,114,242,274] along with a requirement for neuroimaging evidence of vascular change, i.e. MRI hyperintensities.[100,275–277] This is supported by evidence in depressed subjects of increased general vascular pathology and vascular neuropathology that is co-localised with CT and MRI changes[132,278–280] and by a series of studies examining markers of ischaemia-induced inflammation in depression.[134,281–82] A strong and bidirectional relationship between depression and vascular disease has already been suggested in this chapter and is emphasised in the review by Thomas *et al.*[3]

Medication associated with depression

There is a received wisdom that certain medications may be depressogenic. The evidence for this is variable in quality, often based on case report literature, and includes relatively little information from well-controlled studies.[283]

A number of reviews explore this area in more detail. These, among other sources,[284–290] form the basis for Table 3.1 which summarises medications commonly prescribed in the elderly, and their reported associations with altered mood states.

TABLE 3.1 Commonly prescribed medications and effects on mood

Drug group	Specific medications	Strength of relationship
Antihypertensives	Reserpine	Initial antihypertensive agent considered related to depression.
	β-blockers	Possibly related to depression but controlled studies less convincing than earliest reports.
	Calcium channel antagonists	No clear relationship.
	Angiotensin converting enzyme (ACE) inhibitors	Equivocal. Some evidence suggesting elevated mood.
	Methyldopa	No clear relationship.
	Clonidine	No clear relationship.
Lipid lowering	Statins	Specific relationship of statins with mood unclear. Possible relationship between lower cholesterol and violent death including suicide.
Steroids	Glucocorticoids	Associated with both elevated and depressed mood; possible association with psychosis.
	Anabolic steroids generally	Range of mood and behavioural effects: rage, depression, mania, suicidality.
Oestrogen receptor modulators	e.g. Tamoxifen, raloxifene	Evidence for effects on mood equivocal.
Hormone Replacement Therapy	In general	Any effect on mood generally positive: Androgen ± oestrogen > oestrogen > progesterone ± oestrogen.
Analgesics	NSAIDs	Case reports – no controlled studies.
Ulcer healing drugs	H_2 receptor antagonists	Positive case reports; negative findings in specific (small) studies.
Hypnotics/anxiolytics	Benzodiazepines	Confounded by close association of depression and anxiety; expert opinion suggests caution in elderly.
	Barbiturates	
Anticonvulsants	In general (exceptions and additional information below)	Epilepsy-related mood symptoms important confounder. Limited data do not suggest affective change as side-effect.

Drug group	Specific medications	Strength of relationship
	Vigabatrin and topiramate	Vigabatrin possibly associated with depression and psychosis; topiramate possibly associated with lowered mood.
	Valproate, carbamazepine, oxcarbazepine, lamotrigine	Note use of these agents in affective disorders and specifically beneficial effect of lamotrigine in bipolar depression.

Sources: references 283–290.

A logical general conclusion is that, despite lacking or contradictory controlled trial evidence, any temporal association between mood change and altered pharmacotherapy needs to be considered in the round with regard to whether it is causative in that particular patient. Klotyar *et al.*[283] comment that small numbers of relevant reactions may be too infrequent to be detected by most trials, but may be of importance to specific individuals. Reported links between antihypertensive medications and depression must be viewed in the context of the close relationship between depression and vascular disease: might it be that vascular pathology brings together the depression and concurrent antihypertensive treatment, rather than the medication causing depression in all instances? In the elderly these considerations are of particular relevance in view of the increased likelihood of treatment for other age-related conditions and an associated risk of polypharmacy.

Personality and psychosocial factors

Personality

Dysfunctional personality factors (particularly dependent, passive-aggressive and, to a lesser extent, obsessive-compulsive and avoidant traits) have been described as more common in early-onset than late-onset depression.[78] Other work did not find a comparable distinction,[291] but identified lower extraversion scores in both early- and late-onset patients compared to controls.

Psychosocial factors

Whilst some aetiological factors would be expected in any age group (being single, stressful life events, substance misuse, family psychiatric history, poor social networks) others may be more common in elderly populations (widowhood, organic disorders associated with depression, worsening general health, loss of productive roles). Social isolation, lack of social networks and loss of roles have long been recognised as factors important in late-life depression,[292] with evidence that socially less-well-engaged individuals are more likely to be depressed (reviewed in Blazer[44]). Evidence that religious belief may afford some protection against developing depression in later life[293] might also indicate an effect of better support networks and strategies for coping with adverse events associated with old age.

Data regarding life events are not yet extensive. Depression overall in the elderly can be associated with cumulative life events, particularly negative ones and those related to the subject's own health or the death or health of persons close to them. Major events appear to have greatest impact in the initiation of illness, lesser events more commonly acting as maintaining factors or triggers for recurrent episodes.[294–295]

With regard to age of onset, findings differ between samples: People aged over 60 and not depressed in 1984 were re-interviewed 5–10 years later.[296] Depression (by definition late-onset) was associated with loss of a parent of the opposite gender prior to age 20, less religious involvement, reduced social networks, marital difficulties, feeling unappreciated, separation from someone close, and (in men) a move to institutional care. In another community sample,[297] late-onset illness was associated with increased age, widowhood and impaired cognition whereas early-onset illness showed greater association with double depression and comorbid anxiety. Early- and late-onset groups did not differ with respect to family history or experience of general early or late-life events. By contrast, in a secondary care sample[291] increased life events were related to early-onset illness, suggesting possible greater influence of psychological factors in this group than in those with late-onset depression. Early-onset depression is more likely to be associated with marital discord[78] and there is evidence for an association of late-life illness with disability in some[298,299] but not all studies.[297] Late-onset major depression and late-onset dysthymic disorder may be aetiologically closer to one another than are late-onset and early-onset dysthymic disorder, further suggesting a distinction between late- and early-onset problems.[300] Grace and O'Brien[291] found bereavement to be more common in early-onset depression than in controls and more common in controls than in those with late-onset illness. Lack of a confidant(e) was more common in early-onset illness than in controls or late-onset patients.

Overall, an interaction of negative events with personality types and cognitive styles is accepted as increasing vulnerability to depression and strongly predicts depressive episodes in elderly patients in response to stressful life events, often loss events (of support, family, physical health and social networks).[301]

Conclusions

Structural and functional brain change has been implicated in the genesis of late-life affective illness both by direct investigation and by implication from observed associations of affective disorder with organic conditions. Also, there are contrasts between the aetiology of early- and late-onset disorders with regard to both biological and psychosocial factors. A helpful view is that of Baldwin[41] suggesting that depression in the elderly is a condition that is modified by factors that are not present in younger individuals, rather than being an illness subtype in its own right. Within this, however, need to be accommodated evolving concepts such as that of vascular depression which is likely to be of particular relevance in old age. It is important to recognise the effect of other illnesses and related therapeutic interventions (particularly drugs) on mood in the elderly. Contrasts defined by age of onset indicate that patients with late-onset affective disorder are more likely to have illness precipitated by acquired organic factors than are age-matched early-onset patients. For the early-onset group psychosocial factors appear to play a larger part with the more important biological effect being genetic, as demonstrated by the greater influence of family history on susceptibility to depression.

Biological factors that appear to be of importance in depression in the elderly may at first seem disparate – cortisol hyper-secretion, hippocampal atrophy, white matter changes, vascular disease – but, as indicated above, there are important interactions between these such that none can be considered mutually exclusive. In addition, there are important neural circuits and connections that offer explanation of the common effect of anatomical or functional changes at many different sites. Exploration within a bio-psychosocial framework in all cases is essential to comprehensively understand the relevant aetiological factors in late-life affective disorder.

KEY POINTS

▸ Late-life affective disorders must be fully assessed from biological, psychological and social viewpoints to understand their aetiology.

▸ Aetiological factors interact and modify one another.

▸ Information regarding the aetiology of bipolar disorder specifically in late life is limited.

▸ The nature of and balance between biological and psychosocial aetiological factors contrasts between early- and late-onset depressive disorders.

REFERENCES

1 Gottfries CG. Neurochemical aspects on aging and diseases with cognitive impairment. *J Neurosci Res.* 1990; **27**: 541–7.

2 Gottfries CG. Late life depression. *Eur Arch Psychiat Clin Neurosci.* 2001; **251**(Suppl. 2): 1157–61.

3 Thomas AJ, Kalaria RN, O'Brien JT. Depression and vascular disease: what is the relationship? *J Affect Disord.* 2004; **79**: 81–95.

4 Jorm AF, van Duijn CM, Chandra V, *et al.* Psychiatric history and related exposures as risk factors for Alzheimer's disease: a collaborative re-analysis of case-control studies. EURODEM Risk Factors Research Group. *Int J Epidemiol.* 1991; **20**: S43–7.

5 Jorm AF. Is depression a risk factor for dementia or cognitive decline? A review. *Gerontology.* 2000; **46**: 219–27.

6 Jorm AF. History of depression as a risk factor for dementia: an updated review. *Aust NZ J Psychiatr.* 2001; **35**: 776–81.

7 Sapolsky RM. Potential behavioral modification of glucocorticoid damage to the hippocampus. *Behav Brain Res.* 1993; **57**: 175–82.

8 O'Brien JT. The 'glucocorticoid cascade' hypothesis in man. *Br J Psychiatr.* 1997; **170**: 199–201.

9 Shulman KI, Herrmann N. Bipolar disorder in old age. *Can Family Physician.* 1999; **45**: 1229–37.

10 Krishnan KR. Biological risk factors in late life depression. *Biol Psychiatr.* 2002; **52**(3): 185–92.

11 Depp CA, Jin H, Mohamed S, *et al.* Bipolar disorder in middle-aged and elderly adults: is age of onset important? *J Nerv Ment Dis.* 2004; **192**(11): 796–9.

12 Leboyer M, Henry C, Paillere-Martinot ML, *et al.* Age at onset in bipolar affective disorders: a review. *Bipolar Disord.* 2005; **7**(2): 111–18.

13 Shulman KI, Herrmann N. The nature and management of mania in old age. *Psychiatr Clinics Nth Am.* 1999; **22**(3): 649–65.

14 Jacoby R. Manic illness. In: Jacoby R, Oppenheimer C, editors. *Psychiatry in the Elderly.* Oxford: Oxford University Press; 1997. pp. 574–81.

15 Stone K. Mania in the elderly. *Br J Psychiatr.* 1989; **155**: 220–4.

16 Tohen M, Shulman KI, Satlin A. First-episode mania in late life. *Am J Psychiatr.* 1994; **151**(1): 130–2.

17 Young RC, Klerman GL. Mania in late life: focus on age at onset. *Am J Psychiatr.* 1992; **149**(7): 867–76.

18 Shulman KI, Tohen M, Satlin A, *et al.* Mania compared with unipolar depression in old age. *Am J Psychiatr.* 1992; **149**(3): 341–5.

19 Almeida OP, Fenner S. Bipolar disorder: similarities and differences between patients with illness onset before and after 65 years of age. *Int Psychogeriatr.* 2002; **14**(3): 311–22.

20 Krauthammer C, Klerman GL. Secondary mania: manic syndromes associated with antecedent physical illness or drugs. *Arch Gen Psychiatr.* 1978; **35**(11): 1333–9.

21 Shulman K, Post F. Bipolar affective disorder in old age. *Br J Psychiatr.* 1980; **136**: 26–32.

22 Glasser M, Rabins P. Mania in the elderly. *Age Ageing.* 1984; **13**(4): 210–13.

23 Shulman KI. Disinhibition syndromes, secondary mania and bipolar disorder in old age. *J Affect Disord.* 1997; **46**(3): 175–82.

24 Starkstein SE, Robinson RG. Affective disorders and cerebral vascular disease. *Br J Psychiatr.* 1989; **154**: 170–82.

25 Snowdon J. A retrospective case-note study of bipolar disorder in old age. *Br J Psychiatr.* 1991; **158**: 485–90.

26 Soares JC, Mann JJ. The anatomy of mood disorders: review of structural neuroimaging studies. *Biol Psychiatr.* 1997; **41**(1): 86–106.

27 Haldane M, Frangou S. New insights help define the pathophysiology of bipolar affective disorder: neuroimaging and neuropathology findings. *Prog Neuropsychopharmacol Biol Psychiatr.* 2004; **28**(6): 943–60.

28 McDonald C, Zanelli J, Rabe-Hesketh S, *et al.* Meta-analysis of magnetic resonance imaging brain morphometry studies in bipolar disorder. *Biol Psychiatr.* 2004; **56**(6): 411–17.

29 Bruno SD. Neuroimaging of bipolar disorder: emphasis on novel MRI techniques. *Epilepsia.* 2005; **46**(Suppl. 4): 14–18.

30 Hajek T, Carrey N, Alda M. Neuroanatomical abnormalities as risk factors for bipolar disorder. *Bipolar Disord.* 2005; **7**(5): 393–403.

31 Monkul ES, Malhi GS, Soares JC. Anatomical MRI abnormalities in bipolar disorder: do they exist and do they progress? *Aus NZ J Psychiatr.* 2005; **39**(4): 222–6.

32 Strakowski SM, Delbello MP, Adler CM. The functional neuroanatomy of bipolar disorder: a review of neuroimaging findings. *Mol Psychiatr.* 2005; **10**(1): 105–16.

33 Strakowski SM, DelBello MP, Sax KW, *et al.* Brain magnetic resonance imaging of structural abnormalities in bipolar disorder. *Arch Gen Psychiatr.* 1999; **56**(3): 254–60.

34 Altshuler LL, Bartzokis G, Grieder T, *et al.* An MRI study of temporal lobe structures in men with bipolar disorder or schizophrenia. *Biol Psychiatr.* 2000; **48**(2): 147–62.

35 Brambilla P, Harenski K, Nicoletti M, *et al.* MRI investigation of temporal lobe structures in bipolar patients. *J Psychiatr Res.* 2003; **37**(4): 287–95.

36 Lochhead RA, Parsey RV, Oquendo MA, *et al.* Regional brain gray matter volume differences in patients with bipolar disorder as assessed by optimised voxel-based morphometry. *Biol Psychiatr.* 2004; **55**(12): 1154–62.

37 Adler CM, Levine AD, Delbello MP, *et al.* Changes in gray matter volume in patients with bipolar disorder. *Biol Psychiatr.* 2005; **58**(2): 151–7.

38 Lyoo IK, Kim MJ, Stoll AL, *et al.* Frontal lobe gray matter density decreases in bipolar I disorder. *Biol Psychiatr.* 2004; **55**(6): 648–51.

39 Frangou S. The Maudsley Bipolar Disorder Project. *Epilepsia.* 2005; **46**(Suppl. 4): 19–25.

40 McDonald C, Bullmore E, Sham P, *et al.* Regional volume deviations of brain structure in schizophrenia and psychotic bipolar disorder: computational morphometry study. *Br J Psychiatr.* 2005; **186**: 369–77.

41 Baldwin RC. Depressive illness. In: Jacoby R, Oppenheimer C, editors. *Psychiatry in the Elderly.* Oxford: Oxford University Press; 1997. pp. 536–73.

42 Mulsant BH, Ganguli M. Epidemiology and diagnosis of depression in late life. *J Clin Psychiatr.* 1999; **60**(Suppl. 20): 9–15.

43 Wittchen H-U, Knauper B, Kessler RC. Lifetime risk of depression. *Br J Psychiatr.* 1995; **165**(Suppl. 26): S16–22.

44 Blazer DG. Depression in late life: review and commentary. *J Gerontol Series A Biol Sci Med Sci.* 2003; **58**(3): 249–65.

45 Ballard CG, Patel A, Solis M, *et al.* A one-year follow-up study of depression in dementia sufferers. *Br J Psychiatr.* 1996; **168**: 287–91.

46 Ballard C, Holmes C, McKeith I, *et al.* Psychiatric morbidity in dementia with Lewy bodies: a prospective clinical and neuropathological comparative study with Alzheimer's disease. *Am J Psychiatr.* 1999; **156**(7): 1039–45.

47 Chen P, Ganguli M, Mulsant BH, *et al.* The temporal relationship between depressive symptoms and dementia. *Arch Gen Psychiatr.* 1999; **56**: 261–6.

48 Kessing LV, Olsen EW, Mortensen PB, *et al.* Dementia in affective disorder: a case-register study. *Acta Psychiatr Scand.* 1999; **100**(3): 176–85.

49 Rovner BW, Broadhead J, Spencer M, *et al.* Depression and Alzheimer's disease. *Am J Psychiatr.* 1989; **146**(3): 350–3.

50 Reifler BV, Larson E, Teri L, *et al.* Dementia of the Alzheimer's type and depression. *J Am Geriatr Soc.* 1986; **34**(12): 855–9.

51 Burns A, Jacoby R, Levy R. Psychiatric phenomena in Alzheimer's disease. III: Disorders of mood. *Br J Psychiatr.* 1990; **157**: 81–6.

52 Lobo A, Saz P, Marcos G, *et al.* The prevalence of dementia and depression in the elderly community in a southern European population: The Zaragoza study. *Arch Gen Psychiatr.* 1995; **52**(6): 497–506.

53 Zweig RM, Ross CA, Hedreen JC, *et al.* The neuropathology of aminergic nuclei in Alzheimer's disease. *Ann Neurol.* 1988; **24**(2): 233–42.

54 Kral VA. The relationship between senile dementia (Alzheimer type) and depression. *Can J Psychiatr – Revue Canadienne de Psychiatrie.* 1983; **28**(4): 304–6.

55 Reding M, Haycox J, Blass J. Depression in patients referred to a dementia clinic: a three-year prospective study. *Arch Neurol.* 1985; **42**(9): 894–6.

56 Agbayewa MO. Earlier psychiatric morbidity in patients with Alzheimer's disease. *J Am Geriatr Soc.* 1986; **34**(8): 561–4.

57 Bassuk SS, Berkman LF, Wypij D. Depressive symptomatology and incident cognitive decline in an elderly community sample. *Arch Gen Psychiatr.* 1998; **55**(12): 1073–81.

58 Yaffe K, Blackwell T, Gore R, *et al.* Depressive symptoms and cognitive decline in nondemented elderly women: a prospective study. *Arch Gen Psychiatr.* 1999; **56**(5): 425–30.

59 Geerlings MI, Schmand B, Braam AW, *et al.* Depressive symptoms and risk of Alzheimer's disease in more highly educated older people. *J Am Geriatr Soc.* 2000; **48**(9): 1092–7.

60 Geerlings MI, Schoevers RA, Beekman AT, *et al.* Depression and risk of cognitive decline and Alzheimer's disease: results of two prospective community-based studies in the Netherlands. *Br J Psychiatr.* 2000; **176**: 568–75.

61 Paterniti S, Verdier-Taillefer MH, Dufouil C, *et al.* Depressive symptoms and cognitive decline in elderly people: longitudinal study. *Br J Psychiatr.* 2002; **181**: 406–10.

62 Kral VA, Emery OB. Long-term follow-up of depressive pseudodementia of the aged. *Can J Psychiatr – Revue Canadienne de Psychiatrie.* 1989; **34**(5): 445–6.

63 Emery VO, Oxman TE. Update on the dementia spectrum of depression. *Am J Psychiatr.* 1992; **149**(3): 305–17.

64 Alexopoulos GS, Meyers BS, Young RC, *et al.* The course of geriatric depression with 'reversible dementia': a controlled study. *Am J Psychiatr.* 1993; **150**(11): 1693–9.

65 Speck CE, Kukull WA, Brenner DE, *et al.* History of depression as a risk factor for Alzheimer's disease. *Epidemiol.* 1995; **6**(4): 366–9.

66 Devanand DP, Sano M, Tang MX, *et al.* Depressed mood and the incidence of Alzheimer's disease in the elderly living in the community. *Arch Gen Psychiatr.* 1996; **53**(2): 175–82.

67 Kessing LV. Cognitive impairment in the euthymic phase of affective disorder. *Psychol Med.* 1998; **28**(5): 1027–38.

68 Pearlson GD, Rabins PV, Kim WS, *et al.* Structural brain CT changes and cognitive deficits in elderly depressives with and without reversible dementia ('pseudodementia'). *Psychol Med.* 1989; **19**(3): 573–84.

69 Mendez MF, Underwood KL, Zander BA, *et al.* Risk factors in Alzheimer's disease: a clinicopathologic study. *Neurology.* 1992; **42**(4): 770–5.

70 Dufouil C, Fuhrer R, Dartigues JF, *et al.* Longitudinal analysis of the association between depressive symptomatology and cognitive deterioration. *Am J Epidemiol.* 1996; **144**(7): 634–41.

71 Henderson AS, Korten AE, Jacomb PA, *et al.* The course of depression in the elderly: a longitudinal community-based study in Australia. *Psychol Med.* 1997; **27**(1): 119–29.

72 Palsson S, Aevarsson O, Skoog I. Depression, cerebral atrophy, cognitive performance and incidence of dementia: population study of 85-year-olds. *Br J Psychiatr.* 1999; **174**: 249–53.

73 Brown RP, Sweeney J, Loutsch E, *et al.* Involutional melancholia revisited. *Am J Psychiatr.* 1984; **141**(1): 24–8.

74 Burvill PW, Hall WD, Stampfer HG, *et al.* A comparison of early-onset and late-onset depressive illness in the elderly. *Br J Psychiatr.* 1989; **155**: 673–9.

75 Conwell Y, Nelson JC, Kim KM, *et al.* Depression in late life: age of onset as marker of a subtype. *J Affect Disord.* 1989; **17**(2): 189–95.

76 Brodaty H, Peters K, Boyce P, *et al.* Age and depression. *J Affect Disord.* 1991; **23**(3): 137–49.

77 Baldwin RC, Tomenson B. Depression in later life: a comparison of symptoms and risk factors in early and late onset cases. *Br J Psychiatr.* 1995; **167**(5): 649–52.

78 Brodaty H, Luscombe G, Parker G, *et al.* Early and late onset depression in old age: different aetiologies, same phenomenology. *J Affect Disord.* 2001; **66**(2–3): 225–36.

79 Cantillon M, Harwood D, Barker W, *et al.* No association between apolipoprotein E genotype and late-onset depression in Alzheimer's disease. *Biol Psychiatr.* 1997; **41**(2): 246–8.

80 Forsell Y, Corder EH, Basun H, *et al.* Depression and dementia in relation to apolipoprotein E polymorphism in a population sample age 75+. *Biol Psychiatr.* 1997; **42**(10): 898–903.

81 Lopez OL, Kamboh MI, Becker JT, *et al.* The apolipoprotein E epsilon 4 allele is not associated with psychiatric symptoms or extrapyramidal signs in probable Alzheimer's disease. *Neurology.* 1997; **49**(3): 794–7.

82 Schmand B, Hooijer C, Jonker C, *et al.* Apolipoprotein E phenotype is not related to late-life depression in a population-based sample. *Social Psychiatr Psychiatr Epidemiol.* 1998; **33**(1): 21–6.

83 Harwood DG, Barker WW, Ownby RL, *et al.* Factors associated with depressive symptoms in non-demented community-dwelling elderly. *Int J Geriatr Psychiatr.* 1999; **14**(5): 331–7.

84 Papassotiropoulos A, Bagli M, Jessen F, *et al.* Early-onset and late-onset depression are independent of the genetic polymorphism of apolipoprotein E. *Dement Geriatr Cogn Disord.* 1999; **10**(4): 258–61.

85 Ohara K, Nagai M, Suzuki Y, *et al.* Apolipoprotein E epsilon 4 allele and Japanese late-onset depressive disorders. *Biol Psychiatr.* 1999; **45**(3): 308–12.

86 Mauricio M, O'Hara R, Yesavage JA, *et al.* A longitudinal study of apolipoprotein-E genotype and depressive symptoms in community-dwelling older adults. *Am J Geriatr Psychiatr.* 2000; **8**(3): 196–200.

87 Hickie I, Scott E, Naismith S, *et al.* Late-onset depression: genetic, vascular and clinical contributions. *Psychol Med.* 2001; **31**(8): 1403–12.

88 Jackson EJ, Rajah S, Morris C, *et al.* Is apolipoprotein e4 associated with cognitive decline in depression? *Int J Geriatr Psychiatr.* 2001; **16**(4): 436–7.

89 Rigaud AS, Latour F, Moulin F, *et al.* Apolipoprotein E epsilon4 allele and clinically defined vascular depression. *Arch Gen Psychiatr.* 2002; **59**(3): 290–1.

90 Scarmeas N, Brandt J, Albert M, *et al.* Association between the APOE genotype and psychopathologic symptoms in Alzheimer's disease. *Neurology.* 2002; **58**(8): 1182–8.

91 Krishnan KR, Tupler LA, Ritchie JC, Jr., *et al.* Apolipoprotein E-epsilon 4 frequency in geriatric depression. *Biol Psychiatr.* 1996; **40**(1): 69–71.

92 Rigaud AS, Traykov L, Caputo L, *et al.* Association of the apolipoprotein E epsilon4 allele with late-onset depression. *Neuroepidemiol.* 2001; **20**(4): 268–72.

93 Kim DH, Payne ME, Levy RM, *et al.* APOE genotype and hippocampal volume change in geriatric depression. *Biol Psychiatr.* 2002; **51**(5): 426–9.

94 Lavretsky H, Lesser IM, Wohl M, *et al.* Apolipoprotein-E and white-matter hyperintensities in late-life depression. *Am J Geriatr Psychiatr.* 2000; **8**(3): 257–61.

95 Nebes RD, Vora IJ, Meltzer CC, *et al.* Relationship of deep white matter hyperintensities and apolipoprotein E genotype to depressive symptoms in older adults without clinical depression. *Am J Psychiatr.* 2001; **158**(6): 878–84.

96 Ladwig KH, Kieser M, Konig J, *et al.* Affective disorders and survival after acute myocardial infarction: results from the post-infarction late potential study. *Eur Heart J.* 1991; **12**(9): 959–64.

97 Frasure-Smith N, Lesperance F, Talajic M. Depression and 18-month prognosis after myocardial infarction. *Circulation.* 1995; **91**(4): 999–1005.

98 Musselman DL, Evans DL, Nemeroff CB. The relationship of depression to cardiovascular disease: epidemiology, biology, and treatment. *Arch Gen Psychiatr.* 1998; **55**(7): 580–92.

99 Newman SC. The prevalence of depression in Alzheimer's disease and vascular dementia in a population sample. *J Affect Disord.* 1999; **52**(1–3): 169–76.

100 Baldwin RC, O'Brien J. Vascular basis of late-onset depressive disorder. *Br J Psychiatr.* 2002; **180**: 157–60.

101 Wassertheil-Smoller S, Applegate WB, Berge K, *et al.* Change in depression as a precursor of cardiovascular events. SHEP Cooperative Research Group (Systolic Hypertension in the Elderly). *Arch Internal Med.* 1996; **156**(5): 553–61.

102 Ford DE, Mead LA, Chang PP, *et al.* Depression is a risk factor for coronary artery disease in men: the precursors study. *Arch Internal Med.* 1998; **158**(13): 1422–6.

103 Glassman AH, Shapiro PA. Depression and the course of coronary artery disease. *Am J Psychiatr.* 1998; **155**(1): 4–11.

104 Alexopoulos GS, Meyers BS, Young RC, *et al.* 'Vascular depression' hypothesis. *Arch Gen Psychiatr.* 1997; **54**(10): 915–22.

105 Alexopoulos GS, Meyers BS, Young RC, *et al.* Clinically defined vascular depression. *Am J Psychiatr.* 1997; **154**(4): 562–5.

106 Hickie I, Scott E. Late-onset depression: a preventable variant of cerebrovascular disease? *Psychol Med.* 1998; **28**: 1007–13.

107 Conway CR, Steffens DC. Geriatric depression: further evidence for the 'vascular depression' hypothesis. *Curr Opin Psychiatr.* 1999; **12**: 463–70.

108 Rao R, Jackson S, Howard R. Depression in older people with mild stroke, carotid stenosis and peripheral vascular disease: a comparison with healthy controls. *Int J Geriatr Psychiatr.* 2001; **16**(2): 175–83.

109 MacHale SM, O'Rourke SJ, Wardlaw JM, *et al.* Depression and its relation to lesion location after stroke. *J Neurol Neurosurg Psychiatr.* 1998; **64**(3): 371–4.

110 Gonzalez-Torrecillas JL, Mendlewicz J, Lobo A. Effects of early treatment of poststroke depression on neuropsychological rehabilitation. *Int Psychogeriatr.* 1995; **7**(4): 547–60.

111 Morris PL, Robinson RG, de Carvalho ML, *et al.* Lesion characteristics and depressed mood in the stroke data bank study. *J Neuropsychiatr Clin Neurosci.* 1996; **8**(2): 153–9.

112 Morris PL, Robinson RG, Raphael B, *et al.* Lesion location and poststroke depression. *J Neuropsychiatr Clin Neurosci.* 1996; **8**(4): 399–403.

113 Kramer-Ginsberg E, Greenwald BS, Krishnan KRR, *et al.* Neuropsychological functioning and MRI signal hyperintensities in geriatric depression. *Am J Psychiatr.* 1999; **156**(3): 438–44.

114 O'Brien JT, Ames D, Schweitzer I. White matter changes in depression and Alzheimer's disease: a review of magnetic resonance imaging studies. *Int J Geriatr Psychiatr.* 1996; **11**: 681–94.

115 Steffens DC, Helms MJ, Krishnan KR, *et al.* Cerebrovascular disease and depression symptoms in the cardiovascular health study. *Stroke.* 1999; **30**(10): 2159–66.

116 Greenwald BS, Kramer-Ginsberg E, Krishnan KR, *et al.* A controlled study of MRI signal hyperintensities in older depressed patients with and without hypertension. *J Am Geriatr Soc.* 2001; **49**(9): 1218–25.

117 Steffens DC, Krishnan KR, Crump C, *et al.* Cerebrovascular disease and evolution of depressive symptoms in the cardiovascular health study. *Stroke.* 2002; **33**(6): 1636–44.

118 Kim JM, Stewart R, Kim SW, *et al.* Vascular risk factors and incident late-life depression in a Korean population. *Br J Psychiatr.* 2006; **189**: 26–30.

119 Frasure-Smith N, Lesperance F, Talajic M. Depression following myocardial infarction: impact on 6-month survival. *JAMA.* 1993; **270**(15): 1819–25.

120 Frasure-Smith N, Lesperance F, Talajic M. Depression and 18-month prognosis after myocardial infarction. *Circulation.* 1995; **91**(4): 999–1005.

121 Frasure-Smith N, Lesperance F, Juneau M, *et al.* Gender, depression, and one-year prognosis after myocardial infarction. *Psychosom Med.* 1999; **61**(1): 26–37.

122 Glassman AH, O'Connor CM, Califf RM, *et al.* Sertraline treatment of major depression in patients with acute MI or unstable angina. *JAMA.* 2002; **288**(6): 701–9.

123 Kim JM, Stewart R, Shin IS, *et al.* Vascular disease/risk and late-life depression in a Korean community population. *Br J Psychiatr.* 2004; **185**: 102–7.

124 Morgan RE, Palinkas LA, Barrett-Connor EL, *et al.* Plasma cholesterol and depressive symptoms in older men. *Lancet.* 1993; **341**: 75–9.

125 Blazer DG, Burchett BB, Fillenbaum GG. APOE epsilon4 and low cholesterol as risks for depression in a biracial elderly community sample. *Am J Geriatr Psychiatr.* 2002; **10**(5): 515–20.

126 Brown SL, Salive ME, Harris TB, *et al.* Low cholesterol concentrations and severe depressive symptoms in elderly people. *BMJ.* 1994; **308**: 1328–32.

127 Wardle J, Armitage J, Collins R, *et al.* Randomised placebo controlled trial of effect on mood of lowering cholesterol concentration. Oxford Cholesterol Study Group. *BMJ.* 1996; **313**: 75–8.

128 Jones-Webb R, Jacobs DR, Jr., Flack JM, *et al.* Relationships between depressive symptoms, anxiety, alcohol consumption, and blood pressure: results from the CARDIA Study. Coronary Artery Risk Development in Young Adults Study. *Alcoholism: Clin Exp Res.* 1996; **20**(3): 420–7.

129 Rajala U, Keinanen-Kiukaanniemi S, Kivela SL. Non-insulin-dependent diabetes mellitus and depression in a middle-aged Finnish population. *Social Psychiatr Psychiatr Epidemiol.* 1997; **32**(6): 363–7.

130 Stewart R, Prince M, Mann A, *et al.* Stroke, vascular risk factors and depression: cross-sectional study in a UK Caribbean-born population. *Br J Psychiatr.* 2001; **178**(1): 23–8.

131 Baldwin RC. Is vascular depression a distinct sub-type of depressive disorder? A review of causal evidence. *Int J Geriatr Psychiatr.* 2005; **20**(1): 1–11.

132 Thomas AJ, Ferrier IN, Kalaria RN, *et al.* A neuropathological study of vascular factors in late-life depression. *J Neurol Neurosurg Psychiatr.* 2001; **70**(1): 83–7.

133 Thomas AJ, Ferrier IN, Kalaria RN, *et al.* Elevation in late-life depression of intercellular adhesion molecule-1 expression in the dorsolateral prefrontal cortex. *Am J Psychiatr.* 2000; **157**(10): 1682–4.

134 Thomas AJ, Ferrier IN, Kalaria RN, *et al.* Cell adhesion molecule expression in the dorsolateral prefrontal cortex and anterior cingulate cortex in major depression in the elderly. *Br J Psychiatr.* 2002; **181**: 129–34.

135 Pantoni L, Garcia JH. The significance of cerebral white matter abnormalities 100 years after Binswanger's report: a review. *Stroke.* 1995; **26**(7): 1293–301.

136 Pantoni L, Garcia JH. Pathogenesis of leukoaraiosis: a review. *Stroke.* 1997; **28**(3): 652–9.

137 Asnis GM, Sachar EJ, Halbreich U, *et al.* Cortisol secretion in relation to age in major depression. *Psychosom Med.* 1981; **43**(3): 235–42.

138 Rubinow DR, Post RM, Savard R, *et al.* Cortisol hypersecretion and cognitive impairment in depression. *Arch Gen Psychiatr.* 1984; **41**(3): 279–83.

139 O'Brien JT, Ames D, Schweitzer I, *et al.* Clinical and magnetic resonance imaging correlates of hypothalamic-pituitary-adrenal axis function in depression and Alzheimer's disease. *Br J Psychiatr.* 1996; **168**: 679–87.

140 Deuschle M, Schweiger U, Weber B, *et al.* Diurnal activity and pulsatility of the hypothalamus-pituitary-adrenal system in male depressed patients and healthy controls. *J Clin Endocrinol Metab.* 1997; **82**(1): 234–8.

141 Selye H, Tuchweber B. Stress in relation to aging and disease. In: Everitt AV, Burgess JA, editors. *Hypothalamus, pituitary and aging.* Springfield, IL: Charles C Thomas; 1976. pp. 553–69.

142 Carroll BJ, Curtis GC, Davies BM, *et al.* Urinary free cortisol excretion in depression. *Psychol Med.* 1976; **6**(1): 43–50.

143 Carroll BJ, Curtis GC, Mendels J. Cerebrospinal fluid and plasma free cortisol concentrations in depression. *Psychol Med.* 1976; **6**(2): 235–44.

144 Carroll BJ, Curtis GC, Mendels J. Neuroendocrine regulation in depression. II. Discrimination of depressed from nondepressed patients. *Arch Gen Psychiatr.* 1976; **33**(9): 1051–8.

145 Halbreich U, Asnis GM, Zumoff B, *et al.* Effect of age and sex on cortisol secretion in depressives and normals. *Psychiatr Res.* 1984; **13**(3): 221–9.

146 Holsboer F, Gerken A, von Bardeleben U, *et al.* Human corticotropin-releasing hormone in depression: correlation with thyrotropin secretion following thyrotropin-releasing hormone. *Biol Psychiatr.* 1986; **21**(7): 601–11.

147 Catalan R, Gallart JM, Castellanos JM, *et al.* Plasma corticotropin-releasing factor in depressive disorders. *Biol Psychiatr.* 1998; **44**(1): 15–20.

148 Scott LV, Dinan TG. Vasopressin and the regulation of hypothalamic-pituitary-adrenal axis function: implications for the pathophysiology of depression. *Life Sci.* 1998; **62**(22): 1985–98.

149 Sapolsky RM. Glucocorticoids and hippocampal atrophy in neuropsychiatric disorders. *Arch Gen Psychiatr.* 2000; **57**(10): 925–35.

150 Sapolsky RM, Krey LC, McEwen BS. The neuroendocrinology of stress and aging: the glucocorticoid cascade hypothesis. *Endocr Rev.* 1986; **7**(3): 284–301.

151 Kalimi M, Shafagoj Y, Loria R, *et al.* Anti-glucocorticoid effects of dehydroepiandrosterone (DHEA). *Mol Cell Biochem.* 1994; **131**(2): 99–104.

152 Magarinos AM, McEwen BS. Stress-induced atrophy of apical dendrites of hippocampal CA3c neurons: involvement of glucocorticoid secretion and excitatory amino acid receptors. *J Neurosci.* 1995; **69**(1): 89–98.

153 Magarinos AM, McEwen BS, Flugge G, *et al.* Chronic psychosocial stress causes apical dendritic atrophy of hippocampal CA3 pyramidal neurons in subordinate tree shrews. *J Neurosci.* 1996; **16**(10): 3534–40.

154 McEwen BS. Possible mechanisms for atrophy of the human hippocampus. *Mol Psychiatr.* 1997; **2**(3): 255–62.

155 De Kloet ER, Vreugdenhil E, Oitzl MS, *et al.* Brain corticosteroid receptor balance in health and disease. *Endocr Rev.* 1998; **19**(3): 269–301.

156 Trethowen WH, Cobb S. Neuropsychiatric aspects of Cushing's syndrome. *Arch Neurol Psychiatr.* 1952; **67**: 283–309.

157 Jeffcoate WJ, Silverstone JT, Edwards CR, *et al.* Psychiatric manifestations of Cushing's syndrome: response to lowering of plasma cortisol. *Q J Med.* 1979; **48**(191): 465–72.

158 Kelly WF, Checkley SA, Bender DA. Cushing's syndrome, tryptophan and depression. *Br J Psychiatr.* 1980; **136**: 125–32.

159 Kelly WF, Checkley SA, Bender DA, *et al.* Cushing's syndrome and depression: a prospective study of 26 patients. *Br J Psychiatr.* 1983; **142**: 16–19.

160 Murphy BE. Steroids and depression. *J Steroid Biochem Mol Biol.* 1991; **38**(5): 537–59.

161 Dorn LD, Burgess ES, Friedman TC, *et al.* The longitudinal course of psychopathology in Cushing's syndrome after correction of hypercortisolism. *J Clin Endocrinol Metab.* 1997; **82**(3): 912–19.

162 Starkman MN, Gebarski SS, Berent S, *et al.* Hippocampal formation volume, memory dysfunction, and cortisol levels in patients with Cushing's syndrome. *Biol Psychiatr.* 1992; **32**: 756–65.

163 Starkman MN, Giordani B, Gebarski SS, *et al.* Decrease in cortisol reverses human hippocampal atrophy following treatment of Cushing's disease. *Biol Psychiatr.* 1999; **46**(12): 1595–602.

164 De Kloet ER, Kovacs GL, Szabo G, *et al.* Decreased serotonin turnover in the dorsal hippocampus of rat brain shortly after adrenalectomy: selective normalization after corticosterone substitution. *Brain Res.* 1982; **239**(2): 659–63.

165 De Kloet ER, Sybesma H, Reul HM. Selective control by corticosterone of serotonin1 receptor capacity in raphe-hippocampal system. *Neuroendocrinol.* 1986; **42**(6): 513–21.

166 De Bellis MD, Gold PW, Geracioti TD, Jr., *et al.* Association of fluoxetine treatment with reductions in CSF concentrations of corticotropin-releasing hormone and arginine vasopressin in patients with major depression. *Am J Psychiatr.* 1993; **150**(4): 656–7.

167 Dinan TG. Glucocorticoids and the genesis of depressive illness: a psychobiological model. *Br J Psychiatr.* 1994; **164**(3): 365–71.

168 Dinan TG. Noradrenergic and serotonergic abnormalities in depression: stress-induced dysfunction? *J Clin Psychiatr.* 1996; **57**(Suppl. 4): S14–18.

169 Holsboer F, Barden N. Antidepressants and hypothalamic-pituitary-adrenocortical regulation. *Endocr Rev.* 1996; **17**(2): 187–205.

170 Duval F, Mokrani MC, Crocq MA, *et al.* Dopaminergic function and the cortisol response to dexamethasone in psychotic depression. *Prog Neuro-Psychopharmacol Biol Psychiatr.* 2000; **24**(2): 207–25.

171 Young EA, Haskett RF, Grunhaus L, *et al.* Increased evening activation of the hypothalamic-pituitary-adrenal axis in depressed patients. *Arch Gen Psychiatr.* 1994; **51**(9): 701–7.

172 Holsboer F. The rationale for corticotropin-releasing hormone receptor (CRH-R) antagonists to treat depression and anxiety. *J Psychiatr Res.* 1999; **33**(3): 181–214.

173 Owens MJ, Nemeroff CB. Physiology and pharmacology of corticotropin-releasing factor. *Pharmacol Rev.* 1991; **43**(4): 425–73.

174 Holsboer F, Liebl R, Hofschuster E. Repeated dexamethasone suppression test during depressive illness: normalisation of test result compared with clinical improvement. *J Affect Disord.* 1982; **4**(2): 93–101.

175 Greden JF, Gardner R, King D. Dexamethasone suppression tests in antidepressant treatment of melancholia: the process of normalization and test-retest reproducibility. *Arch Gen Psychiatr.* 1983; **40**(5): 493–500.

176 Holsboer-Trachsler E, Stohler R, Hatzinger M. Repeated administration of the combined dexamethasone-human corticotropin releasing hormone stimulation test during treatment of depression. *Psychiatr Res.* 1991; **38**(2): 163–71.

177 Heuser IJ, Schweiger U, Gotthardt U, *et al.* Pituitary-adrenal-system regulation and psychopathology during amitriptyline treatment in elderly depressed patients and normal comparison subjects. *Am J Psychiatr.* 1996; **153**(1): 93–9.

178 Michelson D, Galliven E, Hill L, *et al.* Chronic imipramine is associated with diminished hypothalamic-pituitary-adrenal axis responsivity in healthy humans. *J Clin Endocrinol Metab.* 1997; **82**(8): 2601–6.

179 Murphy BE, Ghadirian AM, Dhar V. Neuroendocrine responses to inhibitors of steroid biosynthesis in patients with major depression resistant to antidepressant therapy. *Can J Psychiatr – Revue Canadienne de Psychiatrie.* 1998; **43**(3): 279–86.

180 Zobel AW, Yassouridis A, Frieboes RM, *et al.* Prediction of medium-term outcome by cortisol response to the combined dexamethasone-CRH test in patients with remitted depression. *Am J Psychiatr.* 1999; **156**(6): 949–51.

181 Starkstein SE, Preziosi TJ, Bolduc PL, *et al.* Depression in Parkinson's disease. *J Nerv Mental Dis.* 1990; **178**(1): 27–31.

182 Starkstein SE, Petrracca G, Chemerinski E, *et al.* Depression in classic versus akinetic-rigid Parkinson's disease. *Mov Disord.* 1998; **13**(1): 29–33.

183 Mayberg HS, Solomon DH. Depression in Parkinson's disease: a biochemical and organic viewpoint. *Adv Neurol.* 1995; **65**: 49–60.

184 Tandberg E, Larsen JP, Aarsland D, Cummings JL. The occurrence of depression in Parkinson's disease. *Arch Neurol.* 1996; **53**: 175–9.

185 McDonald WM, Richard IH, DeLong MR. Prevalence, etiology, and treatment of depression in Parkinson's disease. *Biol Psychiatr.* 2003; **54**: 363–75.

186 Alexander GE, DeLong MR, Strick PL. Parallel organization of functionally segregated circuits linking basal ganglia and cortex. *Ann Rev Neurosci.* 1986; **9**: 357–81.

187 Alexander GE, Crutcher MD. Functional architecture of basal ganglia circuits: neural substrates of parallel processing. *TINS.* 1990; **13**(7): 226–71.

188 Alexander GE, Crutcher MD, DeLong MR. Basal ganglia-thalamocortical circuits: parallel substrates for motor, oculomotor, 'prefrontal' and 'limbic' functions. *Prog Brain Res.* 1990; **85**: 119–46.

189 Cummings JL. Frontal-subcortical circuits and human behavior. *Arch Neurol.* 1993; **50**(8): 873–80.

190 Salloway S, Cummings J. Subcortical disease and neuropsychiatric illness. *J Neuropsychiatr Clin Neurosci.* 1994; **6**(2): 93–9.

191 Mega MS, Cummings JL. Frontal-subcortical circuits and neuropsychiatric disorders. *J Neuropsychiatr Clin Neurosci.* 1994; **6**(4): 358–70.

192 Morris P, Rapoport SI. Neuroimaging and affective disorder in late life: a review. *Can J Psychiatr – Revue Canadienne de Psychiatrie.* 1990; **35**(4): 347–54.

193 Krishnan KRR. Organic bases of depression in the elderly. *Ann Rev Med.* 1991; **42**: 261–6.

194 Baldwin RC. Late life depression and structural brain changes: a review of recent magnetic resonance imaging research. *Int J Geriatr Psychiatr.* 1993; **8**: 115–23.

195 Videbech P. MRI findings in patients with affective disorder: a meta-analysis. *Acta Psychiatr Scand.* 1997; **96**: 157–68.

196 Drevets WC. Functional neuroimaging studies of depression: the anatomy of melancholia. *Ann Rev Med.* 1998; **49**: 341–61.

197 Beyer JL. Volumetric brain imaging studies in the elderly with mood disorders. *Curr Psychiatr Rep.* 2006; **8**(1): 18–24.

198 Dolan RJ, Calloway SP, Mann AH. Cerebral ventricular size in depressed subjects. *Psychol Med.* 1985; **15**(4): 873–8.

199 Zubenko GS, Sullivan P, Nelson JP, *et al.* Brain imaging abnormalities in mental disorders of late life. *Arch Neurol.* 1990; **47**: 1107–11.

200 Beats B, Levy R, Forstl H. Ventricular enlargement and caudate hyperdensity in elderly depressives. *Biol Psychiatr.* 1991; **30**(5): 452–8.

201 Rabins PV, Pearlson GD, Aylward E, *et al.* Cortical magnetic resonance imaging changes in elderly inpatients with depression. *Am J Psychiatr.* 1991; **148**(5): 617–20.

202 Jacoby RJ, Levy R, Bird JM. Computed tomography and the outcome of affective disorder: a follow-up study of elderly patients. *Br J Psychiatr.* 1981; 139: 288–92.

203 Alexopoulos GS, Young RC, Shindledecker RD. Brain computed tomography findings in geriatric depression and primary degenerative dementia. *Biol Psychiatr.* 1992; **31**(6): 591–9.

204 Krishnan KR, McDonald WM, Escalona PR, *et al.* Magnetic resonance imaging of the caudate nuclei in depression: preliminary observations. *Arch Gen Psychiatr.* 1992; **49**(7): 553–7.

205 Greenwald BS, Kramer-Ginsberg E, Bogerts B, *et al.* Qualitative magnetic resonance imaging findings in geriatric depression: possible link between later-onset depression and Alzheimer's disease? *Psychol Med.* 1997; **27**: 421–31.

206 Jacoby RJ, Levy R. Computed tomography in the elderly. 3. Affective disorder. *Br J Psychiatr.* 1980; **136**: 270–5.

207 Coffey CE, Figiel GS, Djang WT, *et al.* Leukoencephalopathy in elderly depressed patients referred for ECT. *Biol Psychiatr.* 1988; **24**(2): 143–61.

208 Lesser IM, Miller BL, Boone KB, *et al.* Brain injury and cognitive function in late-onset psychotic depression. *J Neuropsychiatr Clin Neurosci.* 1991; **3**(1): 33–40.

209 Wurthmann C, Bogerts B, Falkai P. Brain morphology assessed by computed tomography in patients with geriatric depression, patients with degenerative dementia, and normal control subjects. *Psychiatr Res.* 1995; **61**(2): 103–11.

210 Dahabra S, Ashton CH, Bahrainian M, *et al.* Structural and functional abnormalities in elderly patients clinically recovered from early- and late-onset depression. *Biol Psychiatr.* 1998; **44**: 34–46.

211 Jeste DV, Lohr JB, Goodwin FK. Neuroanatomical studies of major affective disorders: a review and suggestions for further research. *Br J Psychiatr.* 1988; **153**: 444–59.

212 Krishnan KRR. Neuroanatomic substrates of depression in the elderly. *J Geriatr Psychiatr Neurol.* 1993; **6**: 39–58.

213 Shima S, Shikano T, Kitamura T, *et al.* Depression and ventricular enlargement. *Acta Psychiatr Scand.* 1984; **70**(3): 275–7.

214 Pantel J, Schroder J, Essig M, *et al.* Quantitative magnetic resonance imaging in geriatric depression and primary degenerative dementia. *J Affect Disord.* 1997; **42**: 69–83.

215 Abas M, Sahakian BJ, Levy R. Neuropsychological deficits and CT scan changes in elderly depressives. *Psychol Med.* 1990; **20**: 507–20.

216 Kumar A, Schweizer E, Jin Z, *et al.* Neuroanatomical substrates of late-life minor depression: a quantitative magnetic resonance imaging study. *Arch Neurol.* 1997; **54**(5): 613–17.

217 Hauser P, Matochik J, Altshuler LL, *et al.* MRI-based measurements of temporal lobe and ventricular structures in patients with bipolar I and bipolar II disorders. *J Affect Disord.* 2000; **60**(1): 25–32.

218 Rabins PV, Aylward E, Holroyd S, *et al.* MRI findings differentiate between late-onset schizophrenia and late-life mood disorder. *Int J Geriatr Psychiatr.* 2000; **15**(10): 954–60.

219 Axelson DA, Doraiswamy PM, McDonald WM, *et al.* Hypercortisolemia and hippocampal changes in depression. *Psychiatr Res.* 1993; **47**(2): 163–73.

220 Dupont RM, Jernigan TL, Heindel W, *et al.* Magnetic resonance imaging and mood disorders: localization of white matter and other subcortical abnormalities. *Arch Gen Psychiatr.* 1995; **52**(9): 747–55.

221 Ashtari M, Greenwald BS, Kramer-Ginsberg J, *et al.* Hippocampal/amygdala volumes in geriatric depression. *Psychol Med.* 1999; **29**: 629–38.

222 Rusch BD, Abercrombie HC, Oakes TR, *et al.* Hippocampal morphometry in depressed patients and control subjects: relations to anxiety symptoms. *Biol Psychiatr.* 2001; **50**(12): 960–4.

223 Coffey CE, Wilkinson WE, Weiner RD, *et al.* Quantitative cerebral anatomy in depression: a controlled magnetic resonance imaging study. *Arch Gen Psychiatr.* 1993; **50**: 7–15.

224 Kumar A, Bilker W, Jin Z, *et al.* Atrophy and high intensity lesions: complementary neurobiological mechanisms in late-life major depression. *Neuropsychopharmacol.* 2000; **22**(3): 264–74.

225 Sheline YI. Hippocampal atrophy in major depression: a result of depression-induced neurotoxicity? *Mol Psychiatr.* 1996; **1**(4): 298–9.

226 Bremner JD, Narayan M, Anderson ER, *et al.* Hippocampal volume reduction in major depression. *Am J Psychiatr.* 2000; **157**(1): 115–18.

227 Mervaala E, Fohr J, Kononen M, *et al.* Quantitative MRI of the hippocampus and amygdala in severe depression. *Psychol Med.* 2000; **30**(1): 117–25.

228 Steffens DC, Byrum CE, McQuoid DR, *et al.* Hippocampal volume in geriatric depression. *Biol Psychiatr.* 2000; **48**(4): 301–9.

229 Frodl T, Meisenzahl EM, Zetzsche T, *et al.* Hippocampal changes in patients with a first episode of major depression. *Am J Psychiatr.* 2002; **159**(7): 1112–18.

230 Bell-McGinty S, Butters MA, Meltzer CC, *et al.* Brain morphometric abnormalities in geriatric depression: long-term neurobiological effects of illness duration. *Am J Psychiatr.* 2002; **159**(8): 1424–7.

231 MacQueen GM, Campbell S, McEwen BS, *et al.* Course of illness, hippocampal function, and hippocampal volume in major depression. *Proc Nat Acad Sci USA.* 2003; **100**(3): 1387–92.

232 Caetano SC, Hatch JP, Brambilla P, *et al.* Anatomical MRI study of hippocampus and amygdala in patients with current and remitted major depression. *Psychiatr Res.* 2004; **132**(2): 141–7.

233 Lloyd AJ, Ferrier IN, Barber R, *et al.* Hippocampal volume change in depression: late- and early-onset illness compared. *Br J Psychiatr.* 2004; **184**: 488–95.

234 O'Brien JT, Lloyd A, McKeith I, *et al.* A longitudinal study of hippocampal volume, cortisol levels, and cognition in older depressed subjects. *Am J Psychiatr.* 2004; **161**(11): 2081–90.

235 Coffey CE, Figiel GS, Djang WT, *et al.* Subcortical hyperintensity on magnetic resonance imaging: a comparison of normal and depressed elderly subjects. *Am J Psychiatr.* 1990; **147**(2): 187–9.

236 Breteler MM, van Swieten JC, Bots ML, *et al.* Cerebral white matter lesions, vascular risk factors, and cognitive function in a population-based study: the Rotterdam Study. *Neurology.* 1994; **44**(7): 1246–52.

237 Erkinjuntti T, Gao F, Lee DH, *et al.* Lack of difference in brain hyperintensities between patients with early Alzheimer's disease and control subjects. *Arch Neurol.* 1994; **51**: 260–9.

238 Christiansen P, Larsson HB, Thomsen C, *et al.* Age dependent white matter lesions and brain volume changes in healthy volunteers. *Acta Radiol.* 1994; **35**(2): 117–22.

239 Ylikoski A, Erkinjuntti T, Raininko R, *et al.* White matter hyperintensities on MRI in the neurologically nondiseased elderly: analysis of cohorts of consecutive subjects aged 55 to 85 years living at home. *Stroke.* 1995; **26**(7): 1171–7.

240 Greenwald BS, Kramer-Ginsberg E, Krishnan KRR, *et al.* MRI signal hyperintensities in geriatric depression. *Am J Psychiatr.* 1996; **153**(9): 1212–15.

241 Iidaka T, Nakajima T, Kawamoto K, *et al.* Signal hyperintensities on brain magnetic resonance imaging in elderly depressed patients. *Eur Neurol.* 1996; **36**: 293–9.

242 O'Brien J, Desmond P, Ames D, *et al.* A magnetic resonance imaging study of white matter lesions in depression and Alzheimer's disease. *Br J Psychiatr.* 1996; **168**: 477–85.

243 Greenwald BS, Kramer-Ginsberg E, Krishnan KRR, *et al.* Neuroanatomic localization of magnetic resonance imaging signal hyperintensities in geriatric depression. *Stroke.* 1998; **29**: 613–17.

244 Skoog I. A review on blood pressure and ischaemic white matter lesions. *Demen Geriatr Cogn Disord.* 1998; **9**(Suppl. 1): 13–19.

245 Schmidt R, Fazekas F, Kapeller P, *et al.* MRI white matter hyperintensities: three-year follow-up of the Austrian Stroke Prevention Study. *Neurology.* 1999; **53**(1): 132–9.

246 de Leeuw FE, de Groot JC, Bots ML, *et al.* Carotid atherosclerosis and cerebral white matter lesions in a population based magnetic resonance imaging study. *Neurology.* 2000; **247**(4): 291–6.

247 de Leeuw FE, de Groot JC, Oudkerk M, *et al.* Atrial fibrillation and the risk of cerebral white matter lesions. *Neurology.* 2000; **54**(9): 1795–801.

248 de Leeuw FE, De Groot JC, Oudkerk M, *et al.* Aortic atherosclerosis at middle age predicts cerebral white matter lesions in the elderly. *Stroke.* 2000; **31**(2): 425–9.

249 Awad IA, Johnson PC, Spetzler RF, *et al.* Incidental subcortical lesions identified on magnetic resonance imaging in the elderly. II. Postmortem pathological correlations. *Stroke.* 1986; **17**(6): 1090–7.

250 Grafton ST, Sumi SM, Stimac GK, *et al.* Comparison of postmortem magnetic resonance imaging and neuropathologic findings in the cerebral white matter. *Arch Neurol.* 1991; **48**(3): 293–8.

251 van Swieten JC, van den Hout JH, van Ketel BA, *et al.* Periventricular lesions in the white matter on magnetic resonance imaging in the elderly: a morphometric correlation with arteriolosclerosis and dilated perivascular spaces. *Brain.* 1991; **114**(2): 761–74.

252 Chimowitz MI, Estes ML, Furlan AJ, *et al.* Further observations on the pathology of subcortical lesions identified on magnetic resonance imaging. *Arch Neurol.* 1992; **49**: 747–52.

253 Fazekas F, Kleinert R, Offenbacher H, *et al.* Pathologic correlates of incidental MRI white matter signal hyperintensities. *Neurology.* 1993; **43**: 1683–9.

254 Firbank MJ, Lloyd AJ, Ferrier N, *et al.* A volumetric study of MRI signal hyperintensities in late-life depression. *Am J Geriatr Psychiatr.* 2004; **12**(6): 606–12.

255 Salloway S, Malloy P, Kohn R, *et al.* MRI and neuropsychological differences in early- and late-life-onset geriatric depression. *Neurology.* 1996; **46**: 1567–74.

256 Hickie I, Scott E, Mitchell P, *et al.* Subcortical hyperintensities on magnetic resonance imaging: clinical correlates and prognostic significance in patients with severe depression. *Biol Psychiatr.* 1995; **37**: 151–60.

257 Figiel GS, Krishnan KRR, Doraiswamy PM, *et al.* Subcortical hyperintensities on brain magnetic resonance imaging: a comparison between late age onset and early onset elderly depressed subjects. *Neurobiol Aging.* 1991; **26**: 245–7.

258 Simpson SW, Jackson A, Baldwin RC, *et al.* Subcortical hyperintensities in late-life depression: acute response to treatment and neuropsychological impairment. *Int Psychogeriatr.* 1997; **3**: 257–75.

259 Baldwin RC, Walker S, Simpson SW, *et al.* The prognostic significance of abnormalities seen on magnetic resonance imaging in late life depression: clinical outcome, mortality and progression to dementia at three years. *Int J Geriatr Psychiatr.* 2000; **15**(12): 1097–104.

260 Barber R, Scheltens P, Gholkar A, *et al.* White matter lesions on magnetic resonance imaging in dementia with Lewy bodies, Alzheimer's disease, vascular dementia, and normal aging. *J Neurol Neurosurg Psychiatr.* 1999; **67**(1): 66–72.

261 O'Brien J, Perry R, Barber R, *et al.* The association between white matter lesions on magnetic resonance imaging and noncognitive symptoms. *Ann New York Acad Sci.* 2000; **903**: 482–9.

262 Curran SM, Murray CM, Van Beck M, *et al.* A single photon emission computerised tomography study of regional brain function in elderly patients with major depression and with Alzheimer-type dementia. *Br J Psychiatr.* 1993; **163**: 155–65.

263 Vasile RG, Schwartz RB, Garada B, *et al.* Focal cerebral perfusion defects demonstrated by 99mTc-hexamethylpropyleneamine oxime SPECT in elderly depressed patients. *Psychiatr Res.* 1996; **67**(1): 59–70.

264 Goodwin GM. Functional imaging, affective disorder and dementia. *Br Med Bull.* 1996; **52**(3): 495–512.

265 Meltzer CC, Smith G, DeKosky ST, *et al.* Serotonin in aging, late-life depression, and Alzheimer's disease: the emerging role of functional imaging. *Neuropsychopharmacol.* 1998; **18**(6): 407–30.

266 Halloran E, Prentice N, Murray CL, *et al.* Follow-up study of depression in the elderly: clinical and SPECT data. *Br J Psychiatr.* 1999; **175**: 252–8.

267 Navarro V, Gasto C, Lomena F, *et al.* Frontal cerebral perfusion dysfunction in elderly late-onset major depression assessed by 99MTC-HMPAO SPECT. *Neuroimage.* 2001; **14**(1): 202–5.

268 Sheline YI, Mintun MA, Moerlein SM, *et al.* Greater loss of 5-HT(2A) receptors in midlife than in late life. *Am J Psychiatr.* 2002; **159**(3): 430–5.

269 Smith GS, Kramer E, Hermann CR, *et al.* Acute and chronic effects of citalopram on cerebral glucose metabolism in geriatric depression. *Am J Geriatr Psychiatr.* 2002; **10**(6): 715–23.

270 Meltzer CC, Price JC, Mathis CA, *et al.* Serotonin 1A receptor binding and treatment response in late-life depression. *Neuropsychopharmacol.* 2004; **29**(12): 2258–65.

271 Aizenstein HJ, Butters MA, Figurski JL, *et al.* Prefrontal and striatal activation during sequence learning in geriatric depression. *Biol Psychiatr.* 2005; **58**(4): 290–6.

272 Krishnan KRR, Hays JC, Blazer DC. MRI-defined vascular depression. *Am J Psychiatr.* 1997; **154**(4): 497–501.

273 Steffens DC, Krishnan KR. Structural neuroimaging and mood disorders: recent findings, implications for classification, and future directions. *Biol Psychiatr.* 1998; **43**(10): 705–12.

274 Simpson S, Baldwin RC, Jackson A, *et al.* Is subcortical disease associated with a poor response to antidepressants? Neurological, neuropsychological and neuroradiological findings in late life depression. *Psychol Med.* 1998; **28**: 1015–26.

275 Krishnan KR, Goli V, Ellinwood EH, *et al.* Leukoencephalopathy in patients diagnosed as major depressive. *Biol Psychiatr.* 1988; **23**(5): 519–22.

276 Krishnan KR, Hays JC, George LK, *et al.* Six-month outcomes for MRI-related vascular depression. *Depress Anxiety.* 1998; **8**(4): 142–6.

277 O'Brien J, Ames D, Chiu E, *et al.* Severe deep white matter lesions and outcome in elderly patients with major depressive disorder: follow up study. *BMJ.* 1998; **317**(7164): 982–4.

278 Lloyd AJ, Grace JB, Jaros E, *et al.* Depression in late life, cognitive decline and white matter pathology in two clinico-pathologically investigated cases. *Int J Geriatr Psychiatr.* 2001; **16**: 281–7.

279 Thomas AJ, Perry R, Barber R *et al.* Pathologies and pathological mechanisms for white matter hyperintensities in depression. *Ann New York Acad Sci.* 2002; **977**: 333–9.

280 Thomas AJ, O'Brien JT, Barber R, *et al.* A neuropathological study of periventricular white matter hyperintensities in major depression. *J Affect Disord.* 2003; **76**(1–3): 49–54.

281 Thomas AJ, Perry R, Kalaria RN, *et al.* Neuropathological evidence for ischemia in the white matter of the dorsolateral prefrontal cortex in late-life depression. *Int J Geriatr Psychiatr.* 2003; **18**(1): 7–13.

282 Thomas AJ, Davis S, Morris C, *et al.* Increase in interleukin-1beta in late-life depression. *Am J Psychiatr.* 2005; **162**(1): 175–7.

283 Kotlyar M, Dysken M, Adson DE. Update on drug-induced depression in the elderly. *Am J Geriatr Pharmacother.* 2005; **3**(4): 288–300.

284 Long TD, Kathol RG. Critical review of data supporting affective disorder caused by nonpsychotropic medication. *Ann Clin Psychiatr.* 1993; **5**(4): 259–70.

285 Zweifel JE, O'Brien WH. A meta-analysis of the effect of hormone replacement therapy upon depressed mood. *Psychoneuroendocrinol.* 1997; **22**(3): 189–212.

286 Patten SB, Neutel CI. Corticosteroid-induced adverse psychiatric effects: incidence, diagnosis and management. *Drug Safety.* 2000; **22**(2): 111–22.

287 Muldoon MF, Manuck SB, Mendelsohn AB, *et al.* Cholesterol reduction and non-illness mortality: meta-analysis of randomised clinical trials. *BMJ.* 2001; **322**(7277): 11–15.

288 Riggs BL, Hartmann LC. Selective estrogen-receptor modulators: mechanisms of action and application to clinical practice. *N Engl J Med.* 2003; **348**(7): 618–29.

289 Yang CC, Jick SS, Jick H. Lipid-lowering drugs and the risk of depression and suicidal behavior. *Arch Intern Med.* 2003; **163**(16): 1926–32.

290 Besag FM. Behavioural effects of the newer antiepileptic drugs: an update. *Expert Opin Drug Safety.* 2004; **3**(1): 1–8.

291 Grace J, O'Brien JT. Association of life events and psychosocial factors with early but not late onset depression in the elderly: implications for possible differences in aetiology. *Int J Geriatr Psychiatr.* 2003; **18**(6): 473–8.

292 Murphy E. Social origins of depression in old age. *Br J Psychiatr.* 1982; **141**: 135–42.

293 Braam AW, Van den Eeden P, Prince MJ, *et al.* Religion as a cross-cultural determinant of depression in elderly Europeans: results from the EURODEP collaboration. *Psychol Med.* 2001; **31**(5): 803–14.

294 Kraaij V, de Wilde EJ. Negative life events and depressive symptoms in the elderly: a life span perspective. *Aging Mental Health.* 2001; **5**(1): 84–91.

295 Brilman EI, Ormel J. Life events, difficulties and onset of depressive episodes in later life. *Psychol Med.* 2001; **31**(5): 859–69.

296 Kivela SL, Kongas-Saviaro P, Laippala P, *et al.* Social and psychosocial factors predicting depression in old age: a longitudinal study. *Int Psychogeriatr.* 1996; **8**(4): 635–44.

297 Janssen J, Beekman AT, Comijs HC, *et al.* Late-life depression: the differences between early- and late-onset illness in a community-based sample. *Int J Geriatr Psychiatr.* 2006; **21**(1): 86–93.

298 Alexopoulos GS, Vrontou C, Kakuma T, *et al.* Disability in geriatric depression. *Am J Psychiatr.* 1996; **153**(7): 877–85.

299 Steffens DC, Hays JC, Krishnan KR. Disability in geriatric depression. *Am J Geriatr Psychiatr.* 1999; **7**(1): 34–40.

300 Devanand DP, Adorno E, Cheng J, *et al.* Late onset dysthymic disorder and major depression differ from early onset dysthymic disorder and major depression in elderly outpatients. *J Affect Disord.* 2004; **78**(3): 259–67.

301 Mazure CM, Maciejewski PK, Jacobs SC, *et al.* Stressful life events interacting with cognitive/personality styles to predict late-onset major depression. *Am J Geriatr Psychiatr.* 2002; **10**(3): 297–304.

Pharmacological management of depression in older people

STEPHEN CURRAN, ANDREW BYRNE AND JOHN P WATTIS

Introduction

Late-life depression is similar to depression at other times of life. However, ageing and other factors may alter the presentation in older people. In particular older people are less likely to complain of sadness compared with younger patients; they are more likely to complain of physical symptoms, memory complaints and anxiety symptoms.[1] In addition, depression in patients with dementia may lead to behavioural disturbance.[2] Consequently, diagnosis can be more difficult and therefore missed and patients may go untreated. Some of the issues to do with diagnosis are discussed in Chapter 2.

Depression also has a significant impact on individual patients, their families and society more generally. In particular, depression is one of the leading causes of disability; it leads to a greater risk of hospitalisation as well as inappropriate bed use and prolonged hospitalisation; it is the single most important predictor of suicide. It also reduces compliance with medical treatments, reduces the patient's quality of life and is an independent predictor of mortality.[1]

Prevalence

Depression is two to three times more prevalent than dementia and is the most common mental health problem among older adults. In a recent community-based study of people aged 65 years and over the prevalence of depression was 8.7% with a higher prevalence in women (10.4%) and was associated with functional disability, comorbid physical illness and social deprivation.[3] Rates of depression in nursing and residential homes and acute medical wards can rise to 45%. Since depressive disorder, disability and dependency are all highly correlated it is important to consider the diagnosis of depression in these settings.[3]

Aetiology

A number of factors can increase the risk of depression occurring, precipitate depression or make the depression more difficult to treat and these issues have been discussed in Chapter 3. However, a brief discussion here emphasises the importance of understanding the aetiology of depression as this can have important implications for treatment and prognosis. *Genetic* susceptibility is less important in depression when onset is in later life and *females* are more susceptible to depression. A *previous history of depression* is an important predisposing factor and *widows*, *widowers* and *divorcees* are more susceptible. *Neurotransmitter* changes are also well recognised in older people including reductions in noradrenaline and serotonin.[5] There are a number of other *brain changes* including cerebral atrophy but it is not entirely clear if this is related to depression. Deep white matter lesions and subcortical grey matter lesions seem to be commoner in late-onset depression. Epidemiological studies have also highlighted an association between *hypertension* and depression as well as other *vascular risk factors* including smoking, excessive alcohol consumption and hypotension. Personality factors are important predisposing factors, particularly *avoidant* and *dependent* personality types. There is a strong association between disability (functional limitation) due to medical conditions and depression and especially with pain.[6] Being a carer of someone who is chronically ill is another important risk factor. Precipitating factors include *life events* such as bereavement, separation, acute physical illness, moving into residential care and chronic stress. A number of *drugs* can also cause or aggravate depression including beta-blockers, methyldopa, reserpine, clonidine, calcium channel blockers, digoxin, codeine, opioids, indomethacin, steroids, L-Dopa, amantadine, tetrabenazine, antipsychotics and benzodiazepines. Some factors can be protective including good *medical care* including general health, nutrition and physical fitness, good *coping behaviours*, e.g. adaptive personality, capacity for confiding relationships and good *social support* including religious/spiritual beliefs.

Association with physical illness

The association between depression and physical illness is complex and is discussed more fully in Chapters 1, 8 and 9. Depression may worsen or cause a physical illness, and a physical illness and certain drugs can cause or exacerbate depression. Pain in particular is an important element. The perception of pain can be improved by improvement of the depression and antidepressants can also directly improve pain symptoms. Depression is an independent risk factor for a number of medical conditions including stroke[7] and heart failure.[8]

Depressive symptoms also add to the disability from physical illness and are associated with physical decline.[9] A number of medical conditions increase the risk of depression including hypo/hyperthyroidism, Cushing's disease, hypercalcaemia, pernicious anaemia, cerebrovascular disease, Parkinson's disease, Alzheimer's disease, SLE, HIV-AIDS, cancer particularly of the lung and pancreas and chronic infections such as brucellosis. In addition, hyponatraemia has been associated with all types of antidepressants but especially with selective serotonin reuptake inhibitors (SSRIs). It typically causes drowsiness and confusion and convulsions when more severe but responds well to stopping the antidepressant.

Mechanism of action

For nearly 40 years, the principal theory to explain the biological basis of depression has been the *monoamine hypothesis*. This theory proposes that depression is due to a deficiency in one or more of three monoamines, namely noradrenaline, serotonin and dopamine in the synaptic clefts of the appropriate neurones. For example, tricyclic antidepressants (TCAs) block the neurotransmitter reuptake pump, causing neurotransmitters to accumulate in the synaptic cleft thus returning the neuron to a 'normal state'. However, despite the fact that neurotransmitter levels return to normal fairly quickly the clinical effect is delayed as is the down-regulation of receptor sensitivity. A related theory is the *monoamine receptor hypothesis*. The consequence of neurotransmitter depletion is that postsynaptic receptors become up-regulated (increased in number) and the degree of up-regulation correlates with the degree of depression. In addition, down-regulation correlates with the onset of antidepressant action.[10]

Classes of antidepressants

Tricyclic antidepressants (TCAs)

All these compounds are inhibitors of noradrenaline uptake with a variable potency of inhibiting serotonin uptake as well. They include amitriptyline, imipramine, dothiepin, doxepin, nortriptyline and lofepramine. Tricyclics can be subdivided into secondary (e.g. nortriptyline) and tertiary amines (e.g. imipramine and amitriptyline). Secondary amines are predominantly noradrenaline reuptake inhibitors.

These drugs are generally well absorbed orally. They are lipophilic and widely distributed in the body. They are metabolised in the liver and some of the metabolites are active antidepressants. The major route of elimination is renal excretion. The lower rates of both hepatic metabolism and decreased renal clearance in this age group may reduce the dosage needed to achieve a given blood level. Some clinicians have recommended plasma level monitoring for TCAs in older patients but this is seldom done in clinical practice. Lofepramine has minimal anticholinergic properties and cardiac toxicity in older patients by comparison with older TCAs but in the authors' experience it can occasionally cause jaundice.

Drugs with a tertiary amine structure tend to produce more antagonism of α_1 adrenergic receptors with subsequent hypotension, blockage of histamine (causing sedation) and cholinergic receptors (causing dry mouth, blurred vision, urinary retention, dizziness, tachycardia, memory impairment and at high and toxic doses, delirium). The tendency to produce orthostatic hypotension is a serious side-effect in older patients leading to an increased risk of falls and limb fracture.

Clinical studies

In a systematic review of 186 randomised controlled trials (RCTs) mainly involving younger people, amitriptyline was found to be less well tolerated than other drugs (mainly SSRIs) but slightly more patients recovered compared with alternative antidepressants.[11] There have also been a small number of double-blind, placebo-controlled trials of antidepressants in older people and most of these are of TCAs.[12,13] There is also some evidence that TCAs may be more effective than SSRIs in treating severe depression in older people.[14]

Patients commenced on TCAs often receive subtherapeutic doses for inadequate periods of time compared with SSRIs.[15] However, a recent Cochrane review found that treatment of depression with low dose tricyclics is justified.[16] In addition, a further Cochrane review of amitryptyline for older people found that it was at least as effective as other TCAs (in therapeutic doses) and newer compounds, especially SSRIs, but patients taking amitriptyline experienced a higher prevalence of side-effects.[17]

Selective serotonin reuptake inhibitors (SSRIs)

SSRIs have a selective effect on serotonin reuptake, making them less likely to cause the side-effects encountered with TCAs. They include fluvoxamine, fluoxetine, paroxetine, sertraline, citalopram and escitalopram. Escitalopram is the therapeutically active S-enantiomer of RS-citalopram.

These drugs are rapidly absorbed from the gut and broken down into several metabolites (often with antidepressant activity) each with different half-lives. All SSRIs are extensively protein-bound. The plasma half-lives of fluvoxamine and fluoxetine are relatively unaffected by age while steady-state plasma concentrations of paroxetine, sertraline and citalopram are higher in the elderly and elimination half-life is longer than for the same dose in adult patients.[18] Paroxetine has also some affinity for muscarinic receptors, making it the most sedative SSRI. Administration of all SSRIs can augment TCA activity, as well as other drugs metabolised by the hepatic cytochrome P450 system. These interactions tend to be dose dependent.

All SSRIs are effective and well tolerated in older depressed patients.[18] They are relatively free of anticholinergic effects and cardiotoxicity, and cause less postural hypotension than TCAs. Their main side-effects include headache, nausea, diarrhoea, insomnia, dizziness and sexual dysfunction. Most SSRIs (not citalopram, escitalopam and sertraline) cause clinically relevant drug–drug interactions through their inhibitory effects on the cytochrome P450 system. Paroxetine, fluoxetine and fluvoxamine have inhibitory effects on cytochrome P450 isoenzymes that can lead to increased plasma levels of antipsychotics and TCAs.[19] The half-lives of sertraline, citalopram and paroxetine are prolonged in the older patients[18] and lower starting doses of paroxetine (10mg/day) and perhaps citalopram may be needed. Elimination of citalopram, fluoxetine, sertraline and fluvoxamine are decreased in hepatic impairment and paroxetine elimination is reduced in renal impairment.

Clinical studies

Wilson *et al.*[13] found that in older people with depression the number needed to treat for a therapeutic response for a TCA was 4 whereas for SSRIs the number was 7. However, only two trials met criteria for the analysis and both of these involved fluoxetine.

One study involving 369 patients (many of whom were over 65 with a mean age of 57.1 years) showed sertraline was well tolerated in patients with major depression and acute MI or unstable angina.[20] Sertraline was also effective and well tolerated in patients with comorbid medical illness in a randomised controlled trial (RCT) (with placebo) involving 752 older patients.[21]

In a more recent long-term study looking at depression in older people, 254 patients were treated with sertraline and entered the treatment (eight weeks) and continuation phases (16–20 weeks) of the study. 113 patients entered the maintenance phase (100 weeks) and were randomised into a double-blind, placebo-controlled continuation/maintenance phase of approximately two years' duration. No significant difference between the sertraline and placebo groups was found in the proportion of recurrences. The authors concluded that sertraline at therapeutic dosage does not provide significant protection against recurrence. However, very small numbers finished the trial.[22]

In a recent RCT involving 319 older patients with major depression, paroxetine controlled-release (CR) was compared with paroxetine immediate-release (IR) and placebo over 12 weeks. Both active treatments were more effective than placebo and responders were 72% (CR), 65% (IR) and 52% for patients on placebo and these were significantly different.[23]

Citalopram is well tolerated in older patients and in a review of 1344 patients from RCTs treated for a minimum of six weeks, bradycardia was significantly more likely in older people (2.4% versus 0.2%) whereas gastrointestinal side-effects, sweating and headache were less prevalent in older patients.[24] A recent eight-week RCT study comparing fluoxetine, escitalopram and placebo in 517 patients found that escitalopram was well tolerated in older people with depression and was as effective as fluoxetine.[25]

The Committee on Safety of Medicines, UK, in 2004 issued general guidance on the use of SSRIs. The report examined SSRIs in both children and adults and focused particularly on suicidal behaviour and withdrawal reactions. In relation to adults the report concluded that:

> From the available clinical trial data, both published and unpublished, a modest increase in the risk of suicidal thoughts and self-harm for SSRIs compared with placebo cannot be ruled out. There is insufficient evidence from clinical trial data to conclude that there is any marked difference between members of the class of SSRIs or between SSRIs and other antidepressants with respect to their influence on suicidal behaviour.

In relation to withdrawal reactions the CSM concluded that all SSRIs may be associated with withdrawal reactions on stopping or reducing treatment but paroxetine seems to be associated with a greater frequency of withdrawal reactions than other SSRIs.[26]

Serotonin and noradrenaline reuptake inhibitors (SNRIs)

Venlafaxine selectively inhibits the uptake of serotonin and noradrenaline and in comparison with TCAs shows no affinity for other neuroreceptors.[27] No dosage adjustments are recommended for older people. Compared with SSRIs, venlafaxine affects the cytochrome P450 enzyme system relatively little. The most common side-effects include nausea, headache, dry mouth, dizziness, constipation and hypertension, although postural hypotension can be a problem in older people and should be monitored. To minimise risk of discontinuation symptoms, the dose of venlafaxine should be gradually tapered over a few weeks period. SSRIs and venlafaxine are also associated with hyponatraemia in older patients.[28]

Clinical studies

Venlafaxine is well tolerated and shows similar efficacy to TCAs. There is evidence that the efficacy of venlafaxine is dose related and that at higher doses (>150 mg daily) venlafaxine is more effective than SSRIs in younger patients with major depression.[29] There have been a number of RCTs of venlafaxine in older people.

In an RCT comparing dothiepin and venlafaxine in 92 older patients with major depression, response to therapy in the venlafaxine group was 60% compared with 53% in the dothiepin group but these were not significantly different. Side-effects were very similar in the two groups and not significantly different.[30] Another RCT that compared venlafaxine, clomipramine and trazodone (n=170) over six weeks found significantly more patients treated with venlafaxine (74%) and clomipramine (69%) improved compared with trazodone (57%) and venlafaxine was better tolerated compared with clomipramine and trazodone.[31]

In a 10-week randomised-controlled, double-blind trial of venlafaxine (up to 150 mg/day) versus sertraline (up to 100 mg/day) in 52 older nursing home patients with major depression, venlafaxine was less well tolerated but there were no significant differences in response to treatment.[32]

However, in a systematic review of eight RCTs, remission rates were significantly higher with venlafaxine compared with an SSRI in a series of studies involving over 2000 patients, but the mean age in all groups was approximately 40 years.[33] In addition, in a recent RCT involving eight older patients, venlafaxine 37.5 mg bd (unlike dothiepin 25–50 mg daily) had no significant effects on cognition or psychomotor performance compared with dothiepin.[34]

In 2004 the Committee on Safety of Medicines[35] issued advice in relation to venlafaxine. It recommended that venlafaxine should only be initiated by specialist mental health practitioners or GPs with a special interest in mental health and there should be appropriate supervision of patients. It further recommended that venlafaxine should not be initiated in patients with heart disease, e.g. cardiac failure, coronary artery disease, patients with ECG abnormalities including QT prolongation, in patients with electrolyte disturbances and in patients with hypertension. Patients currently taking and tolerating venlafaxine and getting clinical benefit should continue to the end of the course. However, in June 2006 the CSM issued new guidance following a review. The new guidance notes that the restriction on who can initiate venlafaxine and the requirement for specialist supervision or shared care arrangements have been removed for doses below 300 mg daily (or venlafaxine XL 225 mg daily). However, in relation to patients with heart disease the recommendation has been amended to 'venlafaxine should not be used in patients with an identified very high risk of a serious cardiac ventricular arrythmia' or in patients with 'uncontrolled hypertension'. The requirement for a baseline ECG has been removed.

More recently, a 24-week open-label study involving 97 elderly (>80 years) depressed patients found remission rates of 57.1%. Venlafaxine (75–225 mg/day) was well tolerated with 7.2% of patients experiencing adverse events, although none was classified as serious.[36]

There is also good evidence that duloxetine is well tolerated and effective in older people with depression. Duloxetine is also a dual uptake inhibitor of both serotonin and noradrenaline with comparable affinities for both systems. A number of studies in younger patients have shown it to be effective with good safety and tolerability.[37] A number of open-label and RCTs have also shown it to be effective and well tolerated in older people with depression.[38,39,40] The active treatment phase of the Raskin study[39] lasted eight weeks and included 311 depressed patients with comorbid pain. As well as significant improvements in response and remission rates compared with placebo significant improvements in pain scores were also observed.

Monoamine oxidase inhibitors (MAOIs)

Traditional MAOIs include phenelzine, isoniazid and tranylcypromine. These bind non-selectively, either irreversibly or almost so, to both Type A and Type B monoamine oxidase enzymes to prevent the destruction of endogenous catecholamines (noradrenaline and dopamine) and the sympathomimetic amine tyramine. Because they lack selectivity, traditional MAOIs can lead to serious side-effects when foods rich in tyramine or other amines are eaten. In addition, these drugs have significant interactions with other drugs that seriously limit their use compared with other antidepressants. However, they may have a place in the treatment of resistant depression,[41] but they are seldom used as first line drugs. There is no good quality data specifically in relation to depression in older people.

Reversible inhibitors of monoamine oxidase (RIMA)

These drugs preferentially inhibit monoamine oxidase A but the inhibition is reversible. Moclobemide is effective and well tolerated and may be a useful alternative for depressed patients with prominent anxiety symptoms.[42] In addition, it may enhance cognition in dementia with depressive symptoms.[43] It lacks anticholinergic and cardiotoxic side-effects but it can cause insomnia and nausea. Drug interactions can occur with sympathomimetics and opiates but unlike traditional MAOIs it requires little or no dietary restrictions. Bonnet[44] has recommended combining moclobemide with another antidepressant, e.g. clomipramine or an SSRI for treatment-resistant depression. However, these combinations are not without risks.

Noradrenaline and serotonin synaptic antagonists (NaSSAs)

Mianserin and mirtazapine are both potent antagonists at α_2-autoreceptors. This leads to an increase in noradrenaline release. These drugs have low affinity for muscarinic, cholinergic and dopamine receptors, resulting in reduced side-effects. Mianserin has fallen out of favour over the past 10 years or so because of the small risk of agranulocytosis necessitating blood monitoring. There is very little published data in older people with depression. Mirtazapine has effects on both the noradrenergic and serotonergic systems. It enhances central noradrenergic and $5HT_1$-receptor mediated serotonergic neurotransmission. It is also an antagonist at α_2 presynaptic autoreceptors and also blocks $5HT_2$ and $5HT_3$ receptors, resulting in increased noradrenergic release. Changes in pharmacokinetics with age are considered minor.[45] The main side-effects of mirtazapine include sedation and weight gain and less commonly mania, convulsions, paraesthesia and reversible agranulocytocis.

Clinical studies

Mirtazapine (maximum 35 mg) has been compared with trazodone (maximum 280 mg) in a placebo-controlled, double-blind trial over six weeks involving 150 older patients with major depression. Significant improvements in depression were observed with both active compounds from week two compared with placebo. However, compared with placebo, both drugs had significantly higher levels of somnolence and dry mouth and trazodone also had higher levels of dizziness, and blurred vision.[46]

A similar study compared mirtazapine with amitriptyline (30–90 mg) in 115 older depressed patients in a double-blind, multi-centre study. Similar clinical benefit was observed with both drugs but the Clinical Global Impression (CGI) was statistically better in the amitriptyline group. Side-effects were noted to be similar in both groups.[47]

In a recent RCT, mirtazapine was compared with paroxetine over eight weeks in 255 older patients with major depression. Mirtazapine had a significantly earlier onset of action and was better tolerated.[48]

Noradrenaline reuptake inhibitors (NARIs)

There is limited evidence that reboxetine has benefit in older people with depression and causes less hypotension and fewer serious side-effects than TCAs.[49] However, renal clearance is reduced in older patients.[50] The pharmacokinetics of reboxetine are linear following both single and multiple oral doses and the plasma half-life is approximately 12 hours. Metabolism is mainly via the liver with only 10% cleared by the kidneys but plasma concentrations are increased in older patients.

In a prospective, uncontrolled, multicentre study of reboxetine involving 160 older patients with major depression over 52 weeks, 104 patients completed the study. The proportion who were rated as either 'much' or 'very much improved' were 15.1% at two weeks and 88% at six weeks with 95.2% at 52 weeks. The drug was well tolerated although nausea (11.9%) and headache (10%) were relatively common.[51] However, because of these side-effects some authors have recommended that older patients should be started on 4 mg/day in two divided doses[50] but use of reboxetine is not recommended in older people in the UK. Controlled trials in older people are still needed.

Herbal remedies

Extracts of the plant *Hypericum perforatum* – usually referred to as St John's wort – have been used for a long time as an unlicensed herbal remedy for depression. However, a recent systematic review concluded that extracts of *Hypericum* are not more effective than placebo for treating mild to moderately severe depressive disorder.[52] However, it can induce a number of drug-metabolising enzymes, lowering the plasma concentration of a number of drugs including coumarins, amitriptyline, carbamazepine, phenytoin, aripiprazole, digoxin and a number of other drugs. When St John's wort is stopped concentrations of these drugs can increase to toxic levels. It also increases the serotonergic effect of SSRIs and duloxetine. The amount of active ingredient also varies in different preparations.

Practical prescribing

Although depression can be successfully treated it is frequently missed and treated with suboptimal doses of antidepressants for inadequate periods of time. A recent study showed that in 193 older people with clinical depression referred to secondary services only one third were adequately treated and one third had been untreated.[53] The treatment of depression in older people invariably needs an integrated approach with pharmacological, social and psychological approaches working together. Patient education is also important as well as treatment for physical illness, good diet and fluid intake, appropriate levels of exercise and close working with family members. Underlying all this is good multi-professional team working. It is also important to undertake an appropriate risk assessment with a specific focus on antidepressant treatment including the risk of accidental and deliberate overdose, the risk of exacerbating any underlying physical illness, the likely effect on the patient's ability to drive or operate other potentially dangerous machinery such as lawnmowers, the risk of falls and compliance.

The optimal treatment of depression in later life is crucial and requires appreciation of a number of factors such as comorbidity, polypharmacy, altered drug kinetics, variable treatment response and increased predisposition to side-effects. Older people need to be thoroughly assessed[54] before commencing antidepressants due to the increased incidence of physical illnesses, changes in pharmacokinetics and increased sensitivity to side-effects. It is also an important opportunity to develop a good rapport with patients to improve understanding of and compliance with medication.

Despite the NICE (2004) recommendation that SSRIs should be used as a 'first line' antidepressant, individual prescribing needs to take into account a number of factors including efficacy, safety, tolerability, real-world efficacy and economic value[55] as well as previous response to treatment and patient preferences. Regular review is also important to monitor compliance, response, side-effects and physical health.

General aspects of management

NICE guidance on management is quite specific and detailed (*see* Box 4.1). According to NICE 'watchful waiting' and 'guided self help' are the best strategies for mild depression. For moderate or severe depression, medication, psychological interventions and social support are appropriate. These can, in the first instance, be delivered in primary care. Where depression is treatment resistant, atypical, recurrent or psychotic or where there is 'significant risk' specialist mental health teams should be involved using medication, complex psychological interventions and/or combined treatments. (In the experience of the authors this includes many older people with moderate and all with severe depression.) Finally, where there is risk to life or severe self-neglect crisis intervention and inpatient care with medication, combined treatments and ECT may be needed.

It is essential that high quality psychological interventions are made available to older people.[56] There is a need for research into the availability of these interventions but a description of them is beyond the scope of this review. A comprehensive account of cognitive behavioural therapy (CBT) with older adults can be found in Laidlaw *et al.*[57]

BOX 4.1 Key points from NICE guidance on the management of depression (modified)[58]

- Screening is justified in high risk subgroups; for example, those with chronic disability or in hospital or residential care.
- Guided self-help (where the patient wants it) or 'watchful waiting' with a further assessment within two weeks is the correct intervention for *mild* depression. Antidepressants are *not* recommended for this group.
- Short-term psychological treatment specifically focused on depression is recommended for mild to moderate depression.
- SSRI antidepressants are the first-choice drugs for uncomplicated moderate depression but other drugs also make a major contribution particularly in more severe or resistant depression.
- Patients should be fully informed about medication, including discontinuation symptoms.
- In severe depression the combination of cognitive behavioural therapy (CBT) with medication should be considered as it is more effective than either treatment alone.
- In recurrent depression continuation of antidepressants for at least two years and CBT both have a role.

In April 2007 NICE issued amended guidance[59] for the management of depression with a view to publishing a full update in late 2007. The key points include those in Box 4.2.

BOX 4.2 Key points from NICE guidance (2007) on the management of depression (modified)[59]

- **Screening**: Screening should be undertaken in primary care and general hospital settings for depression in high-risk groups.
- **Watchful waiting**: Patients with mild depression who do not want an intervention should be further assessed after two weeks.
- **Antidepressants**: Not recommended for the initial treatment of mild depression.
- **Guided self-help**: Patients with mild depression should be offered a guided self-help programme based on CBT.
- **Psychological treatment**: Psychological treatment should be considered for patients with mild-moderate depression.
- **SSRI**: This should be the initial drug treatment of choice.
- **Maintenance**: Patients who have had two or more episodes in the recent past and who have experienced significant functional impairment should continue their antidepressant for two years.
- **Treatment-resistant depression**: Combination with CBT should be considered.

Choosing an antidepressant for older people

Which antidepressant should be used? In a review of 18 meta-analyses of different antidepressants mainly involving younger patients, the main finding was a lack of major difference in efficacy between the newer and older antidepressants. Venlafaxine was found to be superior to SSRIs and SSRIs better tolerated. Interestingly, in older patients dothiepin was found to be better tolerated than SSRIs.[19] In addition, in a recent Cochrane review[60] TCAs, SSRIs and MAOIs were reported to be effective in the treatment of older community patients and inpatients with severe physical illness. At least six weeks of antidepressant treatment was recommended to achieve optimal therapeutic effect. Data from some of the newer drugs such as duloxetine also appear very promising. However, in 2001 a consensus panel looking at the management of depression in older people recommended using either an SSRI or venlafaxine as a first line treatment[61] and NICE[58,59] also recommended starting with an SSRI.

Antidepressants do not help everyone with depression. Although much has been written about how to identify responders this is still difficult in clinical practice and 'trial and error' is still largely the norm. This may become possible in the future with advances in pharmacogenetics. It remains largely a case of balancing information such as efficacy in older people, tolerability and side-effects, the propensity of the drug to worsen an underlying physical illness, the potential to cause drug interactions, availability of different preparations such as liquids and tablets, patient preferences, drug costs as well as published guidance and clinical experience.

TABLE 4.1 Antidepressants, available preparations and indications

Drug	Available types	Indications	Comments
Amitriptyline	Tablets	Depressive illness	Initially 30–75 mg daily increasing to 150–200 mg daily.
Clomipramine	Capsules Tablets Slow release	Depressive illness Phobias OCD	Initially 10 mg gradually increasing to 30–75 mg daily.
Dosulepin	Capsules	Depressive illness	Initially 50–75 mg daily increasing gradually to 150 mg daily.
Imipramine	Tablets	Depressive illness	Initially 10 mg increasing gradually to 30–50 mg daily.
Lofepramine	Tablets	Depressive illness	70–210 mg daily.
Nortriptyline	Tablets	Depressive illness	30–50 mg daily.

(Continued)

Drug	Available types	Indications	Comments
Mianserin	Tablets	Depressive illness	Initially 30 mg daily increased to maximum of 90 mg daily. Check FBC every four weeks during first three months of treatment.
Trazodone	Capsules Tablets	Depressive illness	Initially 100 mg daily increasing to 300 mg.
Phenelzine	Tablets	Depressive illness	Initially 15 mg tds increasing to qds after two weeks if necessary. Usual maintenance dose 15 mg on alternate days.
Isocarboxazid	Tablets	Depressive illness	5–10 mg daily.
Tranylcypromine	Tablets	Depressive illness	10 mg bd increasing to 30 mg daily. Maintenance dose 10 mg daily.
Moclobemide	Tablets	Depressive illness Social phobia	Initially 300 mg daily increasing to maximum of 600 mg daily.
Citalopram	Tablets Drops	Depressive illness Panic disorder	20–40 mg daily.
Escitalopram	Tablets Drops	Depressive illness Panic disorder Social phobia GAD	Initially 5 mg increasing to 10–20 mg daily.
Fluoxetine	Capsules Liquid	Depressive illness Bulimia nervosa OCD	20–40 mg daily.
Paroxetine	Tablets Liquid	Depressive illness OCD Panic disorder Social phobia PTSD GAD	20–40 mg daily.
Sertraline	Tablets	Depressive illness OCD PTSD	Initially 50 mg increasing to 200 mg. Usual maintenance dose 50 mg.

(Continued)

Drug	Available types	Indications	Comments
Flupenthixol	Tablets	Depressive illness Psychoses	Initially 500 µg daily increasing to 2 mg in divided doses.
Venlafaxine	Tablets Modified Release (MR)	Depressive illness GAD	Initially 75 mg daily – maximum 375 mg daily. MR – maximum 225 mg daily.
Duloxetine	Capsules	Depressive illness	60 mg daily.
Mirtazapine	Tablets Orodispersible	Depressive illness	Initially 15 mg daily increasing to 45 mg daily.

PTSD – Post Traumatic Stress Disorder; GAD – Generalised Anxiety Disorder; OCD – Obsessive Compulsive Disorder

Acute treatment

Approximately 70% of patients will respond to an antidepressant[62] but this can be lower in older people with rates of 40–60% being more typical.[63] However, only approximately 50% of patients with major depression achieve remission with their first antidepressant.[64] Several studies have shown that the onset of therapeutic action may take longer in older people and that optimum benefit can take 8–12 weeks after commencing treatment.[65] The general notion of a delayed onset of action for antidepressants has recently been challenged in younger patients[66] but the general consensus remains unchanged, i.e. that antidepressants take several weeks before they start working. When initial treatment with a tricyclic has been ineffective a second antidepressant may take five to six weeks to have an effect.[67] 'Start low; go slow' is a useful guide when prescribing in older people but with the aim of reaching therapeutic dosages. This is less of a problem with newer drugs as patients can be put straight onto a therapeutic dose. Older patients are at high risk of recurrence following a depressive episode, with up to a 70% risk of recurrence within two years of remission.[68] Therefore, after a successful response, continuation of antidepressant medication may be needed for at least two years.

Continuation treatment

How long should an antidepressant be continued for? Antidepresssant drug treatment should be continued for at least 12 months after remission in the elderly.[69,70] If antidepressant treatment is stopped within 6–12 months and substituted with placebo, approximately 50% of patients will relapse. In addition, if treatment is continued for 12 months, 90% will continue to respond. The risk is greater if the patient has had a number of previous episodes, e.g. one (<50%), two (50–90%) and three episodes (>90%).[62] Continuation of drug therapy reduces the risk of relapse after remission. However, patients with recurrent depression should be treated for two years (or more). For patients with delusional depression on antipsychotic medication, it is recommended that this be continued for six months before being tailed off.

Maintenance treatment

When should maintenance therapy be used? This would usually be if there have been two or more previous episodes for younger patients but one or more previous episodes for older patients.[62] The dose of antidepressant should be with the same dose as used to treat the acute episode.[70] Older patients taking dothiepin over a two-year period are 2.5 times less likely to relapse compared with those taking placebo.[69] Reynolds *et al.*[71] found that maintenance therapy with either nortriptyline or paroxetine was effective in 80–90% of older patients over an 18-month period.

In older patients, citalopram prevented recurrence over a period of one to two years, suggesting that protection is not confined to TCAs.[72] However, Wilson *et al.*[13] did not find any benefit from sertraline in prophylaxis. Possibly the dose used was too small. This study cautions against assuming all antidepressants are equally effective in prevention. The case for long-term antidepressant treatment needs to be balanced against adverse effects, which in the case of older antidepressants can include troublesome weight gain and cardiovascular disturbance.

Lithium salts are also widely used for the prophylaxis of recurrent depression despite limited evidence in older patients. A small prospective study by Abou-Saleh and Coppen[73] found that an older subgroup benefited from lithium prophylaxis. However, clearance of lithium is reduced in older patients, so half the standard adult dosage may be required and maintenance levels of 0.5 mmol/L have been suggested. Lithium should be used cautiously with SSRIs because of the risk of serotoninergic neurotoxicity.

Compliance

This is a much neglected area in older people with depression. With the exception of lithium and nortriptyline this can only be assessed by asking patients and carers and doing a 'tablet count' in routine clinical practice. However, compliance aids such as dosset or nomad boxes may be appropriate and can significantly improve compliance. However, tablets which readily absorb water may disintegrate unless the compliance aid is appropriately sealed. A recent study looking at citalopram compliance in 228 older people with depression found that patients could be classed as compliant, unknown compliance and not compliant. However, there was no association between the type of compliance and age, gender, education level, degree of depression, cognitive function or medical comorbidity, though white patients were more likely to be compliant.[74] As well as developing compliance therapy specifically for older people with depression more objective ways of quickly determining compliance need to be developed including blood and salivary drug levels.

Bereavement and dysthymia

Patients experiencing a normal bereavement reaction do not usually require drug treatment unless the bereavement reaction is unusually severe (e.g. psychosis is present) or if the reaction is unduly prolonged, usually more than six months. Supportive measures are usually sufficient.

Dysthymia is a depressive disorder of chronic nature but of less severity than major depression. Symptoms have usually been continuous for at least two years. Patients experience considerable disability and social dysfunction. A recent Cochrane review concluded that antidepressants are effective for the treatment of dysthymia but no differences in terms of efficacy were identified between different classes of drugs including SSRIs, TCAs and MAOIs.[75]

Physical illness

Physically ill patients need a careful assessment and any physical illness needs treatment in its own right. Depression may worsen an underlying physical illness and may increase both morbidity and mortality if left untreated. In addition, physical illness may cause or exacerbate a depressive illness. The choice of antidepressant will depend on a number of factors but an important area is to consider antidepressant side-effects and the likelihood of a specific antidepressant worsening an underlying physical illness. TCAs, for example, can cause sedation, delirium, memory impairment and urinary retention so should be avoided where these are likely to be significant problems. Depression in Parkinson's disease is common and can not only be difficult to diagnose but also difficult to treat. However, there is no consensus about which is the best antidepressant from an efficacy perspective.[76] The newer drugs including SSRIs and SNRIs have fewer side-effects and are used by the authors.

Management of treatment-resistant depression

Treatment resistance is reported in up to 40% of older patients with major depression.[77] There is little evidence to guide the management of depression that has failed to respond to a course of an antidepressant and further research is needed to inform clinical practice. A review of 29 studies concluded that 35–60% of older patients showed a good recovery from a first depressive episode.[78] However, research on treatment-resistant depression in older people is hampered in part by lack of an agreed definition.

The definition of treatment-resistant depression can be confusing. Some have suggested that it is failure to respond to one effective medication at a therapeutic dosage and for an adequate duration.[79] Renwick[80] has suggested that it is the failure to respond to an adequate trial of two antidepressants or an antidepressant and/or ECT. Thase and Rush[81] extended the definition by developing a staging system of treatment resistance based on types of failed treatment.

The first step is to review the diagnosis and ensure that an organic cause has not been missed. Further investigations may be necessary such as an ECG, chest X-ray, EEG or CT head scan. Severe deep white matter lesions on a brain MRI scan[82] and prefrontal dysfunction may predict a poor response to antidepressant treatment.[83] Depression in patients with Alzheimer's disease is more likely to resolve spontaneously without requiring intensive antidepressant treatment compared with patients with vascular dementia who are more likely to have persistent and treatment-resistant depressive symptoms.[84] The presence of a silent cerebral infarction also reduces response to antidepressant treatment.[85]

Where there are maintaining social or environmental factors, psychological therapies may be beneficial as an adjunct to pharmacological treatment. A recent meta-analysis of psychological outreach programmes demonstrated a large effect size (0.7) in depressed older patients (comparable to effect sizes found in younger adults). Cognitive behavioural therapy was found to have a larger effect size than other therapies but also had higher drop-out rates.[86]

It is also important to ensure treatment adequacy in terms of duration and compliance. This has been called a stepped-care approach, meaning that each step of treatment follows a logical sequence rather than a chaotic mishmash.[87] This has been reinforced in a study by Flint and Rifat[67] in which over 80% of patients recovered if a logical process is adopted; for example, starting with a trial of antidepressant monotherapy and eventually moving up to ECT. There is a range of options[88] and these are now briefly reviewed.

Some of the specific drug-related approaches include:

Change the dose of antidepressant

This usually, though not always, means increasing the dose. This may be beneficial for TCAs and venlafaxine but there is little evidence that increasing the dose significantly alters the outcome in the case of SSRIs. At higher doses (>150mg daily) venlafaxine may be more effective than SSRIs in major depression.[89] Blood pressure monitoring is recommended when patients are taking high doses of venlafaxine (>200mg daily).

Increase the length of treatment

Here the therapeutic trial is continued beyond what is usually considered an 'adequate' period of time. There is evidence that an extension to nine weeks or even longer may improve recovery from a depressive episode in older patients,[41] although not if there has been no improvement in the first four weeks.[90]

Switch to a different antidepressant class

Switching between classes of antidepressants has been shown to have modest benefit, although there is little systematic evaluation. The most popular strategy is a change from one antidepressant to another from a different class: for example, from a TCA to an SSRI, or vice versa.[91] Venlafaxine showed some promise in resistant depression but evaluation is mostly confined to clinical experience,[92] or open trials.[93] It has been estimated that the overall success rate for class switching is about 50%.[94]

Augmentation with lithium

Following failure of two classes of antidepressants, traditionally, the next step would be lithium augmentation. As yet there have been no randomised-controlled trials of lithium augmentation in older patients. Flint and Rifat,[94] in an open prospective study, showed a 23% response rate. They also found that 50% of older patients experienced side-effects, including polydipsia, polyuria, tremor, dry mouth and nausea. Fahy and Lawlor[95] followed up a small cohort of older depressed patients who had their long-term lithium augmentation therapy discontinued for varying reasons: 52% relapsed and the longer the length of lithium treatment prior to discontinuation the poorer the outcome. The time needed to judge response to lithium augmentation is approximately two to three weeks.[79]

Austin *et al.*[96] conducted a meta-analysis of five small double-blind trials and found that 18/50 patients augmented with lithium responded compared with 6/49 of those who were given placebo. In another study[97] venlafaxine and lithium augmentation was studied in an open trial in outpatients aged 18–70. At the end of seven weeks' study, 35% of the patients showed a more than 50% reduction in depressive symptoms and the combination was well tolerated.

Other augmentation approaches include use of anticonvulsants, thyroid hormone and L-tryptophan but the evidence base is too weak to make firm recommendations for older patients.

Augmentation with antipsychotics

There is also emerging evidence of benefit for combining antidepressants, mainly SSRIs with an antipsychotic including aripiprazole,[98] olanzapine[99] and risperidone.[100] A recent meta-analysis confirmed the benefits of antipsychotic augmentation for treatment-resistant depression in 1500 younger patients.[101] Augmentation is particularly important when psychotic symptoms are present but there is also emerging evidence for benefit in the absence of psychotic symptoms. However, studies tend to be small and open-label and confined to younger patients and more research is needed in this area with a specific focus in older patients.

Other augmentation strategies

A number of other augmentation strategies have been suggested including omega-3 fatty acids, aspirin, buspirone, dopaminergic agents, reserpine, pindolol and modafinil.[115] There have also been some promising results with raloxifene, a selective oestrogen receptor modulator.[102] However, nearly all this work is limited in scope and has been confined to younger patients.

Combination therapies

A number of combinations have been suggested but overall the evidence base, particularly in older people, is very limited. MAOIs and TCAs combinations (with or without lithium) have been used for decades in resistant cases. A review by Cowen[79] demonstrated how open studies in younger adults have shown failure of each type of drug individually, but with good results when combined. Starting at very low dose, adding in the MAOI and not using imipramine or clomipramine is thought to lessen the risks of hazardous side-effects and interactions. There is no evidence for this combination in older people and both MAOIs and TCAs are being used less compared with several years ago.

Other antidepressant combinations that have been tried include TCAs and SSRIs. Again there are no controlled trials. Cowen[79] suggests that due to the high risk of side-effects, drugs such as clomipramine or venlafaxine (with potent serotonin as well as noradrenaline reuptake inhibition in one medication) may be as effective as TCAs and SSRIs combined. There may be a role for low dose trazodone to augment SSRIs but this may just help the sleep disturbance and further studies are necessary. In one small open-label study in younger patients, 9/15 (60%) responded to a combination of atomoxetine (a noradrenaline reuptake inhibitor) with 'standard' antidepressant treatment after six weeks.[103]

Venlafaxine and mirtazapine has become a popular combination but work in this area has been predominantly open-label and confined to younger patients. In a recent study involving 32 patients with treatment-resistant depression, 50% responded after eight weeks and this had risen to 56% after six months. The main side-effects were sedation (19%) and weight gain (19%).[104] There is clearly a need for further research in this area in older people with depression.

A meta-analysis of tri-iodothyronine augmentation of TCA in mixed age groups showed a response rate of 8% (NNT=13).[105] There are no studies comparing other classes of antidepressants. It should be used cautiously if there is coexisting cardiovascular disease. In younger adults, L-tryptophan has been shown to enhance the combinations of lithium-MAOI and lithium-clomipramine.[106] Again there are no trials in older patients. With the risk of developing eosinophilic myalgic syndrome and possible serotonin syndrome with MAOIs and SSRIs, this combination needs to be used with caution. There is no longer a need to register with the Optimax (tryptophan) Information and Clinical Support (OPTICS) Unit. Pindolol, a beta blocker with 5-HT$_{1A}$-receptor antagonist, had been shown in open studies to augment antidepressants. However, a small double-blind, placebo-cross over trial showed no difference to placebo.[107] Dexamethasone,[108] clonazepam,[109] oestrogen,[110] and methylphenidate[111] have also all been tried but require further research.

Electroconvulsive therapy (ECT)

ECT can be used at any stage alongside the pharmacological management of treatment-resistant depression. SSRIs may increase seizure length in ECT compared with TCAs and may also increase the risk of post-treatment seizures.[112] Shapira *et al.*[113] have shown that the rate of response is more rapid when ECT is given three times a week but memory impairment is more common and suggested that the optimum schedule for bilateral ECT in older patients is twice weekly unless clinical indications require a more rapid antidepressant effect. Unilateral ECT may have an advantage with respect to cognitive side-effects but Krystal *et al.*[114] suggest that moderately suprathreshold unilateral ECT may not be as effective as bilateral ECT for older patients. He found that older patients were more likely to have a rise in seizure threshold and to be non-responders to unilateral ECT. For more information on ECT as well as current thinking on repetitive transcranial magnetic stimulation (rTMS), vagal nerve stimulation (VNS) and magnetic seizure therapy (MST) *see* Chapter 6.

Discontinuing treatment

Antidepressants need to be discontinued slowly (weekly decrements) as all have the potential to cause a withdrawal syndrome.[97] Typical withdrawal symptoms are anxiety, agitation, insomnia, dizziness, low mood, paraesthesia, nausea and diarrhoea. When changing from one antidepressant to another, cross tapering is recommended, though in some cases it is important to ensure one drug was been washed out of the system before another is started, e.g. with SSRIs and MAOIs.

Future developments

An enormous amount of research has been directed towards uncovering specific deficits in serotonin, noradrenaline and dopamine neurotransmitter systems and ways to manipulate these with a view to improving the symptoms of depression. To a very large extent these approaches have been successful, particularly drugs enhancing serotonin and noradrenaline mechanisms. However, patients do not always respond to their first antidepressant and treatment-resistant depression is not uncommon. In addition it is not possible to predict which patient will respond to a particular antidepressant and pharmacogenomics may help with this in the future. In addition, more accurate and objective monitoring of drug levels might help to identify non-responders at an earlier stage rather than having to wait 8–12 weeks before classifying a patient as a non-responder.

A number of other drugs are currently in development but many are still at an early stage or not available in the UK. These include dopamine reuptake inhibitors, 5-HT$_3$ receptor antagonists, corticotropin-releasing factor antagonists, neurokinin (substance P) receptor antagonists, melatonergic agonists and glutamatergic modulators. In addition, most of the focus to date has been on intrasynaptic function. In the future it is likely that developments will shift in part towards intracellular signalling pathways but the latter is still at an early stage. Our own view is that the monoamine hypothesis is very simplistic. The fact that there are multiple interactions between intra- and extra-cellular systems probably means that a drug or drugs which enhances several of these mechanisms is more likely to be beneficial than one which only enhances one. In our view, our understanding of the biological basis of depression remains very limited despite the successes to date.

Conclusions

Depression is common and if not treated results in high morbidity and mortality. Depression in older people generally has a good prognosis. It is therefore important to diagnose the condition and treat systematically. When an antidepressant is indicated, it should be chosen on an individual basis and used at a therapeutic dose for an adequate period. The choice of antidepressant will depend on a number of factors including previous response to treatment, concurrent physical illness and other medications. Pharmacological treatment also needs to be combined with psychosocial interventions. However, further well-planned research is needed into the pharmacological management of depression, especially treatment-resistant, in older people.

REFERENCES

1 Baldwin RC, Chiu E, Katona C, *et al. Guidelines on Depression in Older People: practising the evidence.* London: Martin Dunitz; 2002.
2 Dwyer M, Byrne GJ. Disruptive vocalisation and depression in older nursing home residents. *Int Psychogeriatr.* 2000; **12**: 463–71.
3 McDougall FA, Kvaal K, Matthews FE, *et al. The Medical Research Council Cognitive Function Study.* Cambridge: Psychological Medicine, CUP; 2007.
4 Curran S, Shafiq S. Treatment of depression in older people in care homes. *J Care Serv Manag.* 2007; **1**(2): 155–65.
5 Hindmarch I. Expanding the horizons of depression; beyond the monoamine hypothesis. *Human Psychopharm.* 2001; **16**(3): 203–18.
6 Stahl S, Briley M. Understanding pain in depression. *Human Psychopharm.* 2004; **19**: S9–13.
7 Jonas BS, Mussolino ME. Symptoms of depression as a prospective risk factor for stroke. *Psychosom Med.* 2000; **62**: 463–71.
8 Ariyo AA, Haan M, Tangen CM, *et al.* Depressive symptoms and risks of coronary heart disease and mortality in elderly Americans. *Circulation.* 2000; **102**: 1773–9.
9 Penninx BW, Deeg DJ, van Eijk JT, *et al.* Changes in depression and physical decline in older adults; a longitudinal perspective. *J Affect Disord.* 2000; **61**: 1–12.
10 Stahl, SM. *Psychopharmacology of Antidepressants.* London: Martin Dunitz; 1999. pp. 3–9.
11 Barbui C, Hotopf M. Amitriptyline versus the rest: still the leading antidepressant after 40 years of randomised controlled trials. *Br J Psychiatr.* 2001; **178**: 129–44.
12 Mittman, N, Herrmann, N, Einarson, TR, *et al.* The efficacy, safety and tolerability of antidepressants in late life depression: a meta-analysis. *J Affect Disord.* 1997; **46**: 191–217.
13 Wilson K, Mottram P, Sivanranthan A, *et al.* Antidepressant versus placebo for depressed elderly (Cochrane Review). In: *The Cochrane Library, Issue 2.* Oxford: Update Software; 2001.
14 Navarro V, Gasto C, Torres X, *et al.* Citalopram versus nortriptyline in late-life depression: a 12 week randomised single-blind study. *Acta Psychiatr Scand.* 2001; **103**(6):435–40.

15 Donoghue J, Hylan TR. Antidepressant use in clinical practice: efficacy versus effectiveness. *Br J Psychiatr.* 2001; **179**(Suppl. 42): S9–17.

16 Furukawa T, McGuire H, Barbui C. Low dosage tricyclic antidepressants for depression. *Cochrane Review.* 2004; **3**.

17 Guaiana G, Barbui C, Hotopf M. Amitriptyline versus other types of pharmacotherapy for depression. *Cochrane Review.* 2004; **3**.

18 Baumann P. Care of depression in the elderly: comparative pharmacokinetics of SSRIs. *Int Clin Psychopharm.* 1998; **13**(Suppl. 5): 35–43.

19 Anderson I, Edwards J. Guidelines for choice of selective serotonin reuptake inhibitor in depressive illness. *Adv Psychiatr Treat.* 2001; **7**: 170–80.

20 Glassman AH, O'Connor CM, Califf RM, *et al.* Sertraline treatment of major depression in patients with acute MI or unstable angina. *JAMA.* 2002; **288**(6): 701–9.

21 Sheikh JI, Cassidy EL, Doraiswamy PM, *et al.* Efficacy, safety and tolerability of sertraline in patients with late-life depression. *J Am Geriatr Soc.* 2004; **52**(1): 86–92.

22 Wilson KCM, Mottram PG, Ashworth L, *et al.* Older community residents with depression: long-term treatment with sertraline. *Br J Psychiatr.* 2003; **182**: 492–7.

23 Rapaport MH, Schneider LS, Dunner DL, *et al.* Efficacy of controlled-release paroxetine in the treatment of late-life depression. *J Clin Psychiatr.* 2003; **64**(9):1065–74.

24 Barak Y, Swartz M, Levy D, *et al.* Age-related differences in the side-effect profile of citalopram. *Prog Neuropsychopharmacol Biol Psychiatr.* 2003; **27**(3): 545–8.

25 Kasper S, de Swart H, Friis Andersen H. Escitalopram in the treatment of depressed elderly patients. *Am J Geriatr Psychiatr.* 2005; **13**(10): 884–91.

26 Committee on Safety of Medicines. *Report of the CSM Expert Working Group on the Safety of Selective Serotonin Reuptake Inhibitor Antidepressants.* December 2004. Available from: http://www.mhra.gov.uk

27 Mendlewicz J. Pharmacologic profile and efficacy of venlafaxine. *Int Clin Psychopharmacol.* 1995; **10**(Suppl. 2): S5–13.

28 Kirby D, Harrigun S, Ames D. Hyponatraemia in elderly psychiatric patients treated with SSRIs and venlafaxine: a retrospective controlled study in an in-patient unit. *Int J Geriatr Psychiatr.* 2002; **17**: 231–7.

29 Smith D, Dempster C, Glanvile J, *et al.* Efficacy and tolerability of venlafaxine compared with selective serotonin reuptake inhibitors and other antidepressants: a meta-analysis. *Br J Psychiatr.* 2002; **180**: 396–404.

30 Mahapatra SN, Hackett D. A randomised, double-blind, parallel-group comparison of venlafaxine and dothiepin in geriatric patients with major depression. *Int J Clin Pract.* 1997; **51**(4): 209–13.

31 Smeraldi E, Rizzo F, Crespi G. Double-blind, randomised study of venlafaxine, clomipramine and trazodone in geriatric practice with major depression. *Prim Care Psychiatr.* 1998; **4**: 189–95.

32 Oslin DW, Have TRT, Streim JE, *et al.* Probing the safety of medications in the frail elderly: evidence from a randomised clinical trial of sertraline and venlafaxine in depressed nursing home residents. *J Clin Psychiatr.* 2003; **64**(8): 875–82.

33 Thase ME, Entsuah R, Rudolph RL. Remission rates during treatment with venlafaxine or selective serotonin reuptake inhibitors. *Br J Psychiatr.* 2001; **178**: 234–41.

34 Trick L, Neil S, Una R, *et al.* A double-blind, randomised, 26-week study comparing the cognitive and psychomotor effects and efficacy of 75 mg (37.5 mg bd) venlafaxine and 25mg/50mg of dothiepin in elderly patients with moderate major depression being treated in general practice. *J Psychopharmacol.* 2004; **18**(2): 205–14.

35 Committee on Safety of Medicines. *Safety of Selective Serotonin Reuptake Inhibitor Antidepressants.* 2004. http://www.mhra.gov.uk

36 Baca E, Roca M, Garcia-Calvo C, *et al.* Venlafaxine extended-release in patients older than 80 years with depressive syndrome. *Int J Geriatr Psychiatr.* 2006; **21**(4): 337–43.

37 Hudson JI, Wohlreich MM, Kajdasz DK, *et al.* Safety and tolerability of duloxetine in the treatment of major depressive disorder: analysis of pooled data from eight placebo-controlled clinical trials. *Human Psychopharmacol.* 2005; **20**: 327–41.

38 Wohlreich MM, Mallinckrodt CH, Watkin JG, *et al.* Duloxetine for the long-term treatment of major depressive disorder in patients aged 65 and older: an open-label study. *BMC Geriatrics.* 2004. Available from: http://www.biomedcentral.com/1471-2318/4/11

39 Raskin J, Wiltse C, Dinkel J, *et al.* Duloxetine versus placebo in the treatment of elderly patients with major depression. Presented at the International College of Geriatric Psychoneuropharmacology, Basel, 14–17 October 2004.

40 Nelson JC, Wohlreich MM, Mallinckrodt CH, *et al.* Duloxetine for the treatment of major depressive disorder in older people. *Am J Geriatr Psychiatr.* 2005; **13**(3): 227–35.

41 Georgotas A, McCue R. The additional benefit of extending an antidepressant trial past seven weeks in the depressed elderly. *Int J Geriatric Psychiatr.* 1989; **4**: 191–5.

42 Tourigny-Rivard MF. Pharmacotherapy of affective disorders in old age. *Can J Psychiatr.* 1997; **42**(1): 10–18.

43 Roth M, Montjoy C, Amrein R. Moclobemide in elderly patients with cognitive decline and depression: an international double-blind trial, placebo-controlled trial. *Br J Psychiatr.* 1996; **168**(2):149–57.

44 Bonnet U. Moclobemide: therapeutic use and clinical studies. *CNS Drug Reviews.* 2003; **9**(1): 97–140.

45 Timmer CL, Paanakker JE, van Hal HJM. Pharmacokinetics of mirtazapine from orally administered tablets: influence of age, gender and treatment regimen. *Human Psychopharm.* 1996; **11**: 497–509.

46 Halikas JA. Org 3770 (mirtazapine) versus trazodone: a placebo controlled trial in depressed elderly patients. *Human Psychopharm.* 1995; **10**: 125–33.

47 Hoyberg OJ, Maragakis B, Mullin J, *et al.* A double-blind multi-centre comparison of mirtazapine and amitriptyline in elderly depressed patients. *Acta Psychiatr Scand.* 1996; **93**: 184–90.

48 Schatzberg AF, Kremer C, Rodrigues HE, *et al.* Double-blind, randomised comparison of mirtazapine and paroxetine in elderly depressed patients. *Am J Geriatr Psychiatr.* 2002; **10**(5): 541–50.

49 Katona C, Bercoff E, Chiu E, *et al.* Reboxetine versus imipramine in the treatment of elderly patients with depressive disorders: a double-blind randomised trial. *J Affect Disord.* 1999; **55**: 203–13.

50 Bergmann JF, Laneury JP, Duchene P, *et al.* Pharmacokinetics of reboxetine in healthy, elderly volunteers. *Eur J Drug Metab Pharmacokinet.* 2000; **25**(3–4): 195–8.

51 Aguglia, E. Reboxetine in the maintenance therapy of depressive disorder in the elderly: a long-term open study. *Int J Geriatr Psychiatr.* 2000; **15**: 784–93.

52 Linde K, Mulrow CD. St John's wort for depression. *The Cochrane Library.* 2005; **2**: ID CD000448.

53 Tew JD, Mulsant BH, Houck PR, *et al.* Impact of prior treatment exposure on response to antidepressant treatment in late life. *Am J Geriatr Psychiatr.* 2006; **14**(11), 957–65.

54 Curran S, Nightingale S, Wattis JP. Practical issues in assessing and prescribing psychotropic drugs in older people. In: Curran S, Bullock R, editors. *Practical Old Age Psychopharmacology: a multi-professional approach.* Oxford: Radcliffe Medical; 2005. pp. 47–72.

55 Mendlewicz J. Optimising antidepressant use in clinical practice: towards criteria for antidepressant selection. *Br J Psychiatr.* 2001; **179**(Suppl. 42): S1–3.

56 *Everybody's Business: integrated mental health service for older adults: a service development guide.* London: Care Services Improvement Partnership/Department of Health; 2005. Available from: http://www.everybodysbusiness.org.uk

57 Laidlaw K, Thompson LW, Dick-Siskin L, *et al. Cognitive Behaviour Therapy with Old People.* Chichester: John Wiley and Sons; 2003.

58 National Institute for Clinical Excellence. *Depression: management of depression in primary and secondary care. Clinical Guideline 23.* London: National Institute for Clinical Excellence; December 2004.

59 National Institute for Health and Clinical Excellence. *Depression (amended): management of depression in primary and secondary care. Clinical Guideline 23 (amended).* London: National Institute for Clinical Excellence; 25 April 2007.

60 Wilson K, Mottram P, Sivanranthan A, *et al.* Antidepressants versus placebo for the depressed elderly. *Cochrane Review.* 2004; **3**.

61 Alexopoulos GS, Katz IR, Reynolds CF, *et al.* The expert consensus guideline series. Pharmacotherapy of depressive disorders in older patients. *Postgrad Med.* 2001; October, 1–86.

62 Stahl S. *Essential Psychopharmacology: neuroscientific basis and practical applications.* 2nd ed. Cambridge: CUP; 2000.

63 Williams JW, Mulrow CD, Chiquette E, *et al.* A systematic review of newer pharmacotherapies for depression in adults: evidence report summary. *Ann Intern Med.* 2000; **132**: 743–56.

64 Pridmore S, Turnier SY. Medication options in the treatment of treatment-resistant depression. *Aus NZ J Psychiatr.* 2004; **38**(4): 219–25.

65 Georgotas AMR, Cooper T. Factors affecting the delay of antidepressant effect in responders to nortriptyline and phenelzine. *Psychiatr Res.* 1989; **28**: 1–9.

66 Mitchell AJ. Two-week delay in onset of action of antidepressants: new evidence. *Br J Psychiatr.* 2006; **188**: 105–6.

67 Flint AJ, Rifat SL. The effect of sequential antidepressant treatment on geriatric depression. *J Affect Disord.* 1996; **36**: 95–105.

68 Flint AJ. The optimum duration of antidepressant treatment in the elderly. *Int J Geriatr Psychiatr.* 1992; **7**: 617–19.

69 Old Age Depression Interest Group. How long should the elderly take antidepressants? A double-blind placebo-controlled study of continuation/prophylaxis therapy with dothiepin. *Br J Psychiatr.* 1993; **162**: 75–182.

70 Anderson IM, Nutt DJ, Deakin JFW. Evidence-based guidelines for treating depressive disorders with antidepressants: a revision of the 1993 British Association for Psychopharmacology guidelines. *J Psychopharmacol.* 2000; **14**(1): 3–20.

71 Reynolds CF, III, Perel JM, Frank E, *et al.* Three-year outcomes of maintenance nortriptyline treatment in late-life depression: a study of two fixed plasma levels. *Am J Psychiatr.* 1999; **156**(8): 1177–81.

72 Appelberg B. Long-term citalopram prevents recurrent depression in the elderly and is well tolerated. *Evid Based Ment Health.* 2002; **6**(1): 24.

73 Abou-Saleh MT, Coppen A. The prognosis of depression in old age: the case for lithium therapy. *Br J Psychiatr.* 1983; **170**: 285–7.

74 Bogner HR, Lin JY, Morales KH (2006) Patterns of early adherence to the antidepressant citalopram among older primary care patients: the prospect study. *Int J Psychiatr and Med.* 2006; **36**(1): 103–19.

75 Lima MS, Moncrieff J. Drugs versus placebo for dysthymia. *The Cochrane Library.* 2005; **3**: CD001130.

76 Shabnam GN, Kho TC, Ce CHR. Therapies for depression in Parkinson's disease. *Cochrane Database Systematic Review.* 2003; **3**: CD003465.

77 Flint AJ. Treatment-resistant depression in late life. *CNS Spectrums.* 2002; **7**(10): 733–8.

78 Angst J. A regular review of long term follow-up of depression. *BMJ.* 1997; **315**: 1143–6.

79 Cowen PJ. Pharmacological management of treatment-resistant depression. *Adv Psychiatr Treat.* 1998; **4**: 320–7.

80 Renwick RA. Treatment resistant depression. *Psychiatr J Univ Ottawa.* 1985; **46**: 576–84.

81 Thase ME, Rush AJ. Treatment resistant depression. In: Bloom FE, Kupfer DJ, editors. *Psychopharmacology: the fourth generation of progress.* New York: Raven Press; 1997. pp. 1081–1215.

82 O'Brien J, Barber B. Neuroimaging in dementia and depression. *Adv Psychiatr Treat.* 2000; **6**: 109–19.

83 Kalayam B, Alexopoulos GS. Prefrontal dysfunction and treatment response in geriatric depression. *Arch Gen Psychiatr.* 1999; **56**(8): 713–18.

84 Li YS, Meyer JS, Thornby J. Longitudinal follow-up of depressive symptoms among normal versus cognitively impaired elderly. *Int J Geriatr Psychiatr.* 2001; **16**(7): 718–27.

85 Yamashita H. Clinical features and treatment response of patients with major depression and silent cerebral infarction. *Neuropsychobiol.* 2000; **44**(4): 182.

86 Cujpers P. Psychological outreach programmes for the depressed elderly: a meta-analysis of effects and dropout. *Int J Geriatr Psychiatr.* 1998; **13**(1): 41–8.

87 Guscott R, Grof P. The clinical meaning of refractory depression: a review for the clinician. *Am J Psychiatr.* 1991; **148**: 695–704.

88 Baldwin RC. Treatment resistant depression in the elderly: a review of treatment options. *Reviews in Clin Gerontol.* 1996; **6**: 343–8.

89 Einarson TR, Arikian SR, Casciano J, *et al.* Comparison of extended release Venlafaxine, selective serotonin reuptake inhibitors, and tricyclic antidepressants in the treatment of depression: a meta-analysis of randomised controlled trials. *Clin Ther.* 1999; **21**: 296–308.

90 Mottram P, Wilson KCM, Ashworth L, *et al.* The clinical profile of older patients' response to antidepressants: an open trial of sertraline. *Int J Geriatr Psychiatr.* 2002; **17**: 574–8.

91 Akiskal HS. An approach to chronic and 'resistant' depressions: evaluation and treatment. *J Clin Psychiatr.* 1985; **46**: 32–6.

92 Bowskill RJ, Bridges PL. Treatment-resistant affective disorders. *Br J Hosp Med.* 1997; **57**: 171–2.

93 Nierenberg AA, Feighner JP, Rudolph R *et al.* Venlafaxine for treatment-resistant unipolar depression. *J Clin Psychopharm.* 1994; **14**: 419–23.

94 Flint AJ, Rifat SL. A prospective study of lithium augmentation in antidepressant-resistant geriatric depression. *J Clin Psychopharm.* 1994; **14**: 353–6.

95 Fahy S, Lawlor BA. Discontinuation of lithium augmentation in an elderly cohort. *Int J Geriatr Psychiatr.* 2001; **16**(10): 1004–9.

96 Austin MPV, Souza FGM, Goodwin GM. Lithium augmentation in antidepressant-resistant patients: a quantitative analysis. *Br J Psychiatr.* 1991; **159**: 510–14.

97 Hoencamp E, Haffmans PMJ, Dijken WA, *et al.* Lithium augmentation of venlafaxine: an open-label trial. *J Clin Psychopharm.* 2000; **20**: 538–43.

98 Simon JS, Nemeroff CB. Aripiprazole augmentation of antidepressants for the treatment of partially responding and non-responding patients with major depressive disorder. *J Clin Psychiatr.* 2005; **66**(10): 1216–20.

99 Shelton RC, Williamson DJ, Corya SA, *et al.* Olanzapine/fluoxetine combination for treatment-resistant depression; a controlled study of SSRI and nortriptyline resistance. *J Clin Psychiatr.* 2005; **66**(10): 1289–97.

100 Rapaport MH, Gharabawi GM, Canuso CM, *et al.* Effects of risperidone augmentation in patients with treatment-resistant depression; results of open-label treatment followed by double-blind continuation. *Neuropsychopharmacol.* 2007; **32**(5): 1208.

101 Papakostas GI, Shelton RC, Smith J, *et al.* Augmentation of antidepressants with atypical antipsychotic medications for treatment-resistant major depressive disorder: a meta-analysis. *J Clin Psychiatr.* 2007; **68**(6): 826–31.

102 Sugiyama N, Sasayama D, Amano N. Remarkable antidepressant augmentation effect of raloxifene, a selective oestrogen receptor modulator in a partial responder to fluvoxamine: a case report. *J Clin Psychiatr.* 2007; **68**(4): 636–7.

103 Carpenter LL, Milosavljevic N, Schecter JM, *et al.* Augmentation with open-label atomoxetine for partial or nonresponse to antidepressants. *J Clin Psychiatr.* 2005; **66**(10): 1234–8.

104 Hannan N, Hamzah Z, Omoniyi H, *et al.* Venlafaxine-mirtazapine combination in the treatment of persistent depressive illness. *J Psychopharm.* 2006; **May**: 226–231.

105 Aronson R, Offman HJ, Joffe RT, *et al.* Triiodothyronine augmentation in the treatment of refractory depression: a meta-analysis. *Arch Gen Psychiatr.* 1996; **53**: 842–8.

106 Hale A, Proctor AW, Bridges PK. Clomipramine, tryptophan and lithium in combination for resistant endogenous depression: seven case studies. *Br J Psychiatr.* 1987; **151**: 213–17.

107 Moreno FA, Gelenberg AJ, Bachar K, *et al.* Pindolol augmentation of treatment-resistant depressed patients. *J Clin Psychiatr.* 1997; **58**(10): 437–9.

108 Bodani M, Sheehan B, Philpot M. The use of dexamethasone in elderly patients with antidepressant-resistant depressive illness. *J Psychopharm.* 1999; **13**(2): 196–7.

109 Morishita S, Aoki S. Clonazepam in the treatment of prolonged depression. *J Affect Disord.* 1999; **53**(3): 275–8.

110 Stahl SM. Basic psychopharmacology of antidepressants part 2: oestrogen as an adjunct to antidepressant treatment. *J Clin Psychiatr.* 1998; **59**(4): 15–24.

111 Emptage RE, Semla TP, Gonzales L, *et al.* Depression in the medically ill elderly: a focus on methylphenidate. *Ann Pharmacother.* 1996; **30**(2): 151–7.

112 Curran S. Effect of paroxetine on seizure length during electroconvulsive therapy. *Acta Psychiatr Scand.* 1995; **12**(2): 239–40.

113 Shapira B, Tubi N, Drexler H, *et al.* Cost and benefit in the choice of ECT schedule: twice versus three times weekly ECT. *Br J Psychiatr.* 1998; **172**: 44–8.

114 Krystal AD, Coffey CE, Weiner RD, *et al.* Changes in seizure threshold over the course of electroconvulsive therapy affect therapeutic response and are detected by ictal EEG ratings. *J Neuropsychiatr Clin Neurosci.* 1998; **10**(2):178–86.

115 Lam JY, Freeman MK, Cates ME. Modafinil augmentation for the residual symptoms of fatigue in patients with a partial response to antidepressants. *Ann Pharmacother.* 2007; **41**(6), 1005–12.

Pharmacological treatment of bipolar affective disorder in old age

NAILA JAWAID AND ROBERT BALDWIN

Introduction

Although only about 10% of new onset cases of bipolar affective disorder (BPD) occur after the age of 50,[1] matched to similarly aged older patients with unipolar depression, BPD is associated with higher morbidity and greater use of mental health services.[2] With demographic changes to the age structure of the population inevitably there will more BPD in later life. About a quarter of late-onset cases of mania are associated with cerebral disorder,[3] especially right hemisphere lesions, making late-life mania a heterogeneous condition and hence a particular challenge to manage.

Definitions

Table 5.1 lists the American Psychiatric Association criteria for a manic episode.[4] For a hypomanic episode criterion A must be present for four days; under criterion D the change in mood is discernable to others but does not cause major impairment. Bipolar I disorder is characterised by repeated manic episodes often with bouts of major depression. Bipolar II disorder occurs when patients have recurrent major depression with hypomanic episodes. For a diagnosis of BPD in DSMIV only one manic episode is required, whereas the European nomenclature[5] requires two episodes of either mania or hypomania. When four or more episodes of illness occur within a 12-month period, a person is said to have **rapid-cycling** bipolar disorder.

Other types of BPD have been proposed. Type III denotes hypomanic episodes occurring in association with antidepressants and/or psychostimulants and type IV with 'hyperthymic' personality. Recurrent depression without discrete hypomania but with mixed hypomanic episodes (agitation, irritability, racing thoughts) has been proposed as a Type V.[6] Akiskal and colleagues[7] have recently proposed a type VI in which mood instability develops in the sixth or seventh decade with a slow progression to neurocognitive deficits, irritability, agitation and poor sleep. They highlight the overlap of this presentation with some cases of agitation in Alzheimer patients.

TABLE 5.1 Criteria for manic episode (American Psychiatric Association)[4]

A.	A distinct period of abnormally and persistently elevated, expansive, or irritable mood, lasting at least one week (or any duration if hospitalisation is necessary).
B.	During the period of mood disturbance, three (or more) of the following symptoms have persisted (four if the mood is only irritable) and have been present to a significant degree.

    1   Inflated self-esteem or grandiosity.

    2   Decreased need for sleep (e.g. feels rested after only three hours of sleep).

    3   More talkative than usual or pressure to keep talking.

    4   Flight of ideas or subjective experience that thoughts are racing.

    5   Distractibility (i.e. attention too easily drawn to unimportant or irrelevant external stimuli).

    6   Increase in goal-directed activity (either socially, at work or school, or sexually) or psychomotor agitation.

    7   Excessive involvement in pleasurable activities that have a high potential for painful consequences (e.g. engaging in unrestrained buying sprees, sexual indiscretions, or foolish business investments).

C.	The symptoms do not meet criteria for a mixed episode.
D.	The mood disturbance:

    1   is sufficiently severe to cause marked impairment in occupational functioning, usual social activities or relationships with others,

    2   necessitates hospitalisation to prevent harm to self or others, or

    3   has psychotic features.

E.	The symptoms are not due to the direct physiological effects of a substance (e.g. a drug of abuse, a medication, or other treatment) or a general medical condition (e.g. hyperthyroidism).

Course and outcome

About half of patients with late-onset BPD have a previous history of depression, often with a latency period of many years.[8] The prognosis of BPD is thought to worsen with age due to the time between episodes of illness becoming shorter as the patient ages.[9] Although manic episodes are very disabling, as much morbidity and functional disturbance in bipolar I and bipolar II arise from depression as from manic or hypomanic episodes.[10]

Treatment principles

The principles of managing late-life BPD are the same as at other times of adult life. Modifications largely arise because of changes with age in pharmacokinetics and pharmacodynamics resulting in altered drug handling. These affect starting and therapeutic dosages of drugs, propensity to side-effects and likelihood of drug interactions.

Treatment phases are divided into acute treatment for mania, hypomania or mixed states, acute treatment of bipolar depression, and long-term treatment (including the treatment of rapid cycling disorder). In practice, a majority of patients will have early-onset BPD. Drug treatment is the mainstay of management in BPD and is the focus of this chapter. However, other interventions such as education about BPD, sleep hygiene, advice about travel across international time zones, psychosocial interventions and electroconvulsive therapy are important. Information about all treatment modalities is available in the current guidelines for BPD, listed in Table 5.2. At present no specific guidelines exist for geriatric bipolar disorders, although Young and colleagues have provided a useful review.[13]

The 2006 NICE guidelines on BPD[12] recommend an annual physical health review to ensure that the following are assessed each year: lipid levels, plasma glucose, weight, smoking status, alcohol use and blood pressure.

The first part of the chapter describes currently available medications for BPD and the second part their application in the phases of treatment.

TABLE 5.2 Guidelines available online for the management of bipolar affective disorder

- American Psychiatric Association (2002)[11]

  http://www.psych.org/psych_pract/treatg/pg/bipolar_revisebook_index.cfm
- British Association of Psychopharmacology (2003)[9]

  http://www.bap.org.uk/consensus/bipolar_disorder.html
- National Institute for Health and Clinical Excellence (NICE) (2006)[12]

  http://www.nice.org.uk/page.aspx?o=CG38

Part 1: Medications used in bipolar affective disorder
Mood stabilisers

'Mood stabiliser' broadly refers to an agent that is effective in acute and long-term treatment of either mania or depression without having significant adverse effects on the opposite pole of BPD. The main members are: lithium, anticonvulsants and antipsychotic drugs. Although anticonvulsants do not have any clear advantage over lithium, they do offer an alternative for patients who cannot take or tolerate lithium. With the exception of some data regarding valproate, the efficacy of anticonvulsants such as carbamazepine, oxcarbazepine, lamotrigine, gabapentin and topiramate has not been established in older BPD patients. Table 5.3 summarises key data for the three most commonly used mood stabilisers.

Lithium

Mode of action

Differences in response to lithium in elderly patients are usually explained by the effect of age-related physiological changes, comorbid conditions, altered renal clearance and concurrent use of other medication. Lithium is readily and completely absorbed and peak level reached in one to two hours. Although absorption of lithium is generally unchanged by the ageing process, the volume of distribution and renal clearance of lithium is substantially different in older adults.[14] The half-life of lithium can vary considerably but on average it is in the region of 22–24 hours and increases with long-term use by 25–30%. It is excreted mostly unchanged by the kidneys. Reduced renal clearance, leading to higher lithium levels, can occur in patients with hypertension, congestive heart failure or renal disease.

The mode of action of lithium is largely unknown. It acts as a highly reactive cation and influences chemical processes at the level of membrane neurophysiology by stabilising electrolyte balance. It has also been shown to increase the neuronal uptake of catecholamines and potentiate serotonergic and noradrenergic function as well as acting on so-called messenger systems.[15] It is not yet clear precisely how these effects on intracellular communication translate into therapeutic benefit. Prior to commencing lithium, routine investigation should include renal function, electrolytes, thyroid function tests, blood glucose and an electrocardiogram (ECG).[16] Recommended starting dose in elderly patients is around 100–200 mg daily.

Lithium has a narrow therapeutic index and perhaps because of this over recent years there has been decline in its use and its replacement with valproate without much supporting evidence.[17]

Efficacy

There have been no definitive randomised controlled studies of lithium treatment of elderly manic patients. Young and colleagues[13] summarised four studies (n=137) and reported that 66% improved regardless of lithium concentration. In a retrospective casenote study Chen et al.[18] compared lithium (n=30) with valproate (n=29) in older manic patients. The percentage of patients improved was significantly greater in the lithium group than in the valproate group (67% vs. 38%). However, there was more improvement in the valproate group when serum levels were 65–90 mcg/mL and for lithium when levels were > or =0.8 mmol/L.

Response to lithium is generally poor in rapid cycling, psychotic mania and mixed affective state, although in the above study[18] comparison of patients with mixed manic states showed a response of two-thirds in both lithium and valproate-treated groups.

Evidence of the efficacy of lithium in maintenance treatment of older BPD patients is limited to naturalistic studies. Young et al.[13] found four studies amounting to 101 elderly patients but could come to no firm conclusions.

In the NICE BPD guidelines of 2006[12] lithium levels of 0.6 to 0.8 mmol/L were recommended for adults requiring maintenance lithium for the first time and up to 1.0 mmol/L where the patient had been exposed to lithium before and residual symptoms were present. In the absence of specific recommendations for lithium augmentation in later life, this remains pragmatic guidance. Based on experience, some Old Age Psychiatrists use lower dosages but the evidence to support this is mixed.[13] Blood should ideally be taken 10–14 hours post dose. The serum level should be measured after five to seven days and then weekly for every dose change until the level is stable, after which it should be repeated at three-monthly intervals. Renal and thyroid function should be monitored six-monthly or as indicated by patient's clinical condition.[12] Weight should also be monitored.

Adverse effects

Polydipsia, polyuria, tremor, dry mouth and subjective memory impairment are the most frequent side-effects. In the longer term, hypothyroidism may occur and this may necessitate treatment with thyroxine. Nephrotoxicity is another long-term complication. A small proportion of patients develop irreversible reduction in urinary concentrating capacity after long-term treatment[19] and renal changes may include interstitial fibrosis and tubular atrophy. There are reports of psoriasis being exacerbated. The sick sinus syndrome may occur in older adults with compromised sinus node function. In a cross-sectional study, Roose *et al.*[20] reported that more than half of older patients treated with maintenance lithium had electrocardiogram abnormalities such as conduction defects.

Clinically significant drug interactions with lithium involve drugs commonly used in elderly patients such as thiazide diuretics, ACE inhibitors and non-steroidal anti-inflammatory drugs, which can increase serum lithium concentration. In a study of 10,615 Canadian residents aged 66 and older receiving lithium, 3.9% were admitted to hospital at least once for lithium toxicity over a 10-year period.[14] There was an especially high risk in the first month of initiating treatment with a loop diuretic or angiotensin-converting enzyme (ACE) inhibitor but not for thiazide diuretics or nonsteroidal anti-inflammatory drugs (NSAIDs).

Lithium neurotoxicity (vomiting, diarrhoea, confusion, myoclonic jerks, cardiac arrhythmias, ataxia, dysarthria, convulsions, coma and in some cases death) can occur at levels above 1.2mmol/L but in older subjects at levels considered therapeutic in younger adults, perhaps especially where there is underlying brain damage. Above 2.5 mmol/L haemodialysis may be required. The risk of neurotoxicity increases with calcium channel blockers, carbamazepine, methyldopa and neuroleptics and there is an increased risk of renal toxicity with metronidazole and verapamil.

Lithium should not be discontinued abruptly. Downward titration should occur for a minimum of four weeks and optimally three months.[12] If it has to be stopped suddenly, cover should be given with another mood stabiliser such as valproate.

Valproate
Mode of action
Valproate is available in the UK in three forms: sodium valproate, valproic acid and semisodium valproate, the last having a product licence for the treatment of acute mania in the UK. Randomised controlled trials have shown valproate to be effective in the treatment of mania.[21,22] It is believed to affect the function of the neurotransmitter GABA (as a GABA transaminase inhibitor) in the human brain, making it an alternative to lithium salts in the treatment of BPD. Absorption is rapid and peak levels are attained in 30–60 minutes. Protein binding is up to 95% and half-life varies with the preparation but is in the range of 5–20 hours. It is metabolised partly via the microsomal cytochrome P450 system and partly via mitochondrial oxidation. Serum level monitoring is supposedly of limited use compared with lithium and carbamazepine and is not routinely recommended, although there is a little evidence for an optimum window as discussed in the preceding section.[16] Target dosages are in the range of 500–1500 mg per day in divided doses.

Efficacy
Valproate has a broad spectrum of activity in mania, mixed affective states,[23] rapid cycling bipolar disorders and secondary mania, which is particularly relevant to older patients.[24] Divalproex (DVP, combined sodium valproate and valproic acid) is increasingly prescribed for elderly people in preference to lithium on the grounds that it is safer and better tolerated than lithium in older patients,[23,25] although the evidence to support this is weak.[17] Nevertheless, unlike other anticonvulsants valproate can serve as a sole antimanic drug.[26]

Young and colleagues[13] summarised the results from five studies (n=137). The dose of DVP was 250–2250 mg and overall 59% of patients showed some degree of improvement.

A combination of valproate and lithium may be more effective in elderly patients with a poor response to either drug.[27,28] Valproate was also effective in a case series of older bipolar patients with rapid cycling.[28]

Adverse effects
Common side effects are sedation, dyspepsia and tremor. In the long term weight gain and hair loss can occur. Benign increases in hepatic transaminases can occur or rarely hepatotoxicity and reversible thrombocytopaenia or leucopenia. In older adults sedation and gait disturbance can be problematic.[17] Many side-effects are dose related. Potential drug interactions with aspirin, phenytoin, fluoxetine and carbamazepine can occur[16] while lamotrigine metabolism can be inhibited, necessitating lower starting doses of the latter. Liver function, blood count and weight should be monitored at the outset and at six months.[12] Overdosage is usually non-lethal.

Carbamazepine
Mode of action

Carbamazepine acts by stabilising sodium channels in neurons so that brain cells are less excitable. Following slow and rather erratic absorption, peak levels are attained in four to six hours. The half-life averages 7–24 hours and the main site of metabolism is the liver by the enzyme epoxide hydroxylase. This enzyme can be inhibited by the co-administration of other drugs such as valproate or lamotrigine, hence caution is required if either combination is contemplated. Carbamazepine levels can be increased by co-administration of fluoxetine, some antibiotics and calcium channel blockers.

Adverse effects

Side-effects are common, more so in older patients, and include drowsiness, diplopia, impaired motor coordination and stomach upset. Carbamazepine can slow intra-cardiac conduction and produce arrhythmias. Mild hyponatraemia (more common in older patients), thrombocytopaenia, leucopenia or altered liver enzymes can occur. Overdosage can be lethal, with onset characterised by neurological signs. Tolerability to the drug is related to dose and titration intervals. Carbamazepine has a greater propensity for drug–drug interactions than other mood stabilisers, which is of particular concern in the elderly. Prior to commencing carbamazepine, carry out liver enzyme tests, electrolytes and a full blood count. Starting doses are typically 100 mg once or twice daily, with average daily dosages of 400–800 mg to achieve blood levels of 4–12 ug/L.[11] Serum monitoring at least six-monthly is recommended.

Lamotrigine
Mechanism of action

Lamotrigine, a phenyltriazine derivative, is an anticonvulsant with efficacy in the prevention of mood disorders in adult patients with bipolar I disorder.[29] The mechanism of action may be related to the inhibition of sodium and calcium channels in presynaptic neurons and subsequent stabilisation of the neuronal membrane. Lamotrigine is metabolised in the liver and primarily eliminated via hepatic glucoronide conjugation. In elderly patients the clearance is reported to decrease by 37% and the volume of distribution by 12%.[30] It is generally well tolerated and, unlike lithium, does not appear to cause body weight increase, nor does it require monitoring of serum levels.[29] In retrospective case studies lamotrigine showed reasonable tolerability and modest clinical improvement in 19 out of 20 nursing home patients who were treated with it for agitated and aggressive behaviour in a range of medical and psychiatric diagnoses.[31] The starting dose is 25 mg (half if the patient is taking valproate) for two weeks, increasing over weeks three and four by 50 mg with further 50 mg increments as needed.

Lamotrigine delays the time to relapses of depressive episodes[29] and is effective in the treatment of acute episodes of depression but not for acute mania in patients with bipolar disorder.[9]

Adverse effects

The most common side-effects are headache, nausea and insomnia. The slow titration interval is to avoid serious rash (Stevens Johnson syndrome). Interactions with valproate and carbamazepine may occur.

TABLE 5.3 Mood stabilisers used in bipolar disorder in older people

Drug	Investigations prior to prescribing	Side-effects	Average daily dosages	Target serum levels
Lithium	Renal function Electrolytes ECG Thyroid function Blood glucose (preferably fasting)	Polyuria, gastrointestinal upset, tremor, neurological disturbance (toxicity), weight gain, oedema, psoriatic rash	400 mg (slow release)	0.6–0.8 mEq/L
Valproate	Liver enzymes Full blood count ECG (if history or clinical condition suggests[12])	Sedation, nausea, unsteadiness, tremor, weight gain	500–1500 mg	65–90 µg/mL (not definitely established)
Carbamazepine	Liver enzymes Full blood count ECG (if history or clinical condition suggests[12])	Sedation, ataxia, nystagmus, blurred vision, agranulo-cytosis, hyponatraemia	400–800 mg	4–12 µg/L (levels for epilepsy)

Antipsychotics

Antipsychotics are widely used in elderly psychiatric disorders. Atypical antipsychotics that are licensed for use in BPD in the UK are olanzapine, risperidone and quetiapine. In mania, olanzapine is usually administered at 10–15 mg daily, risperidone 1–6 mg and quetiapine 150–600 mg. It is to be expected that in manic patients who are frail or with organic brain damage or suspected underlying dementia (secondary mania) dosages will need to be at the lower end and that there is more likelihood of adverse effects when dosages are increased.

The newer atypicals are preferred to the older drugs on grounds of safety and tolerability rather than efficacy. Refractory cases may respond to off-licence use of clozapine but this drug is poorly tolerated in older patients.

Olanzapine

Mode of action

Olanzapine is a $5HT_2$ and D_2 receptor blocker. It is licensed as both an antipsychotic and a mood stabiliser. Olanzapine has minimal effects on serum prolactin and may be associated with lower incidence of sexual dysfunction compared to other antipsychotics. It can elevate serum cholesterol and triglycerides, more so than other atypical antipsychotics. Its levels are decreased by 1A2 inducers, notably cigarette smoking, and increased by 1A2 inhibitors, such as fluvoxamine and cimetidine.

Adverse effects

Sedation, weight gain and hyperglycaemia (not always related to weight gain) are the main problems. These are especially important in older patients who may be placed at increased risk of diabetes, falls, worsening dyspnoea from pulmonary disease or aggravation of arthritis in weight-bearing joints. Weight gain can occur early on. Orthostatic hypotension, Parkinsonian side-effects (less often than with risperidone) and anticholinergic side effects may occur. Tardive dyskinesia is a risk, but as with other atypical drugs it is considerably less than with older neuroleptics. Liver transaminases are occasionally elevated. Prior to commencement liver enzymes and random glucose should be checked and thereafter at six-monthly intervals.

Risperidone

Mode of action

Risperidone is a benzisoxazole derivative with high affinity for serotonin, dopamine and alpha 1 and 2 adrenergic receptors. Oral risperidone is rapidly absorbed, reaching maximum plasma concentration after one to two hours. It is largely hydroxylated by the cytochrome P450 2D6 enzyme. The elimination half-life is about 20 hours. Excretion is mostly through the urine. Clearance is reduced in elderly people and in those with renal impairment.

Adverse effects

Common side-effects affecting more than 10% of patients are extrapyramidal side-effects, somnolence, weight gain, headache, dizziness, dyspepsia and constipation. Plasma glucose is less affected by risperidone in trials in patients with mania. Prolactin levels should be checked prior to commencement in patients with low libido or sexual dysfunction.

Quetiapine

Quetiapine is reasonably well tolerated in elderly patients. The most common adverse effects observed with quetiapine are postural hypotension, dizziness and somnolence. The potential for reduced renal clearance means that quetiapine should be introduced at lower doses and titrated at a relatively slower rate.[32] This also helps reduce postural hypotension.

Aripiprazole

Aripiprazole is a partial agonist of D_2 receptors which operates through reducing dopamine effects when too high via competitive inhibition while maintaining adequate dopamine function when levels are low through its agonist effects. It is well absorbed and has a half-life of 75 hours. There are potential interactions via P450 metabolism with paroxetine and fluoxetine (raising aripiprazole levels) but so far the incidence of extra-pyramidal and metabolic adverse effects seems low. Its current licence is for schizophrenia but in the US it is also licensed for BPD and this may occur in the UK eventually.

Part 2: Practical pharmacological management of older people with bipolar disorder

The following is a synthesis from the three guidelines in Table 5.2 and the recommendations of Young et al.[13]

Acute treatment of mania or mixed episode

For psychotic patients and severe cases in general, treatment with an antipsychotic or valproate should be initiated. Appreciable clinical improvement may not be apparent until 10–14 days. For very disturbed patients orodispersible forms of some antipsychotics are available. Benzodiazepines (such as lorazepam) are often used to control acute agitation but should be used with extreme care in older patients because of the risks of falls. For less ill patients lithium can be considered or carbamazepine. If the patient is already on an antidepressant, this should be tapered and discontinued.

Where the patient is already on an antimanic drug but has relapsed, then compliance should be ascertained and the highest tolerated dose given. If this is unsuccessful combined treatment can be given; for example, an antipsychotic and a mood stabiliser.

For non-responsive patients substance misuse, psychosocial stressors, physical health problems, comorbid disorders, such as anxiety or severe obsessional symptoms, and inadequate adherence to medication should be addressed. For severe or prolonged mania electroconvulsive therapy (ECT) can be given considered in accordance with 2003 NICE guidelines on ECT.[33]

Secondary mania

If possible offending drugs (such as L-dopa or corticosteroids) should be discontinued or reduced. Thyroid abnormality should be corrected. For organic brain disease, the acute episode should be treated as above but anticipating increased sensitivity to adverse effects. However, divalproex sodium was not found to be very effective in controlling symptoms of mania associated with dementia in a sample of nursing home residents.[34] Thereafter ongoing treatment will depend on the underlying pathology but pragmatically a tapered withdrawal can be considered after a period of euthymia of approximately six months.

Bipolar depressive episode

Older patients are at an increased risk of becoming depressed after an episode of mania. For mild depression, watchful waiting with a review in two weeks is recommended. For moderate depression a psychological intervention, if available, may be preferable to antidepressant medication or augmentation of an existing non-antipsychotic mood stabiliser with quetiapine can be tried.[12] Antidepressant treatment should be given with an antimanic drug such as lithium, valproate or an antipsychotic and not given as monotherapy. Selective serotonin reuptake inhibitors (SSRIs) are associated with less risk of switching to a manic state than are tricyclic antidepressants. If the patient has psychotic depressive symptoms an antipsychotic drug should be added and, again subject to NICE guidance, ECT can be considered. Unlike unipolar depression, the role of antidepressants in the long-term management of BPD is limited. The risk of a relapse may be high in the first six months of recovery but generally the antidepressant should be tapered off as soon as possible.

At present there is insufficient evidence to recommend initial treatment with lamotrigine, lithium or valproate in less severely depressed older BPD patients, although there is some evidence to support this in mixed-aged patients.[9] In particular, if an antidepressant in the past has destabilised BPD then lamotrigine can be considered as an alternative.[9]

Prevention of episodes: maintenance treatment

In 2006, olanzapine and lithium have product licences for use in prophylaxis. Long-term treatment is now recommended after a severe manic episode,[9] two or more episodes of bipolar I or in bipolar II patients who have disabling episodes or at high risk of recurrence. Monotherapy is preferred and lithium has the largest evidence base in the prevention of both manic and depressive poles of BPD but is somewhat more effective for mania. It may take six months before efficacy can be established. Where tolerance is poor, valproate is an alternative which can address both poles. Olanzapine is more effective in preventing manic episodes and lamotrigine depressive episodes. Carbamazepine is a less attractive alternative because its greater propensity for pharmacological interactions, a particular problem in older patients, but it has a licence for the prevention of relapses unresponsive to lithium.

In patients who do not respond to monotherapy or who experience breakthrough symptoms, a second drug can be added. For patients troubled mainly with manic episodes this should be a second antimanic agent but where depression predominates other combinations such as an antidepressant and lamotrigine can be considered. Lamotrigine monotherapy can be considered in patients who have bipolar II disorder with frequent depressive relapses.[9]

Long-acting antipsychotic drugs ('depots') are not recommended for prophylaxis but may have a limited role in patients who have responded well to oral antipsychotics but are poorly adherent. There is a risk of extra-pyramidal side-effects, including tardive dyskinesia.

For all patients considered for long-term treatment a weight gain management programme should be available.

Rapid cycling BPD

This is difficult to treat. Lithium may be less effective in rapid cycling BPD. Nevertheless, lithium in combination with divalproex has been used successfully in geriatric rapid cycling disorder[28] with a suggestion that divalproex sodium might even increase the efficacy of lithium hence allowing treatment with lower lithium concentration. It is also important to identify and treat hypothyroidism, taper off antidepressants and address comorbidity from substance misuse and alcohol excess. Trials of treatment should generally last six months to establish efficacy with diary keeping by the patient.

Bipolar disorder and suicide

For patients identified by admission to hospital, rates of suicide are approximately 10% over long-term follow-up,[9] although naturalistic studies suggest that patients receiving long-term treatments, perhaps especially lithium, have lower rates.[9,35] The vast majority of suicides occur during depressive relapses or mixed states. Long-term lithium treatment is associated with reduction of suicide risk but there is a paucity of data regarding suicide among elderly bipolar patients. In one small retrospective study (n=32) elderly bipolar patients treated with a mood stabilisers and an antidepressant had a lower level of attempting suicide compared to control subjects.[36] This should be replicated in larger samples.

KEY POINTS

▶ Bipolar disorder in later life is associated with high morbidity and mental health service utilisation.
▶ Bipolar depression causes as much or greater morbidity as manic episodes and is a risk factor for suicide in bipolar patients.
▶ Most bipolar patients seen in later life have an early onset of illness; those with a late onset should be carefully investigated for underlying systemic or neurological disorder.
▶ There are few good clinical trials of older patients with bipolar disorder; lithium has the most evidence in later life although the risk of toxicity increases with age and certain co-prescribed medication.
▶ Perhaps because of this recent years have seen valproate replace lithium in later life but this is a practice-based change rather than an evidence-based one.

REFERENCES

1 Sajatovic M. Aging-related issues in bipolar disorder: a health services perspective. *J Geriatr Psychiatr Neurol.* 2002; **15**: 128–33.

2 Bartels SJ, Forester B, Miles KM, *et al.* Mental health service use by elderly patients with bipolar disorder and unipolar major depression. *Am J Geriatr Psychiatr.* 2000; **8**(2): 160–6.

3 Stone K. Mania in the elderly. *Br J Psychiatr.* 1989; **155**: 220–4.

4 American Psychiatric Association. *Diagnostic and Statistical Manual of Mental Disorders (DSM-IV).* 4th ed. Washington, DC; American Psychiatric Association; 2004.

5 World Health Organization. *The ICD-10 Classification of Mental and Behavioural Disorders: Research Criteria.* Geneva: World Health Organization; 1993.

6 Akiskal HS, Pinto O, The evolving bipolar spectrum: prototypes I, II, III, IV. *Psychiatr Clinics Nth Am.* 1999; **22**: 517–34.

7 Akiskal HS, Pinto O, Lara DR. Bipolarity in the setting of dementia: bipolar type VI? *Medscape Prim Care.* 2005; **6**(2): 1–4.

8 Shulman K, Post F. Bipolar affective disorder in old age. *Br J Psychiatr.* 1980; **136**: 26–32.

9 Goodwin GM, for the Consensus Group of the British Association for Psychopharmacology. Evidence-based guidelines for treating bipolar disorder: recommendations from the British Association for Psychopharmacology. *J Psychopharm.* 2003; **17**(2): 149–73.

10 Judd LL, Akiskal HS, Schettler PJ, *et al.* Psychosocial disability in the course of bipolar I and II disorders: a prospective, comparative, longitudinal study. *Arch Gen Psychiatr.* 2005; **62**(12): 1322–30.

11 American Psychiatric Association. Practice guidelines for the treatment of patients with bipolar disorder. *Am J Psychiatr.* 2002; **159**(Suppl. 4): S1–50.

12 National Institute for Health and Clinical Excellence. *Bipolar Disorder: the management of bipolar disorder in adults, children and adolescents, in primary and secondary care. Clinical Guideline 38.* London: National Institute for Health and Clinical Excellence; July 2006.

13 Young RC, Gyulai L, Mulsant BH, *et al.* Pharmacotherapy of bipolar disorder in old age. *Am J Geriatr Psychiatr.* 2004; **12**: 342–57.

14 Juurlink MM, Mamdani A, Kopp A, *et al.* Drug-induced lithium toxicity in the elderly: a population-based study. *J Am Geriatr Soc.* 2004; **52**(5): 794–8.

15 Manji H, Potter WZ, Leox RH. Signal transduction pathways: molecular targets for lithium's action. *Arch Gen Psychiatr.* 1995; **52**: 531–43.

16 Sajatovic M. Treatment of bipolar disorder in older adults. *Int J Geratr Psychiatr.* 2002; **17**: 865–73.

17 Shulman KL, Rochon P, Sykora K. Changing prescription patterns for lithium and valproic acid in old age: shifting practice without evidence. *BMJ.* 2003; **326**: 960–1.

18 Chen ST, Altshuler LL, Melnyk KA, *et al.* Efficacy of lithium vs. valproate in the treatment of mania in the elderly: a retrospective study. *J Clin Psychiatr.* 1999; **60**: 181–5.

19 Gitlin M. Lithium and the kidney: an update review. *Drug Safety.* 1999; **20**: 231–43.

20 Roose SP, Bone S, Haidorfer C, *et al.* Lithium treatment in older patients. *Am J Psychiatr.* 1979; **136**(6): 843–4.

21 Bowden CL, Brugger AM, Swann AC. Efficacy of divalproex sodium vs. lithium and placebo in the treatment of mania. *JAMA.* 1994; **271**: 918–24.

22 Freeman TW, Clothier JL, Pazzaglia P. A double-blind comparison of valproate and lithium in the treatment of acute mania. *Am J Psychiatr.* 1992; 149: 108–11.

23 Puryear LJ, Kunik ME, Workman R. Tolerability of divalproex sodium in elderly psychiatric patients with mixed diagnoses. *J Geriatr Psychiatr Neurol.* 1995; **8**: 234–7.

24 Khouzam HR, Emery PE, Reaves B. Secondary mania in late life. *J Am Geriatr Soc.* 1994; **42**(1): 85–7.

25 Noaghiul S, Natayan M, Nelson JC. Divalproex treatment of mania in elderly patients. *Am J Geriatr Psychiatr.* 1998; **6**(3): 257–62.

26 Mordecai DJ, Sheikh JI, Glick ID. Divalproex for the treatment of geriatric bipolar disorder. *Int J Geriatr Psychiatr.* 1999; **14**: 494–96.

27 Goldberg JF, Sacks MH, Kocsis JH. Low-dose lithium augmentation of divalproex in geriatric mania [letter]. *J Clin Psychiatr.* 2000; **61**: 304.

28 Schneider AL, Wilcox CS. Divalproate augmentation in lithium-resistant rapid cycling mania in four geriatric patients. *J Affect Disord.* 1998; **47**: 201–5.

29 Goldsmith DR, Wagastaff AJ, Ibbotson T. Lamotrigine: a review of its use in bipolar disorder. *Drugs.* 2003; **63**(19): 2029–50.

30 Posner J, Holdrich T, Crome P. Comparison of lamotrigine pharmacokinetics in young and elderly healthy volunteers. *J Pharm Med.* 1991; **1**: 121–8.

31 Aulakh JS, Hawkins JW, Athwal HS. Tolerability and effectiveness of lamotrigine in complex elderly patients. *J Geriatr Psychiatr Neurol.* 2005; **18**(1): 8–11.

32 Jaskiw GE, Thyrum PT, Fuller MA. Pharmacokinetics of quetiapine in elderly patients with selected psychotic disorders. *Clin Pharmacokinet.* 2004; **43**(14): 1025–35.

33 National Institute for Clinical Excellence. *The Clinical Effectiveness and Cost Effectiveness of Electroconvulsive Therapy (ECT) for Depressive Illness, Schizophrenia, Catatonia and Mania. Technology Appraisal 59.* London: National Institute for Clinical Excellence; April 2003.

34 Tariot PN, Schneider LS, Mintzer JE. Safety and tolerability of divalproex sodium in the treatment of signs and symptoms of mania in elderly patients with dementia: results of a double-blind, placebo-controlled trial. *Current Therapeutic Res.* 2001; **62**(1): 51–67.

35 Angst F, Stassen HH, Clayton PJ, *et al.* Mortality of patients with mood disorders: follow-up over 34–38 years. *J Affect Disord.* 2002; **68**: 167–81.

36 Aizenberg D, Olmer A, Barak Y. Suicide attempts amongst elderly bipolar patients. *J Affect Disord.* 2006; **91**(1): 91–4.

CHAPTER 6

Electricity, magnetism and mood

SUSAN MARY BENBOW

Introduction

Using electricity to elicit a seizure as a means of treating severe depressive illness must seem perplexing, if not frankly bizarre, to people who have no experience of electroconvulsive therapy (ECT), but ECT remains a treatment with a useful and important role in modern psychiatric practice. In contrast, the use of pills to treat depression carries little stigma, is widely accepted, indeed often expected, and the name of at least one current antidepressant has entered our everyday language. The BBC website[1] has an article on 'Prozac for pooches' to greet the launch of 'a new drug to treat dogs suffering from depression', and elsewhere we learn that 'an Environment Agency report suggests so many people are taking the drug (i.e. Prozac) nowadays it is building up in rivers and groundwater'.[2] A trawl of the Internet rapidly reveals that, unlike the antidepressant referred to above, stigma and controversy still cling to ECT after over 60 years of research and practice. It is vitally important that mental health professionals are clear about the role of ECT, in order to make it available to patients when appropriate, and to assist them in being open and informative with patients and their families who are considering this treatment option.

The electrical induction of seizures as a treatment for mental illness has a history which goes back to 1938 when Ugo Cerletti, an Italian neuro-psychiatrist, in collaboration with Lucio Bini, treated an acutely ill psychotic patient with a series of electroshocks, which led to the man's recovery.[3] Over ensuing decades the indications for ECT have been established, its safety has dramatically improved, and its administration has become technically much more refined.

This chapter starts by covering the following areas of importance to treating older adults with affective disorders with ECT:

- indications
- concurrent physical illness
- administration of treatment
- side-effects
- efficacy
- maintenance treatment.

There is exciting work ongoing at the moment to investigate other non-pharmacological treatments for depression: of particular interest are transcranial magnetic stimulation (TMS), vagal nerve stimulation (VNS) and magnetic seizure therapy (MST). The chapter concludes with an overview of these developing new treatments and their current status in psychiatric practice.

Indications for ECT

Diagnosis

The main diagnostic indication for ECT in older adults is severe depressive illness. A survey in the early 90s[4] found that old age psychiatrists regarded ECT for older people with depressive illness as the treatment of choice in the following situations:

- failure to respond to antidepressive drugs
- previous episodes known to have responded to ECT but not to antidepressive drugs
- psychotic symptoms
- severe agitation
- high suicidal risk.

A majority of responding old age psychiatrists reported that they found ECT useful often in depressive psychosis. This fits with reports in the literature of a favourable outcome for this group following treatment with ECT.[5] In schizoaffective disorder and depression with some dementia over 50% found the treatment to be appropriate sometimes. Nearly 50% found ECT to be rarely appropriate in manic excitement. Since then NICE has published its technology appraisal of ECT[6] which recommends that ECT should be used

> only to achieve rapid and short-term improvement of severe symptoms after an adequate trial of other treatment options has proven ineffective and/or when the condition is considered to be life-threatening, in individuals with
>
> - severe depressive illness
> - catatonia
> - a prolonged or severe manic episode.

NICE[6] states that the risks associated with ECT may be 'enhanced' in older adults and recommends that clinicians should exercise 'particular caution' when considering ECT. Any decision to recommend ECT to an older adult will involve careful consideration of potential risks and benefits: it would be inappropriate to deprive people of the option of having ECT purely because of their age.

The NICE Clinical Guideline on Depression, *Management of depression in primary and secondary care*,[7] places ECT under inpatient care, where the focus is on risk to life and severe self-neglect. Depressive illness with dementia is mentioned under special patient characteristics, where the Guideline notes that depression in people with dementia should be treated in the same way as depression in other older adults. The NICE Clinical Guideline on Bipolar Disorder[8] states that ECT should be considered for concurrent depressive and psychotic symptoms, 'if depression is severe'. Beale and Kellner[9] pointed out that ECT is often included so near the bottom of treatment algorithms that patients might have to undertake several years of treatment before ECT is considered. They noted that people might have years of suffering as a result and raise a controversial but thought-provoking question: given response rates to anti-depressive drugs and ECT, why save the best till last?

The impact of NICE's publications on the use of ECT for older adults, and whether clinical practice has changed over recent years, is not clear. It is likely that the majority of older people treated with ECT are treated under NICE's category of severe depressive illness, and that older adults with prolonged or severe manic episodes are a small group treated with ECT.

Age

Age in itself does not constitute a contraindication to ECT and older adults are major users of ECT services.[10] There is ongoing debate about why this might be the case, and the mental health charity MIND, arguing that older women are over-represented among the population of people treated with ECT, has campaigned for a scaling down of its use.[11] There are, however, several reasons why older adults might be major users of ECT.

> * Older people might be more likely to suffer from illnesses which respond to ECT: refusal to eat/ drink, severe psychosis, melancholic features, and stupor might be more common in older age groups.
> * Concern about comorbid medical or neurological conditions might lead to preferential use of ECT, in order to take advantage of the more rapid response to ECT in comparison with drug treatments.
> * Depressive illness in later life might be more likely to be drug-resistant.[12]
> * Older adults might be more sensitive to the side-effects of some antidepressive drugs.
> * Older people may have more positive attitudes towards ECT or find it a more acceptable treatment option.
> * Older depressed adults may respond to ECT better than younger adults.[13]

➤ Flint and Gagnon[14] state that there is a positive association between advancing age and the efficacy of ECT, which they relate not to ageing itself but to clinical factors in late-life depressive illness.

ECT and concurrent physical illness

ECT is used successfully to treat people with a wide range of concurrent physical illnesses and the American Psychiatric Association (APA) states that there are no absolute contraindications to its use.[15] Cardiovascular and neurological problems may be of particular concern, and are more likely to coexist alongside affective disorders in older adults. The principles of management in all patients with physical comorbidity are as follows.

➤ Fully assess and treat underlying illnesses prior to ECT.
➤ Seek appropriate medical and anaesthetic opinions prior to treatment.
➤ Consider ways of decreasing risk prior to commencing treatment.
➤ Fully discuss with patient and family the risks and ways of minimising them.

In some cases ECT may need to be administered in an environment offering a rapid response to cardiac complications, e.g. in a coronary care unit or theatre ante-room.

People with established cardiovascular disease are at increased risk of cardiac complications during ECT.[16] Blood pressure and heart rate fall, and then rise rapidly, during the passage of the electrical stimulus. Intracranial pressure undergoes a sudden brief rise, and cerebral blood flow and cerebrovascular permeability increase. Sinus bradycardia is a consequence of vagal stimulation and sometimes periods of asystole, or electrical silence, occur. A sympathetically mediated tachycardia follows rapidly, and can result in cardiac ischaemia. Takada *et al.*[17] assessed the cardiac effects of ECT in 38 people aged over 50 and found transient increases in blood pressure and heart rate, plus a decrease in heart rate variability, but there were no serious adverse clinical effects. Subconvulsive stimuli have been shown to produce longer periods of bradycardia, which may be a concern when people with established heart disease are being treated using a dose titration protocol to determine seizure threshold.[18,19] Beta blockers are a risk factor for longer periods of asystole during ECT,[20] and glycopyrrolate, or other vasolytic drugs, may be used to attenuate the bradycardia.[21] Despite these changes, most cardiovascular complications are transient and allow successful completion of the treatment course.[22] The APA states that, in general, people with cardiovascular disease can be safely treated with ECT.[15]

Conditions which may present higher cardiac risks during ECT are likely to be similar to those causing concern in relation to other surgical interventions.[23] These include recent myocardial infarct,[21,24] severe valvular heart disease,[25,26] clinically significant cardiac dysrhythmias,[21] unstable angina,[21] uncompensated congestive cardiac failure[26] and some aneurysms.[27,28] ECT appears to be safe in people on long-term warfarin,[29] and those with an implanted cardiac device.[30]

People with space-occupying brain lesions are at high risk of neurological deterioration if treated with ECT.[31] This is thought to be due to the aggravation of already raised intracranial pressure.[32] Despite this, ECT has been used safely for people with small, slow-growing cerebral tumours without raised intracranial pressure, and people with a wide range of neurological conditions have been treated successfully with ECT. This includes people with cerebrovascular diseases,[33] epilepsy,[34] cerebral lupus,[34] various dementias,[35,36] learning disabilities,[37,38] following stroke,[39] and post craniotomy.[40]

Administration of ECT

A number of technical aspects of treatment are relevant when ECT is administered to older adults with affective disorders.

Seizure threshold may rise with increasing age, potentially increasing the difficulty of eliciting effective seizures in older people.[41,42,43] ECT clinic protocols are designed to take into account the wide range of seizure thresholds in people presenting for treatment, and choice of anaesthetic agent needs to do so too.[44] High seizure thresholds are likely to be more of a problem for older men.[41,42,43]

Following the withdrawal of methohexitone from routine ECT anaesthesia in the UK, clinics have used several different anaesthetic agents. The effect of propofol on seizure length, and its possible effect on seizure threshold, needs to be taken into account in choosing an anaesthetic drug, although its popularity is increasing.[45] Benbow, Shah and Crentsil[46] argue that the selection of anaesthetic drug should be tailored to the individual being treated with ECT. Etomidate might be the drug of choice when the electrical dose needed for an individual (using another induction agent) is at the maximum level for the ECT machine in use, or when there are side-effects with an alternative induction agent, or when the person has severe cardiac disease.

Another important issue to consider when treating older adults is electrode placement. The two common placements are bilateral (usually bitemporal) and unilateral ECT.[44,47] There is some literature on the use of bifrontal ECT for older adults.[48] Theoretically, electrode placement avoiding the temporal regions might minimise the cognitive side-effects of bilateral treatment, but, although Little and colleagues[48] found bifrontal ECT to be clinically effective in a retrospective study of a small group of older people, they reported cognitive side-effects in 36%, undermining the argument in favour of using bifrontal ECT. Scott recommends the bitemporal position for bilateral ECT in the *ECT Handbook*.[44]

Unilateral ECT is probably underused in the UK. The APA[15] recommends that choice of unilateral or bilateral placement for an individual should be based on the balance of risks and benefits, and should be made by the ECT psychiatrist in consultation with others, but notes that the evidence for the use of unilateral ECT is in relation to depressive disorders, rather than other conditions. Bilateral ECT has continued to be popular in the UK but the most recent Royal College of Psychiatrists guidelines[44] are probably more in line with the APA's recommendations, and changes in practice in the UK may lead to an increase in the use of unilateral treatment. In mania bilateral ECT is preferable.[49]

A number of authors[16,50,51,52,53,54] have reported that increasing age is related to more complications, poor health status and greater number of medications. Sobin et al.[55] reported a similar relationship between pre-existing cognitive impairment and scores on memory impairment after treatment. Thus close monitoring of physical and cognitive state is recommended for older adults undergoing a course of ECT.[56] People who are known to have memory problems prior to a course of ECT are likely to be at risk of developing cognitive side-effects during treatment[57] and modifications to treatment technique might be helpful, e.g. choice of anaesthetic drug, consideration of unilateral treatment, changes to concurrent medication. In UK clinics the ECT consultant will advise prescribing psychiatrists on these technical issues.

Adverse effects of ECT

Mortality

The APA Task Force Report[15] estimated the ECT-related mortality rate as 1 per 10,000 patients or 1 per 80,000 treatments. Against this must be set the risks involved in not having ECT, and, for some people, morbidity and mortality rates with ECT may be lower than with some antidepressive drug treatments.[58] In addition, Abrams[59] pointed out that the death rate associated with ECT is lower than the spontaneous death rate in the general population of the United States. Thus, despite the fact that ECT is often used for older adults with concurrent major medical illnesses, it is regarded as a low risk procedure with a mortality rate similar to that of anaesthesia for minor surgical procedures.[58,60] The main areas of concern are cardiovascular and pulmonary complications[61] – potentially causes of death and serious morbidity. ECT clinic protocols and procedures aim to identify people who are at high risk, to ensure that they are carefully assessed and, wherever possible, actively treated to minimise risk prior to ECT, and that they are closely monitored during the administration of ECT in an appropriate treatment setting which will allow rapid intervention if complications occur.[56]

Some drug treatments lower seizure threshold: this has been used therapeutically by administering caffeine or theophylline to people who have very high seizure thresholds.[15] Concurrent medical conditions may also lower seizure threshold, e.g. electrolyte imbalance.[62] Prolonged seizures and status epilepticus are more likely to occur in these groups, and non-convulsive status epilepticus following ECT may be difficult to diagnose. One advantage of routine EEG monitoring is to show whether or not seizure activity has ceased.[63]

Effect on cognitive functions

Adverse effects are a major concern, and the effect of ECT on cognitive function is a particular concern when treating older adults. During pre-ECT assessment any factors which place an individual at increased risk of adverse effects will be identified and discussed with them and their families, along with any means to decrease the risk. For example, a person with concurrent Alzheimer's disease, who, along with other people with a dementia, would be regarded as having an increased risk of developing cognitive side-effects during a course of ECT,[31,64] might be advised to have unilateral rather than bilateral treatment, in order to minimise the effect on cognition. In contrast a person with existing cardiac disease, who is assessed as at high risk of cardiac complications during treatment, might be treated in a cardiac care unit with specialist staff present and advised to have bilateral ECT, rather than unilateral, in order to minimise the number of anaesthetics required over the course of treatment.[56]

Many people having ECT are concerned about its potential effect on their memory. ECT can affect memory for events which occurred before treatment, retrograde amnesia, and memory for events which take place after treatment, anterograde amnesia. New learning and non-memory cognitive functions (e.g. intelligence, judgement, abstraction, etc.) are unaffected. The most prominent cognitive side-effects occur immediately post-ictally, when people experience a variable period of disorientation, associated with impaired attention, memory and praxis.[65] These effects are normally short-lived. People taking concurrent psychotropic drugs, and those with pre-existing cognitive impairment or neurological conditions, are at increased risk of developing acute confusional states between treatments. When this occurs, modifications to treatment technique may lessen the confusion. Post-ictal delirium[66] is rare, and presents with restlessness, aggression or agitation in the early stages of recovery: it responds to benzodiazepine treatment.

The relationship between ECT and memory is complicated: depressive illness and many psychotropic drugs affect memory,[3] and ECT technique affects both type and severity of adverse cognitive effects. Increased cognitive side-effects are associated with the following treatment parameters:
➤ sine wave treatment (now obsolete in UK practice)
➤ bilateral electrode placement
➤ high stimulus intensity in relation to individual seizure threshold
➤ short inter-ECT interval
➤ some concomitant drug treatments (including lithium)
➤ high doses of anaesthetic medication.

Thus technical aspects of ECT which might be expected to decrease cognitive adverse effects include:
➤ changing sine wave to brief pulse stimulation
➤ using unilateral (rather than bilateral) electrode placement
➤ lowering stimulus intensity in relation to individual seizure threshold
➤ lengthening the inter-ECT interval
➤ decreasing or stopping relevant concomitant drug treatments
➤ reducing anaesthetic drug doses (where possible).

Cognitive side-effects of ECT have been extensively studied: the Systematic Review of the Efficacy and Safety of Electroconvulsive Therapy[47] and the American Psychiatric Task Force Report[15] both reviewed the literature on this topic. In the case of older adults with severe depressive illness, they may well have problems on memory testing prior to treatment, and tests of memory carried out after ECT may show improvement, presumably because the memory deficits associated with depression have improved in response to treatment.[67,68] Weiner[69] highlighted the complex relationship between objective and subjective memory impairment. Although a small proportion of people complain of persisting memory difficulty after treatment and may have persisting loss of memory for events during the period before, during and after ECT,[70,71] objective memory impairment (as demonstrated on objective tests) is generally reversible after conclusion of the ECT course.

Other adverse effects

Some people suffer from headaches, muscular aches, drowsiness, weakness, nausea and anorexia post ECT, but these are usually mild and respond to symptomatic treatments.[72] If a person experiences recurrent headaches after ECT, they may benefit from prophylactic treatment, e.g. with aspirin or a non-steroidal anti-inflammatory drug, immediately after ECT. Rarely, adverse psychological reactions to ECT develop, and may involve the person developing an intense fear of treatment.[73] Support and information is critical in preventing and managing this side-effect of treatment, and is, in any case, good practice.

Efficacy of ECT

It is useful to consider treatment response (short-term prognosis) and relapse and recurrence (longer-term prognosis) separately.

Treatment response (short term)

Van der Wurff et al.[74] reviewed the efficacy of ECT in depressed older adults, but found that of 121 studies only four provided randomised evidence. They identified 10 naturalistic prospective studies which gave immediate response rates to treatment ranging from 55% to 85%, and 14 retrospective studies, which gave immediate response rates varying from 48% complete recovery to 92% improvement. The authors concluded that results of naturalistic and retrospective studies show 'impressive response rates' for immediate treatment outcome, despite the fact that many of these older people treated with ECT had failed to respond to antidepressive drugs; they stressed, however, that this is based on non-randomised evidence.

Longer-term prognosis (relapse and recurrence)

Longer-term efficacy of ECT in older adults with depression is less well established. Older people with depressive illness have a shorter interval to recurrence after treatment of an index episode, and some authors argue that depression in older adults is equally responsive to initial treatments but has a poorer long-term course.[75] Van der Wurff and colleagues[74] were unable to draw conclusions about the longer-term efficacy of ECT. Huuhka et al.[76] reported a 43% rehospitalisation rate at 12 months. Flint and Gagnon,[14] in their review of naturalistic studies of the use of ECT in late-life depressive illness, concluded that 50% of patients or more will relapse within 6 to 12 months post ECT. The clinical implication of these findings is that more prolonged antidepressive treatment will be needed following a course of ECT and, in practice, combination treatments should be considered, e.g. use of a mood stabiliser in combination with an antidepressive drug, or pharmacological and psychological treatment combinations.

In an interesting paper, McCall et al.[77] recently reported that ECT is associated with improved health-related quality of life, both within a few days of completing a course of treatment and at 24 week follow-up, and argue that their findings support an association between ECT and net health benefit in depressed people whose illnesses remit.

Continuation treatment following ECT

The high relapse rate among older adults with depressive illness following a good short-term response highlights the need for ongoing treatment at the end of the course. This continuation treatment aims to prevent relapse in a group which can reasonably be regarded as at high risk of relapse. The optimal approach to continuation of treatment following ECT is open to debate (and awaits further research). It would be logical to approach individual treatment plans following ECT by considering the options for pharmacological, psychological and social treatments, bearing in mind past treatment history. Many clinicians would aim to change antidepressive drugs which an individual has not responded to prior to ECT to an alternative, or consider using a combination of treatments in people who have a history of repeated episodes of depressive illness.

The use of continuation ECT in the UK is controversial. NICE[6] stated that maintenance ECT is not recommended in depressive illness, on the grounds that they consider longer-term risks and benefits have not been established. The existing literature relies on case reports and naturalistic descriptions. Continuation ECT is used to prevent early relapse after an index episode of illness (commonly over the first six months of remission), and maintenance ECT is used to prevent further episodes.[78] The APA[15] recommended that ECT facilities should offer continuation ECT in the following circumstances:

* history of ECT responsive illness
* patient preference for ECT or resistance/intolerance of drug treatment
* the patient is able and willing to comply with the treatment plan.

In the *ECT Handbook*, Barnes[78] offers a sample protocol, but notes that there are no evidence-based guidelines for its use.

Developing treatments

Repetitive transcranial magnetic stimulation (rTMS)

rTMS is a treatment for depressive illness using subconvulsive stimuli to target specific regions of the brain which might be involved in depression and to spare areas likely to be involved in side-effects. It relies on pulses of electro-magnetic currents which are excitatory at high frequency (>5 Hz) and usually inhibitory at low frequency (1 Hz). Early studies were promising but the efficacy of rTMS is modest in treatment of depressive illness so far and only a small percentage of patients achieve remission with a high rate of early relapse. The role of rTMS in older adults with depressive illness is not yet established,[79,80] and one systematic review[81] concluded that the bulk of available evidence showed no effect on depressive symptoms in older adults. Work continues to develop rTMS, but it is not available in routine clinical practice in the UK.

Vagal nerve stimulation (VNS)

VNS is used in the treatment of intractable epilepsy, and involves surgical implantation of a stimulator attached to the vagal nerve. Adverse effects include hoarseness, throat pain and abnormal wound healing. It has been used for treatment-resistant unipolar and bipolar depressive illness,[82] but is still under development and definitive evidence of its efficacy is still lacking.[82,83]

Magnetic seizure therapy (MST)

MST uses transcranial magnetic stimulation to induce a seizure. In theory it should have advantages over ECT as it allows potentially greater control over the site and extent of stimulation. It has been suggested that it might be more acceptable to patients and have less effect on cognitive function, but it is still under development and a clinical role for MST remains to be established.[84]

The future?

New treatments are being developed which use non-convulsive stimuli or novel means of inducing a seizure, but their clinical roles are not yet established. Thus, despite the wide range of pharmacological agents available to treat affective illness in older adults, ECT continues to have an important role in psychiatric practice.

KEY POINTS

- ▸ The main indication for ECT in older adults is severe depressive illness but it is still used occasionally for severe/drug-resistant mania.
- ▸ Concurrent physical illness (especially cardiovascular or pulmonary) may increase the risk of complications during treatment.
- ▸ The adverse effect of ECT on cognitive function is of particular concern for older people.

▶ Immediate treatment response rates to ECT in older people are high but longer-term efficacy is less well established.

▶ Novel treatments under development do not currently offer alternatives to ECT in clinical practice.

REFERENCES

1 http://news.bbc.co.uk/2/hi/health/256487.stm. Accessed 20 September 2006.

2 http://news.bbc.co.uk/1/hi/health/3545684.stm. Accessed 20 September 2006.

3 Fink M. *Electroshock: restoring the mind.* New York: Oxford University Press; 1999.

4 Benbow SM. Old age psychiatrists views on the use of ECT. *Int J Geriatr Psychiatr.* 1991; **6**: 317–22.

5 Birkenhager TK, Renes J-W, Pluijms EM. One-year follow-up after successful ECT: a naturalistic study in depressed inpatients. *J Clin Psychiatr.* 2004; **65**: 87–91.

6 National Institute for Clinical Excellence. *Guidance on the use of electroconvulsive therapy. Technology Appraisal 59.* London: National Institute for Clinincal Excellence; 2003

7 National Institute for Clinical Excellence. *Management of depression in primary and secondary care. Clinical Guideline 23.* London: National Institute for Clinincal Excellence; 2004.

8 National Institute for Clinical Excellence. *The management of bipolar disorder in adults, children and adolescents in primary and secondary care. Clinical Guideline 38.* London: National Institute for Clinincal Excellence; 2006.

9 Beale MD, Kellner CH. ECT in treatment algorithms: no need to save the best for last. *J ECT.* 2000; **16**: 1–2.

10 Benbow SM. The use of ECT for older adults. In: Scott AIF, editor. *ECT Handbook.* 2nd ed. London: The Royal College of Psychiatrists; 2005. pp. 74–8.

11 Cobb A. *Older Women and ECT.* London: MIND; 1995.

12 Prudic J, Sackeim HA, Devanand DP. Medication resistance and clinical response to electroconvulsive therapy. *Psychiatr Res.* 1990; **31**: 287–96.

13 O'Connor MK, Knapp R, Husain M, *et al.* The influence of age on the response of major depression to electroconvulsive therapy; a CORE report. *Am J Geriatr Psychiatr.* 2001; **9**: 382–90.

14 Flint AJ, Gagnon N. Effective use of electroconvulsive therapy in late-life depression. *Can J Psychiatr.* 2002; **47**: 734–41.

15 American Psychiatric Association. *The Practice of Electroconvulsive Therapy: recommendations for treatment, training and privileging.* 2nd ed. Washington, DC: American Psychiatric Association; 2001.

16 Burke WJ, Rubin EH, Zorumski CF, *et al.* The safety of ECT in geriatric psychiatry. *J Am Geriatr Soc.* 1987; **35**: 516–21.

17 Takada JY, Da Luz PL, Giorgi DMA, *et al.* Assessment of the cardiovascular effects of electroconvulsive therapy in individuals older than 50 years. *Braz J Med Biol Res.* 2005; **38**: 1349–57.

18 Dolinski SY, Zvara DA. Anesthetic considerations of cardiovascular risk during electroconvulsive therapy. *Convuls Ther.* 1997; **13**: 157–64.

19 Abrams R. Electroconvulsive therapy in the medically compromised patient. *Psychiatr Clin Nth Am.* 1991; **14**: 871–85.

20 McCall WV. Asystole in electroconvulsive therapy: report of four cases. *J Clin Psychiatr.* 1996; **5**: 199–203.

21 Applegate RJ. Diagnosis and management of ischaemic heart disease in the patient scheduled to undergo electroconvulsive therapy. *Convuls Ther.* 1997; **13**: 128–44.

22 Zielinski RJ, Roose SP, Devanand DP, *et al.* Cardiovascular complications of ECT in depressed patients with cardiac disease. *Am J Psychiatr.* 1998; **150**: 904–9.

23 Dolinski SY, Zvara DA. Anesthetic considerations of cardiovascular risk during electroconvulsive therapy. *Convuls Ther.* 1997; 13: 157–64.

24 Magid M, Lapid MI, Sampson SM, *et al.* Use of electroconvulsive therapy in a patient 10 days after myocardial infarction. *J ECT.* 2005; **21**: 182–5.

25 Rasmussen KG. Electroconvulsive therapy in patients with aortic stenosis. *Convuls Ther.* 1997; **13**: 196–9.

26 Rayburn BK. Electroconvulsive therapy in patients with heart failure or valvular heart disease. *Convuls Ther.* 1997; **13**: 145–56.

27 Bailine SH, Sciano A, Millman B. ECT treatment of a patient with aortic aneurysms. *J ECT.* 2005; **21**: 178–79.

28 Gardner MW, Kellner CH, Hood DE, *et al.* Safe administration of ECT in a patient with a cardiac aneurysm and multiple cardiac risk factors. *Convuls Ther.* 1997; **13**: 200–3.

29 Mehta V, Mueller PS, Gonzalez-Arriaza HL, *et al.* Safety of electroconvulsive therapy in patients receiving long-term warfarin therapy. *Mayo Clin Proc.* 2004; **79**: 1396–401.

30 Dolenc TJ, Barnes RD, Hayes DL, *et al.* Electroconvulsive therapy in patients with cardiac pacemakers and implantable cardioverter defibrillators. *Pacing Clin Electrophysiol.* 2004; **27**: 1257–63.

31 Krystal AD, Coffey CE. Neuropsychiatric considerations in the use of electroconvulsive therapy. *J Neuropsychiatr Clin Neurosci.* 1997. **9**: 283–92.

32 Abrams R. Electroconvulsive therapy in the high-risk patient. In: Abrams R, editor. *Electroconvulsive Therapy.* 3rd ed. Oxford: Oxford University Press; 1997. pp. 81–113.

33 Bader GM, Silk KR, Dequardo JR, *et al.* Electroconvulsive therapy and intracranial aneurysm. *Convuls Ther.* 1995; **11**: 139–43.

34 Hsiao JK, Messenheimer JA, Evans DL. ECT and neurological disorders. *Convuls Ther.* 1987; **3**: 121–36.

35 Weintraub D, Lippmann SB. ECT for major depression and mania with advanced dementia. *J ECT.* 2001; **17**: 65–7.

36 Rao V, Lyketsos CG. The benefits and risks of ECT for patients with primary dementia who also suffer from depression. *Int J Geriatr Psychiatr.* 2000; **15**: 729–35.

37 Thuppal M, Fink M. Electroconvulsive therapy and mental retardation. *J ECT.* 1999; **15**: 140–9.

38 Aziz M, Maixner DF, Dequardo J, *et al.* ECT and mental retardation: a review and case reports. *J ECT.* 2001; **17**: 149–52.

39 Gustafson Y, Nilsson I, Mattsson M, *et al.* Epidemiology and treatment of post-stroke depression. *Drugs Aging.* 1995; **7**: 298–309.

40 Gursky JT, Rummans TA, Black JL. ECT administration in a patient after craniotomy and gamma knife surgery: a case report and review. *J ECT.* 2000; **16**: 295–9.

41 Coffey CE, Lucke J, Weiner RD, *et al.* Seizure threshold in electroconvulsive therapy. 1. Initial seizure threshold. *Biol Psychiatr.* 1995; **37**: 713–20.

42 Sackeim HA, Decina P, Prohovnik I, *et al.* Seizure threshold in electroconvulsive therapy: effects of sex, age, electrode placement, and number of treatments. *Arch Gen Psychiatr.* 1987; **44**: 355–60.

43 Boylan LS, Haskett RF, Mulsant BF, *et al.* Determinants of seizure threshold in ECT: benzodiazepine use, anesthetic dosage and other factors. *J ECT.* 2000; **16**: 3–18.

44 Scott AIF. Practical administration of ECT. In: Scott AIF, editor. *ECT Handbook.* 2nd ed. London: The Royal College of Psychiatrists; 2005. pp. 144–58.

45 Bowly CJ, Walker HAC. Anaesthesia for ECT. In: Scott AIF, editor. *ECT Handbook.* 2nd ed. London: The Royal College of Psychiatrists; 2005. pp. 124–35.

46 Benbow SM, Shah P, Crentsil J. Anaesthesia for electroconvulsive therapy: a role for etomidate. *Psychiatr Bull.* 2002; **26**: 351–3.

47 UK ECT Review Group. Efficacy and safety of electroconvulsive therapy in depressive disorders: a systematic review and meta-analysis. *Lancet.* 2003; **361**(9360): 799–808.

48 Little JD, Atkins MR, Munday J, *et al.* Bifrontal electroconvulsive therapy in the elderly: a 2-year retrospective. *J ECT.* 2004; **20**: 139–41.

49 Whitehouse AM. The use of ECT in the treatment of mania. In: Scott AIF, editor. *ECT Handbook.* 2nd ed. London: The Royal College of Psychiatrists; 2005. pp. 25–9.

50 Alexopoulos GS, Shamoian CJ, Lucas J, *et al.* Medical problems of geriatric psychiatric patients and younger controls during electroconvulsive therapy. *J Am Geriatr Soc.* 1984; **32**: 651–4.

51 Fraser RM, Glass IB. Recovery from ECT in elderly patients. *Br J Psychiatr.* 1978; **133**: 524–28.

52 Fraser RM, Glass IB. Unilateral and bilateral ECT in elderly patients: a comparative study. *Acta Psychiatr Scand.* 1980; **62**: 13–31.

53 Gaspar D, Samarasinghe LA. ECT in psychogeriatric practice: a study of risk factors, indications and outcome. *Comp Psychiatr.* 1982; **23**: 170–5.

54 Tomac TA, Rummans TA, Pileggi TS, *et al.* Safety and efficacy of electroconvulsive therapy in patients over age 85. *Am J Geriatr Psychiatr.* 1997; **5**: 126–30.

55 Sobin C, Sackeim HA, Prudic J, *et al.* Predictors of retrograde amnesia following ECT. *Am J Psychiatr.* 1995; **152**: 995–1001.

56 Benbow SM. Safe ECT practice in people with a physical illness. In: Scott AIF, editor. *ECT Handbook.* 2nd ed. London: The Royal College of Psychiatrists; 2005. pp. 68–73.

57 Zervas IM, Calev A, Jandorf L, *et al.* Age-dependent effects of electroconvulsive therapy on memory. *Convuls Ther.* 1993; **9**: 39–42.

58 Sackeim HA. The use of electroconvulsive therapy in late-life depression. In: Salzman C, editor. *Geriatric Psychopharmacology.* 3rd ed. Baltimore, MD: Williams and Wilkins; 1998. pp. 262–309.

59 Abrams R. The mortality rate with ECT. *Convuls Ther.* 1992; **13**: 125–7.

60 Weiner RD, Coffey CE, Krystal AD. Electroconvulsive therapy in the medical and neurologic patient. In: Stoudemire A, Fogel BS, Greenberg D, editors. *Psychiatric Care of the Medical Patient.* 2nd ed. New York: Oxford University Press; 2000. pp. 419–28.

61 Nuttall GA, Bowersox MR, Douglass SB, *et al.* Morbidity and mortality in the use of electroconvulsive therapy. *J ECT.* 2004; **20**: 237–41.

62 Finlayson AJ, Vieweg WV, Wiley WD, *et al.* Hyponatraemic seizure following ECT. *Can J Psychiatr.* 1989; **34**: 463–4.

63 Benbow SM, Benbow J, Tomenson B. Electroconvulsive therapy clinics in the United Kingdom should routinely monitor electro-encephalographic seizures. *J ECT.* 2003; **19**: 217–20.

64 Griesemer DA, Kellner CH, Beale MD, *et al.* Electroconvulsive therapy for treatment of intractable seizures: initial findings in two children. *Neurology.* 1997; **49**: 1389–92.

65 Sackeim HA. Acute cognitive side-effects of ECT. *Psychopharmacol Bull.* 1986; **22**: 482–4.

66 Devanand DP, Briscoe KM, Sackeim HA. Clinical features and predictors of post-ictal excitement. *Convuls Ther.* 1989; **5**: 140–6.

67 Coleman EA, Sackeim HA, Prudic J, *et al.* Subjective memory complaints before and after electroconvulsive therapy. *Biol Psychiatr.* 1996; **39**: 346–56.

68 Bosboom PR, Deijen JB. Age-related cognitive effects of ECT and ECT-induced mood improvement in depressive patients. *Depress Anxiety.* 2006; **23**: 93–101.

69 Weiner RD. Retrograde amnesia with electroconvulsive therapy: characteristics and implications. *Arch Gen Psychiatr.* 2000; **57**: 591–2.

70 Lisanby SH, Maddox JH, Prudic J, *et al.* The effects of electroconvulsive therapy on memory of autobiographical and public events. *Arch Gen Psychiatr.* 2000; **57**: 581–90.

71 Sackeim HA, Prudic J, Devanand DP, *et al.* A prospective, randomized, double-blind comparison of bilateral and right unilateral electroconvulsive therapy at different stimulus intensities. *Arch Gen Psychiatr.* 2000; **57**: 425–34.

72 Benbow SM, Crentsil J. Subjective experience of ECT. *Psych Bull.* 2004; **28**: 289–91.

73 Fox HA. Patients' fear of and objection to electroconvulsive therapy. *Hosp Community Psychiatry.* 1993; **44**: 357–60.

74 Van der Wurff FB, Stek ML, Hoogendijk WJG, *et al.* The efficacy and safety of ECT in depressed older adults: a literature review. *Int J Geriatr Psychiatr.* 2003; **18**: 894–904.

75 Mitchell AJ, Subramaniam H. Prognosis of depression in old age compared to middle age: a systematic review of comparative studies. *Am J Psychiatr.* 2005; **162**: 1588–601.

76 Huuhka M, Korpisammal L, Haataja R, *et al.* One-year outcome of elderly inpatients with major depressive disorder treated with ECT and antidepressants. *J ECT.* 2004; **20**: 179–85.

77 McCall WV, Prudic J, Olfson M, *et al.* Health-related quality of life following ECT in a large community sample. *J Affect Disord.* 2006; **90**: 269–74.

78 Barnes R. The use of ECT as a continuation or maintenance treatment. In: Scott AIF, editor. *ECT Handbook.* 2nd ed. London: The Royal College of Psychiatrists; 2005. pp. 79–81.

79 Gershon AA, Dannon PN, Grunhaus L. Transcranial magnetic stimulation in the treatment of depression. *Am J Psychiatr.* 2003; **160**: 835–45.

80 Mosimann UP, Schmitt W, Greenberg BD, *et al.* Repetitive transcranial magnetic stimulation: a putative add-on treatment for major depression in elderly patients. *Psychiatr Res.* 2004; **126**: 123–33.

81 Frazer CJ, Christensen H, Griffiths KM. Effectiveness of treatments for depression in older people. *Med J Aus.* 2005; **182**: 627–32.

82 Nemeroff CB, Mayberg HS, Krahl SE, *et al.* VNS therapy in treatment-resistant depression: clinical evidence and putative neurobiological mechanisms. *Neuropsychopharmacol.* 2006; **31**: 1345–55.

83 Rush AJ, Marangell LB, Sackeim HA, *et al.* Vagus nerve stimulation for treatment-resistant depression: a randomized, controlled acute phase trial. *Biol Psychiatr.* 2005; **58**: 347–54.

84 Lisanby SH. Update on magnetic seizure therapy: a novel form of convulsive therapy. *J ECT.* 2002; **18**: 182–88.

CHAPTER 7

Psychotherapy with older people

IAN ANDREW JAMES

Introduction

The literature on treating depression in older people informs us that they can not only benefit from psychotherapy,[1,2] but in some situations may show better outcomes than their younger counterparts.[3] The present chapter provides a brief review of the area, guiding the reader to texts that offer specific guidance on the use of psychotherapies with older people. Prior to discussing the different forms of psychotherapy from an evidence-based perspective, an overview of the nature of depression is presented, highlighting the difficulties faced by patients and therapists during treatment. A number of the evidence-based treatments are then described, followed by a review of the adaptations required to treat older people. In the final section, a case example is used to illustrate some therapeutic processes. The patient described in the case study was treated using interpersonal therapy (IPT); however, a cognitive behaviour therapy (CBT) framework is provided by way of contrast.

Nature of depression

The nature of depression may be conceptualised in terms of a number of domains. For the purposes of the present discussion, the focus will be on: neurotransmitters, brain localisation, information-processing biases, intrapsychic features, and interpersonal changes.

Neurotransmitters have been discussed in detail in other chapters within this book, as these are generally the targets of psychotropic medication. In contrast, less attention has been paid to the changes frequently found in brain functioning as observed by scanning techniques.[4] Of particular interest to therapists[5] are the changes occurring within the frontal lobes, leading to dys-executive symptoms as these have a direct influence on therapeutic processes. The frontal lobes, situated in the anterior of the brain, govern many high-level intellectual processes including problem-solving skills, conscious processing, and abilities to sustain and shift attention. Disruption to this area as a result of low affect may lead to a deterioration of these processes, but also to changes in personality (disinhibition, irritability, egocentricity, loss of insight); behaviour (loss of initiative) and emotions (lability, anxiety, frustration, anger).[6] Psychometric studies of people experiencing depression also reveal marked information-processing deficits. Some of these deficits can be related directly to frontal lobe dysfunction, but others, such as marked memory problems, demonstrate the more diffuse impact of depression.[7] In addition to these features, depression often leads to changes in people's self-image, their view of the world and of themselves. Such intrapsychic changes tend to be negatively biased, and the emerging perceptions tend not to be open to rational re-evaluation. Furthermore, depression typically interferes with people's abilities to maintain interpersonal networks, and those suffering from depression may often begin to avoid others or fail to find pleasure in other people's company.

TABLE 7.1 The experience of depression: features that need to be acknowledged during treatment

low mood	sleep disturbance
comorbid anxiety	concrete thinking
negative thinking	lack of motivation
hopelessness	memory biases
withdrawal/avoidance	negative information biases (catastrophising, magnifying)
low sense of worth	interpersonal difficulties
agitation	behavioural features (withdrawal)
poor concentration	
poor attention	
poor problem solving	
other executive problems	

The utility of conceptualising depression in terms of these different domains helps one to appreciate some of the experiences a person with depression is coping with when he/she comes for treatment. These experiences have been summarised in Table 7.1. Thus, from a therapist's perspective, it is important to appreciate that any therapy offered must take account of the executive and memory difficulties, the poor motivation, limited attentional capacity, biased thinking and interpersonal difficulties. In short, one must choose a therapeutic model that has the appropriate rationale, structure and process features to deal with the symptoms of depression.

Some of the potential therapies that could be offered are described in the following sections.

Therapeutic models

There are a host of different forms of therapy aimed at treating the affective disorders.[8] The effect-size of 0.78 for psychological interventions in relation to placebo or no intervention compares favourably with medication.[9] Indeed, a recent review of 89 controlled studies demonstrated that psychotherapy and pharmacotherapy were similarly effective for the treatment of depression in older people. Further, in less severe forms of presentation, psychotherapy may be more effective.[10] Figure 7.1 presents a genealogy of the psychotherapies; it does not attempt to detail the complexities within each of the schools. For example, psychoanalytic therapy is not differentiated into its main sub-schools: Freudian, Jungian, Kleinian or Adlerian. While most psychotherapies can trace their ancestry back to Freud,[11] many of them are now radically different in terms of theory and structure from the analytic framework. Some of the approaches have developed out of dissatisfaction with existing models; for example Beck, the originator of CBT, became unhappy with the psychoanalytic approach. Others have attempted to combine 'key' aspects of divergent models (e.g. cognitive analytic therapy[12]). Each approach has its own advocates. However, the National Institute for Health and Clinical Excellence[13] guidelines support the use of only a few of the psychotherapeutic treatments in relation to depression.

NICE advocate using a stepped-care approach for the treatment of depression, suggesting that the brief and simpler treatments should be offered prior to any of the more intensive and invasive approaches in cases of mild to moderate depression. Thus for mild to moderate depression, self-help programmes and problem-solving/brief therapies are suggested. For the more severe presentations, CBT and interpersonal therapy (IPT) are recommended, usually in conjunction with the appropriate pharmacological treatments. Psychodynamic therapy[14] is suggested for the complex comorbid conditions that may present along with the depression. The NICE guidelines, although criticised for omitting studies on older people,[15] are broadly in keeping with the conclusions of three systematic reviews conducted on the use of psychotherapies for older people.[2,16,17] The recommendations of these reviews are similar to those offered for 'working-aged' adults, apart from their greater emphasis on the potential benefits of reminiscence and life-review therapies[18] and family and group therapies.[19]

Nature of the different therapies

The various therapies target different aspects of depression in order to promote change. In Table 7.2, a number of evidence-based interventions are described for the treatment of depression in older people. Their inclusion is based on the guidance suggested by NICE,[35] and the reviews of effective treatments of older

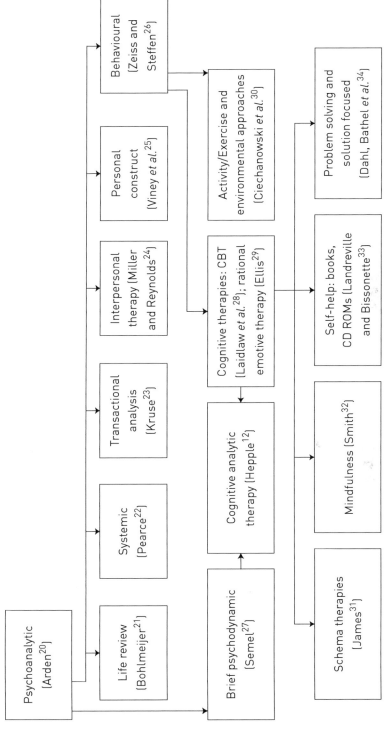

FIGURE 7.1 Family tree of common therapies with key references relevant to working with older people.

TABLE 7.2 Evidence-based psychotherapies for treating older people

Type of therapy	Mechanism of change	Suitability criteria and training	Evidence for older adults
CBT: The chaotic experience of depression is conceptualised, assessed and treated in terms of four interrelated features, aka the depressive cycle: depressogenic thoughts, behaviours, physical sensations and feelings. Particular attention is paid to the role of negative thinking and often to the core beliefs that underpin them. It is hypothesised that dysfunctional core beliefs are formed in childhood, and function as 'Achilles' heels' with respect to the adult, making her vulnerable to depression under the appropriate setting conditions.	The patient is socialised to the model. Once having developed an understanding of the depression in terms of the cycle, the patient is helped to re-evaluate her thoughts and dysfunctional belief systems. Behavioural and educational programmes are used to both disrupt problematic actions and facilitate new learning.	Suitability: Safran and Segal[37] provided empirical evidence for 10 suitability factors (e.g. ability to access thoughts, emotions, acceptability of the model, adherence in session, homework compliance, etc.) Training: There are a large number of courses around the UK. The 'gold standard' courses are typically nine months long, part-time diploma/MSc programmes. The trainees receive weekly supervision and teaching.	1,2,3,4,5* A large no. of quality studies, conducted by a number of different research groups.
IPT: People are social beings, and disruptions to people's social networks can both trigger and maintain depression. This model conceptualises the onset of depression in terms of losses, resulting from one of four sources: grief (death), life transitions, disputes, social skills deficits. The approach attempts to re-establish good social skills and networking that may have triggered and/or become disrupted as a result of the depression.	The onset of the depression is identified, and the subsequent changes to the patient's interpersonal network are assessed. The impact of the changes are acknowledged and 'mourned' where appropriate. Problem-solving techniques are then employed to re-establish or create a fulfilling and worth-enhancing social life.	Suitability: No specific suitability criteria set. Originally designed specifically for unipolar depression, although currently used for a wider range of affective disorders. Training: Initial training involves a three to four-day teaching programme, followed by a term of structured supervised work that provides 'Practitioner' status.	1,2,3,4,5* Moderate evidence, but little support for use as a stand-alone therapy.

Type of therapy	Mechanism of change	Suitability criteria and training	Evidence for older adults
Self-help: Self-help programmes are based on 'written materials' (books leaflets), audio- or video-taped material or computer programs designed to meet therapeutic needs. The programmes can be supported by either face-to-face or 'phone contact with a therapist, and may be delivered on an individual or group basis. The latter versions are usually termed 'guided self-help' programmes.[38]	These are usually based on CBT principles and include guidance on CBT change techniques.[39]	Suitability: NICE guidelines recommend its use for mild to moderate depressive disorders. Training: None specified, although specific packages are named, e.g. NICE support use of 'Beating the Blues' computer package.	2,4* Relatively little evidence in the older people area.
Psychoanalysis: Early negative experiences retard emotional development, resulting in the expression of immature impulses and desires. This produces conflicts between reality and the patient's ideals and standards. The resulting tensions, feelings of helplessness and depression invoke protective mechanisms (e.g. repression, projection, reaction formation). These protective mechanisms themselves tend to become dysfunctional, interfering with the person's decision making abilities. Hence, the patient may perceive himself as acting maturely, although the emotional processing of the situation is that of a child.	The aim of every session is to put the patient in touch with as much of his true feelings as he can bear.[40] This is done by careful inspection of the patient's past, promoting insight regarding the manner in which impulses and desires are impacting on attitudes, actions, goals and relationships. Main goal is to increase awareness and insight into the unconscious processes leading an individual to repeat past experiences and to institute corrective experiences through the interaction between client and therapist.[41]	Suitability: Thus the therapist needs to judge: i. The degree to which the patient is already in touch with his true feelings; ii. The nature of the hidden feelings of which he is not aware; iii. How close these feelings are to the surface; iv. The degree of anxiety with which they are invested; v. The patient's capacity to bear it.[42] It is recommended for trauma, grief and adjustment disorders.[43] Training: Due to the interpersonal stance of the therapist, it is necessary to undertake specialist training which usually involves personal psychoanalysis and the supervised treatment of a number of patients.	1,2,4* Evidence in terms of brief analytic form of the therapy. A small number of studies, conducted mainly by one group of researchers.

(Continued)

Type of therapy	Mechanism of change	Suitability criteria and training	Evidence for older adults
Psychoanalysis [continued] The evidence base mainly comes from brief psychoanalytic therapy (BDT) trials. BDT is generally limited to 15–20 sessions.			
Life review therapy: Sometimes referred to as reminiscence therapy, involves undertaking a structured evaluative approach of a patient's history. However, caution is needed as meta-analytic studies have failed to identify a unitary approach.[21]	Mechanisms are unclear; however, life review often emphasises the need for past evaluation, with resolution of past conflicts. Knight[44] suggests some similarities with grief work.	Suitability: Developmentally appropriate for older people with and without dementia. Training: Regular workshops from various sources throughout country.	1,2,4,5* A small number of studies, requiring replication.

*1 Randomised trials; 2 Comparisons with other therapies/placebo/wait-lists; 3 Comparisons with antidepressants; 4 Use as stand-alone therapy; 5 Use with people with dementia people provided by Scogin *et al.*[17] and Mackin and Arean.[16] As one can see, the mechanisms of change differ markedly between the various methods, ranging from re-evaluating thoughts to problem solving and promoting insight. Even so, they have all been shown to be effective in the treatment of geriatric depression. Of note, when the psychotherapeutic treatments have been compared head to head, there is often little evidence to suggest that any one is better than the other.[36] Some clinicians have suggested that such equivalence reflects the important role of 'therapeutic alliance' as being the primary mechanism of change; its role may be more relevant when working with older people.[28] Despite this notion of equivalence, it is important to stress that the quality of evidence regarding treatment effectiveness with respect to older people is poor, with only CBT interventions having been assessed thoroughly.

Adaptations for older adults

A number of texts have been written on how to adapt therapy for older people.[2,45,46] Such guides generally suggest the use of a slower-paced approach, shorter sessions, a more concrete communication style, and repeated presentation of key materials/concepts. They often also suggest that one should employ strategies to support people's sensory impairments and memory deficits (tape recordings, bibliotherapy, cue cards and pictures), and encourage the assistance of families and advocates in the treatment programmes.[47] Laidlaw *et al.*[28] stress the importance of spending time socialising the patient into the therapeutic model, and consider it helpful initially to use an educative approach. It is relevant to note, however, that based on the depression-related deficits outlined in Table 7.1, the adaptations just described for older people seem appropriate for the treatment of anyone suffering with depression.[28] To reinforce this issue, presented below are a list of strategies written for a general text on depression.[5] As one will see, there is much overlap with these adaptations previously suggested for working with older people.

The following therapeutic strategies were developed to deal with the deficits outlined in Table 7.1.

Poor concentration – Reduce complexity of therapeutic material, shorten sessions, only cover a few topics within a session, use frequent feedback. Frequently check patient's understanding of the material covered, and pace session according to patient's needs. Use therapeutic breaks within session.

Poor attention – Provide feedback frequently and summarise and chunk relevant information. Elicit feedback. Use simple diagrams and use written materials to reinforce concepts, but avoid being abstract. Remove any environmental distractors (e.g. may need to close windows to prevent extraneous noises).

Poor memory – Prevent overloading of the patient's short-term memory. Ensure that information is provided in a paced manner. Repeat main therapeutic concept frequently to help consolidate material and facilitate encoding. Avoid blaming the patient for an inability to recall either positive events or coping strategies from the past, as such difficulties are a feature of their executive problems.

Poor problem solving – Reduce problems into component parts in order to simplify tasks. Patients may need a great deal of guidance until they can engage in a more collaborative approach. Use behavioural experiments to re-energise problem-solving skills. The experiments need to be set up sensitively, so even if the patient is unable to carry out activities, he/she will learn something about his/her depression from having attempted to engage in them. Keep tasks simple; it is important that therapists acknowledge their roles in the therapeutic problems (e.g. 'The reason you had difficulties was because I didn't explain last week's homework task well').

Case illustration

The next section provides a case study of a man suffering from late-onset depression who was treated using IPT.[48] The IPT formulation is presented alongside a CBT framework in order to highlight the differences in the conceptualisations. These two models have been selected owing to current levels of evidence supporting their use.[49]

CASE HISTORY 7.1

Background to the case: Mr M, a 71-year-old widower, had a seven-month history of depression and 18-month history of mild-moderate cognitive difficulties resulting from a cerebrovascular accident. On initial psychometric assessment, Mr M scored in the moderate to severe depression ranges on both the Beck Depression Inventory[50] and the Hopelessness Scale.[51] He also showed deficits in memory and on tests requiring sustained attention and concentration. Initially, he attended the hospital's Elderly Day Unit (EDU) for a full assessment and to provide social contact. Unfortunately, he found it difficult to settle, stating that he preferred the company of 'real blokes' – men who could talk about football. In a discussion with his family, his daughter said that he was very lonely and was desperate to meet 'like-minded' people. His daughter, with her two teenagers, had tried to help lift the loneliness by cohabiting with her father. Unfortunately, this had resulted in major intergenerational conflicts.

Prior to the present difficulties Mr M had been a market trader, travelling all over the North East of England with his stall. He was forced to retire at the age of 70, when his family recognised his memory difficulties. He was a widower of 10 years' standing, with two sons and two daughters. His sons were former employees of their father in the family business. They had recently taken over his stalls and expanded his business. He had a history of heavy alcohol use, although a stomach disorder had curtailed his drinking. This abstinence was problematic, however, as his social life was centred around the local pub. It is noteworthy that he was not prepared to go to the pub and drink non-alcoholic beverages.

Owing to his good level of insight, it was decided to engage him in therapy. Mr M's difficulties can readily be formulated within a CBT model (*see* Figure 7.2); such a framework is presented below.

CBT perspective

Figure 7.2 represents Mr M's CBT conceptualisation. The background features (i.e. personality, history, etc.) provide a context to his current mood state. His interpretation and reaction to the trigger (his son's visit) was influenced by his biased style of thinking – and this was affected by the degree of impairment resulting from both his vascular problems and affective states (*see* Table 7.1). Owing to his problem-solving difficulties, his ability to effectively deal with the triggering situation was lessened. Indeed, in the current situation he was unable to think of his son's visit in a balanced way; he interpreted the event as the son feeling sorry for him and used this as further confirmation of his own uselessness. Thus, Mr M's sense of self-efficacy was reduced, leading him to feel depressed and consequently causing him to withdraw even more. The latter feature is compounded by the fact that he thinks that he is not going to meet any 'like-minded' people, and so he thinks that there is no point in attempting to socialise.

Based on the above formulation, an integrated set of cognitive and behavioural strategies would need to be developed for Mr M in order to promote his sense of worth. For example, the CBT work would typically attempt to (1) educate him about the thinking biases maintaining his depression, (2) increase the flexibility of his thinking, which at present is rigid and inflexible, (3) help him to accept the changes in his life (e.g. de-couple his association between worth and work), and (4) assist him to develop some new goals and mechanisms by which to obtain a sense of worth (e.g. develop his growing interest in computers; renew his interest in snooker, a game he had previously excelled at). The behavioural work would encourage him to start interacting with others. In the actual case, when one examined his interests more widely, it was evident that he liked gardening; a topic that he was prepared to speak about with others – even women. The behavioural work would also try to motivate him to re-establish his visits to the local pub. Such work would clearly require him to re-evaluate his current inflexible view: '*If you can't drink ale, you can't go to the pub*'.

The next section examines the utility of the IPT conceptual framework for Mr M.

Interpersonal therapy (IPT) perspective

In IPT, depression is viewed as a medical illness. The patient is recommended to take up the 'sick role', providing him with allowances such as relief from certain obligations (e.g. looking after the grandchildren), but also expecting him to participate actively in therapy and work towards recovery. Attempts are also made to link the depressed feelings to the patient's interpersonal context.[52] In the case of

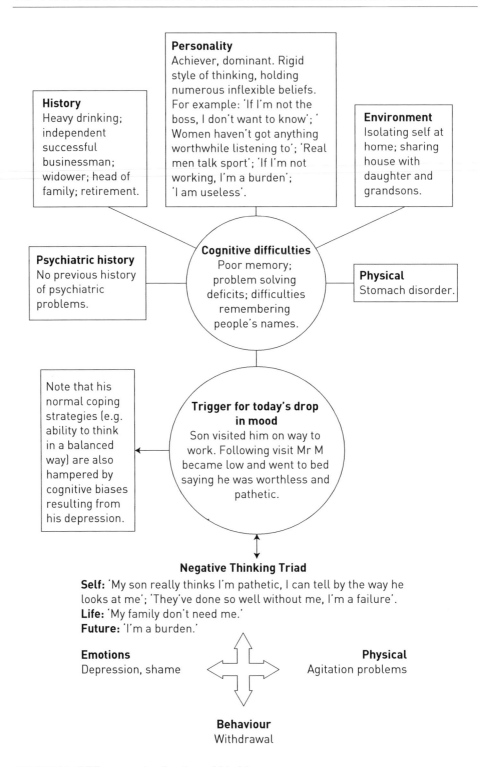

FIGURE 7.2 CBT conceptualisation of Mr M.

Mr M, the first step was to identify a 'focus' or key domain (i.e. the domain most strongly associated with the *start* of the depression). In IPT there are four potential domains: transitions, grief (death), interpersonal conflict, interpersonal deficits. A description of the material relevant to each domain is described below.

Transitions: Mr M was experiencing difficulties in both accepting retirement and coping with the new living arrangements. In addition, his decision to stop drinking alcohol had removed his main form of socialising. Note that he had not become depressed after becoming aware of his memory difficulties, suggesting this was not key to the onset of the depression. On balance, the transition that seemed to be the most strongly associated with the start of the depression was the retirement. As a consequence of this transition, Mr M had experienced a series of losses: the structure provided by his work; his status within the family; social contacts at work and in the pub.

Grief: Mr M had not recently experienced any actual deaths that could explain this depressive episode.

Interpersonal conflict: Some conflicts had developed at home between him, his daughter and her family. However, as the depression preceded the cohabitation, it was not considered a focus area.

Interpersonal deficits: Mr M had a rigid and domineering style, but, despite this, he had been able to make and maintain friendships prior to his depression. So this was not regarded as a key domain. However, it is relevant to note that owing to his memory problems, Mr M had lost some confidence in his ability to communicate effectively.

As one can see there is a great deal of inter-domain overlap. However, in IPT, a single domain is usually agreed upon as being central to the depression. Once having established a main conceptual focus, a framework is developed (*see* Figure 7.3), which forms the basis of the interventions.

When focusing on transitional difficulties, the main goals of therapy are typically: the mourning of the loss(es) of the old role; helping the patient to see the new role as positive, and trying to restore self-esteem within the demands of the new role.[53] In the case of Mr M, who was actually treated using IPT, a treatment plan was collaboratively set with the help of the family. The first treatment strategy was an attempt to resolve the interpersonal losses that he had experienced since retiring. Mr M's family agreed to meet regularly at the house, or pub, and consult him about work and family matters. It was stressed that it was important that his sons visited, and demonstrated that they respected their father's views. The family also contacted some of his old friends, who had also retired, and found that they had started to spend some of their time at the local social club. Indeed, it transpired that two of his mates went to play snooker at the club. The first target was therefore to encourage him to attend this club. A further goal was to resolve the difficulties with the living arrangements. After a number of unsuccessful strategies had been abandoned, the most effective solution to the dilemma was to designate certain areas of the house as 'no-go' zones for the grandchildren.

Pre-morbid
Active lifestyle; meeting many people through work.
A dominant individual, successful businessman, head of family.
Socialising by drinking alcohol with people in the pub.
Rigid thinker, and often inflexible in his attitudes.

Ongoing decline in health and cognitive status
(memory problems, sensitivity to alcohol).

Transition
Retirement

Consequence
No longer meeting people.
Collapse of his interpersonal network associated with work.
Loss of status within family.
Social withdrawal and avoidance.

Feelings
Depressed, hopeless, bored, apathetic, shameful.

Other important factors occurring as a consequence of depression
- Daughter moved in, and major difficulties occurring with grandchildren.
  - Sons busy building business, and rarely visit their father.

> It is relevant to note that although the memory difficulty was an important feature, it was regarded as a contextual issue in terms of Mr M's low mood. The actual trigger to the depression was his retirement, and the associated interpersonal consequences.

FIGURE 7.3 IPT conceptualisation for Mr M.

It is relevant to note that the type of interventions used with Mr M would be wholly in keeping with a CBT approach. Indeed, one could argue that any good CBT treatment programme would have addressed the interpersonal issues discussed above. However, it would be incorrect to label the present work as CBT, owing to the fact that the patient was not socialised to the cognitive framework, and the treatment was not underpinned by the cognitive rationale.

In the present case, IPT was the treatment of choice based on the following four reasons.
1 He scored poorly on the Safran and Segal[37] CBT suitability scale – issues of rigidity and acceptance of the cognitive rationale were problematic.
2 IPT provided a better way of representing his interpersonal difficulties. For

example, it highlighted the conflicts associated with him both wanting and rejecting company, and the family problems to do with his grandchildren.

3   He seemed to display a high level of insight into his interpersonal problems. Indeed, despite his memory difficulties and problems generalising material from session to session, Mr M was aware that part of his difficulty was his reluctance to re-engage in social activities. Hence, while he sometimes struggled to recall the specifics of what had been talked about in the previous sessions, due to the fact that the focus was always interpersonal, he could quickly reorient himself. To this end, he did not need to be socialised into a new way of understanding his dilemma; he already had good insight in this respect. Hence, the focus of treatment could quickly move to increasing his social support, rather than helping him to understand why he felt so bad.

4   IPT was also used because it is a relatively simple model compared to CBT. As mentioned earlier, a good CBT formulation is likely to incorporate many, although not all, of the aspects identified in IPT. However, in some situations the simpler approach offered by IPT is an advantage. Despite this, one must be a little cautious about professing IPT's general utility, as an analysis of the two approaches suggests that many of the effective ingredients of IPT are cognitive-behavioural in nature.[54] Albon and Jones's study suggested that although the foci between CBT and IPT were clearly different, the nature of the interactions between the therapist and patient within the therapy may be very similar.[54]

The case example illustrates the use of CBT and IPT, but clearly other forms of psychotherapy could have been employed, each formulating the case in a different manner. For those interested in comparing and contrasting formulation models used with older people, a number of texts now exist in the area.[55,56] The case also illustrates that the interventions developed for older adults are rather similar to those used with other patient populations.

Conclusion

This chapter has examined the evidence-based therapies used for treating depression in older people. From the findings of a number of critical reviews, it is clear that psychotherapy can be effective. Research also informs us that it is both valued by older adults[57] and often preferred to antidepressants.[58,59] Despite such a positive perspective, it is evident that more controlled trials are needed to test the efficacy of the treatments, and particularly their long-term impacts. A limitation of this chapter, and of the topic area in general, has been the lack of attention paid to the more complex presentations. For example, bipolar depression has not been discussed. It is relevant to note, however, there is a growing psychotherapeutic literature on this topic[60] providing patients with education, monitoring techniques and relapse prevention strategies. However, as yet there is relatively little evidence that much can be done psychotherapeutically during the acute phase of the illness. In addition, this chapter has not addressed depression associated with comorbid conditions, including dementia[47,61] and physical health problems (diabetes, heart disease, asthma, arthritis).[62] It is also relevant to note that most of the studies outlined in this review have been conducted within academic settings, which raises questions to their applicability to clinical contexts. It follows that more research is required in relevant field settings.

On a systemic level, more work is needed to educate patients, the public and health professionals about depression in old age. Despite some people's perspectives, depression is not a natural consequence of becoming 'old'. In addition to improving people's knowledge bases, increased efforts are needed to remove some of the barriers to treatment. For example, in many situations basic practical difficulties should be addressed, including improving transportation and making better use of outreach programmes. Furthermore, there is clearly a need to target specific groups who are currently under-represented in our clinics. As such, strategies need to be implemented regarding some of the cultural issues and communication difficulties that may facilitate the greater use of psychotherapeutic services.

KEY POINTS

▶ The psychotherapies are effective at improving depression in older people.
▶ Recent evidence suggests that psychotherapy is as effective as pharmacotherapy in the treatment of depression, and may be more effective in the treatment of mild unipolar depression.
▶ The NICE unipolar depression guidelines favour cognitive behaviour therapy and interpersonal therapy for the treatment of mild to moderate presentations, but the guidelines do not provide detailed guidance for older people.
▶ There is a dearth of good quality, rigorous studies in the area.

REFERENCES

1 Hartman-Stein P. An impressive step in identifying evidence-based psychotherapies for geriatric depression. *Clin Psychol Sci and Pract.* 2005; **12**(3): 238–41.
2 Zalaquett CP, Stens A. Psychosocial treatments for major depression and dysthymia in older adults: a review of the research literature. *J Couns Dev.* 2006; **84**(2): 192–201.
3 Walker DA, Clarke M. Cognitive behavioural psychotherapy: a comparison between younger and older adults in two inner city mental health teams. *Aging Ment Health.* 2001; **5**(2): 197–9.
4 Drevets WC, Raichle ME. *Positron Emission Tomographic Imaging Studies of Human Emotional Disorders.* Cambridge, MA: MIT Press; 1995.
5 James IA, Reichelt FK, Carlsonn-Mitchell P, *et al.* Executive functioning in depression. *J Cogn Psychother.* In press. (Also available from Centre for the Health of the Elderly, Newcastle General Hospital, Westgate Rd, Newcastle upon Tyne, NE4 6BE, UK.)
6 Gazzaniga MS, Ivry RB, Mangun GR. *Cognitive Neuroscience: the biology of the mind.* New York; London: Norton; 2002.
7 Cassens G, Wolfe L, Zola M. The neuropsychology of depressions. *J Neuropsychiatr Clin Neurosci.* 1990; **2**(2): 202–13.

8   Murphy F. Provision of psychotherapy services for older people. *Psychiatr Bull.* 2000; **24**: 184–7.

9   Scogin F, McElreath L. Efficacy of psychosocial treatments for geriatric depression: a quantitative review. *J Consult Clin Psychol.* 1994; **62**: 69–74.

10 Pinquart M, Duberstein PR, Lyness JM. Treatments for later-life depressive conditions: a meta-analytic comparison of pharmacotherapy and psychotherapy. *Am J Psychiatr.* 2000; **163**: 1493–1501.

11 Freud S. On psychotherapy. In: Strachey J (trans). *The Complete Psychological Works of Sigmund Freud, Vol. 6.* London: Hogarth; 1953.

12 Hepple J. Cognitive analytic therapy. In: Hepple J, Pearce J, Wilkinson P, editors. *Psychological Therapies with Older People.* London: Brunner-Routledge; 2002.

13 National Institute for Clinical Excellence. *Depression: management of depression in primary and secondary care. Clinical Guideline 23.* London: National Institute for Clinical Excellence; 2004. Available from: http://www.nice.org.uk/CG023

14 Garner J. Psychodynamic work with older people. *Adv Psychiatr Treat.* 2002; **8**: 128–37.

15 Malone D, Mitchell AJ. *NICE Guidelines for Depression 2004: gaps in the evidence.* 2007. Available at: http://bmj.com/cgi/eletters/330/7486/267

16 Mackin RS, Arean PA. Evidence-based psychotherapeutic interventions for geriatric depression. *Psychiatr Clin Nth Am.* 2005; **28**: 805–20.

17 Scogin F, Welsh D, Hamson A, *et al.* Evidence based psychotherapies for depression in older adults. *Clin Psychol Sci Pract.* 2005; **12**: 222–37.

18 Gatz M, Fiske A, Fox L, *et al.* Empirically validated psychological treatments for older adults. *J Ment Health Aging.* 1998; **4**: 9–46.

19 Qualls SH. Family therapy with older clients. *J Clin Psychol.* 1999; **55**: 977–90.

20 Arden M. Psychodynamic therapy. In: Hepple J, Pearce J, Wilkinson P, editors. *Psychological Therapies with Older People.* London: Brunner-Routledge; 2002.

21 Bohlmeijer E, Smit F, Cuipers P. Effects of reminiscence and life review on late-life depression: a meta-analysis. *Int J Geriatr Psychiatr.* 2003; **18**: 1088–94.

22 Pearce J. Systemic therapy. In: Hepple J, Pearce J, Wilkinson P, editors. *Psychological Therapies with Older People.* London: Brunner-Routledge; 2002.

23 Kruse TL. Transactional analysis and the elderly: teaching TA in a senior center. *Trans Anal J.* 1985; **15**(2): 146–51.

24 Miller M, Reynolds CF. Interpersonal psychotherapy. In: Hepple J, Pearce J, Wilkinson P, editors. *Psychological Therapies with Older People.* London: Brunner-Routledge; 2002.

25 Viney L, Benjamin Y, Preston C. An evaluation of personal construct therapy for the elderly. *Br J Med Psychol.* 1989; **62**: 35–41.

26 Zeiss A, Steffen A. Behavioural and cognitive-behavioural treatments: an overview of social learning. In: Zarit S, Knight B, editors. *A Guide to Psychotherapy and Aging.* Washington, DC: American Psychological Association; 1996.

27 Semel VG. Modern psychoanalytic treatment of the older patient. In: Zarit S, Knight B, editors. *A Guide to Psychotherapy and Aging.* Washington, DC: American Psychological Association; 1996.

28 Laidlaw K, Thompson L, Dick-Siskin L, *et al. Cognitive Therapy with Older People.* Chichester John: Wiley; 2003.

29 Ellis A. Rational emotive therapy and cognitive behaviour therapy for elderly people. *J Rational-emotive Cog Behav Ther.* 1999; **17**(1): 5–18.

30 Ciechanowski P, Wagner E, Schmaling K, *et al.* Community-integrated home-based depression treatment in older adults: a randomised controlled trial. *J Am Med Assoc.* 2004; **29**(13): 1569–77.

31 James IA. Older people's perspectives: implications for Schema Theory. *Clin Psychol and Psychother.* 2003; **10**: 133–43.

32 Smith A. Clinical uses of mindfulness training in older people. *Behav Cog Psychother.* 2004; **32**(4): 385–8.

33 Landreville P, Bissonette L. Effects of cognitive bibliotherapy for depressed older adults with a disability. *Clin Gerontol.* 1997; **17**: 35–55.

34 Dahl R, Bathel D, Carreon C. The use of solution-focused therapy with an elderly population. *J System Ther.* 2000; **19**(4): 45–55.

35 National Institute for Clinical Excellence. *Computerised Cognitive Behaviour Therapy for Depression and Anxiety (Review). Technology Appraisal 97.* London: National Institute for Clinical Excellence; 2006. Available from: http://www.nice.org.uk/CG023

36 Davies C, Collerton D. Psychological therapies for depression with older adults: a qualitative review. *J Ment Health.* 1997; **6**(4): 335–44.

37 Safran JD, Segal ZV. *Interpersonal Processes in Cognitive Therapy.* New York: Basic Books; 1990.

38 Scogin F, Jamison C, Gochneaur K. Comparative efficacy of cognitive and behavioural bibliotherapy for mildly and moderately depressed older adults. *J Consult Clin Psychol.* 1989; **57**: 403–7.

39 Cuipers P. Bibliotherapy in unipolar depression: a meta-analysis. *J Behav Ther Exp Psychiatr.* 1997; **28**: 139–47.

40 Malan DH. *Individual Psychotherapy and the Science of Psychodynamics.* London: Butterworths; 1979.

41 Nordhus IH, Nielsen GH. Brief dynamic psychotherapy with older adults. *J Clin Psychiatr.* 1999; **55**: 935–47.

42 Clare AW. Interpretative psychotherapies. In: Kendell RE, Zealley A, editors. *Companion to Psychiatric Studies.* 5th ed. Edinburgh: Churchill Livingstone; 1993.

43 Kennedy GJ, Tanenbaum S. Psychotherapy with older adults. *Am J Psychother.* 2000; **54**: 386–407.

44 Knight B. Overview of psychotherapy with the elderly: the contextual, cohort-based, maturity-specific-challenge model. In: Zarit S, Knight B, editors. *A Guide to Psychotherapy and Aging.* Washington, DC: American Psychological Association; 1996.

45 Dick L, Gallacher-Thompson D, Thompson L. Cognitive-behavioural therapy. In: Woods RT, editor. *Handbook of the Clinical Psychology of Ageing.* Chichester: Wiley and Sons; 1996.

46 Glantz M. Cognitive therapy with the elderly. In: Freeman A, Simon K, Beutler L, *et al.,* editors. *Comprehensive Handbook of Cognitive Therapy.* New York: Plenum Press; 1989.

47 Teri L, Gallagher-Thompson D. Cognitive-behavioural interventions for treatment of depression in Alzheimer's patients. *Gerontologist.* 1991; **31**(3): 413–16.

48 James IA, Postma K, Mackenzie L. Using and IPT conceptualisation to treat a depressed person with dementia. *Behav Cog Psychother.* 2003; **13**(4): 451–6.

49 Hepple J, Wilkinson P, Pearce J. Psychological therapies with older people. In: Hepple J, Pearce J, Wilkinson P, editors. *Psychological Therapies with Older People.* London: Brunner-Routledge; 2002.

50 Beck AT, Ward CH, Mendelson M, *et al.* An inventory for measuring depression. *Arch Gen Psychiatr.* 1961; **4**: 561–71.

51 Beck AT, Weissman A, Lester D, *et al.* The measurement of pessimism: the hopelessness scale. *J Consult Clin Psychol.* 1974; **42**(6): 861–5.

52 Hinrichsen GA, Clougherty KF. *Interpersonal Psychotherapy for Older Adults.* Washington, DC: American Psychological Association; 2006.

53 Weissman MM, Markowitz JC, Klerman G, *et al. Comprehensive Guide to Interpersonal Psychotherapy.* New York: Basic Books; 2000.

54 Albon JS, Jones EE. Validity of controlled clinical trials of psychotherapy: findings from the NIMH treatment of depression collaborative research program. *Am J Psychiatr.* 2002; **159**(5): 775–83.

55 Hepple J, Wilkinson P, Pearce J. *Psychological Therapies with Older People.* London: Brunner-Routledge; 2002.

56 Zarit S, Knight B. *A Guide to Psychotherapy and Aging.* Washington, DC: American Psychological Association; 1996.

57 Landreville P, Landry J, Baillargeon L, *et al.* Older adults' acceptance of psychological and pharmacological treatments for depression. *J Geront B Psychol Sci Soc Sci.* 2001; **56**(5): 285–91.

58 Unutzer J, Katon W, Callahan CM, *et al.* Collaborative care management of late-life depression in the primary care setting: a randomised controlled trial. *JAMA.* 2003; **28**(22): 2836–45.

59 Rokke P, Scogin F. Depression treatment preferences in younger and older adults. *J Clin Geropsychol.* 1995; **1**: 243–57.

60 Scott J. *Overcoming Mood Swings: a self-help guide using cognitive behavioural techniques.* London: Robinson; 2001.

61 James IA. Using a cognitive rationale to conceptualize anxiety in people with dementia. *Behav Cog Psychother.* 1999; **27**: 345–51.

62 Robinson P. Implementing a primary care depression clinical pathway. In: Cummings NA, O'Donohue WT, Ferguson KE, editors. *Behavioural Health as Primary Care: beyond efficacy to effectiveness.* Reno, NV: Context Press; 2003. pp. 69–94.

CHAPTER 8

Depression in physically ill older patients

GRAHAM MULLEY

Introduction

Depression is the commonest mental illness in old age. In 2001–02, there were 9.8 million visits by older people to office-based physicians in the USA for depression.[1] In the UK, one in six older medical inpatients are depressed (Geriatric Depression Score – GDS – of 7 or more out of 15).[2] The mean prevalence in over sixty-fives living at home is about 12%. In the UK, the National Service Framework (Standard 7) for Older People recognised that 10–15% of people over 65 have depression. It recommended that primary care trusts should ensure that every general practice uses an agreed protocol to diagnose, treat and care for patients with depression.

Although there are few community studies large enough to tell us the precise incidence in old age, it is apparent that the incidence differs markedly in different cities and countries. High rates of depression are found in Amsterdam, Berlin, London, Munich and Verona. Lower rates occur in Dublin, Liverpool, Iceland and Zaragoza.[3] Depression is commoner in women and Asians, and less prevalent in those with a sense of spirituality. It does not increase in prevalence with age, though its severity and associated suicide risk may worsen with advancing years.

The causes are heterogeneous: there are probably interactions between susceptibility (gene products) and a precipitant (in the external environment).[4] Social factors such as loss of status, wealth, intimacy and life opportunities can be important. There may also be developmental, psychological and biological factors. It can be difficult to recognise the disease, particularly if the patient has medical comorbidity. The biological signposts to the disease are less helpful than in younger, healthier people: disturbances of sleep, appetite, weight, libido, and bowel motility can have a variety of physical causes. The non-biological features are therefore usually more helpful: low mood, lethargy, anxiety, irritability, hypochondriasis, regression, crying and pessimism. Geriatricians miss the diagnosis in a half of patients admitted to an acute geriatric unit (in one study, the consultant in old age psychiatry diagnosed depression in 67 out of 155 consecutive admissions, the geriatrician 29 of them).[5]

There is no sharp demarcation between a 'case' and a 'non-case'. Depression is a continuum, ranging from feeling sad to experiencing major depression. The word 'depression' is used for the understandable demoralisation in the face of adversity; grief; persistently negative thoughts and the full-blown clinical syndrome of depression.

Depression can be reversed by treatment (though some cases of severe depression do not always respond so well). However, many people with the disease may receive no treatment. In others, the therapy may be delayed and adherence to the drug regimen may be poor.

The effects of depression are legion: it can cause disability and handicap; increase mortality, exacerbate coexisting illnesses, place a burden on the family and causes much unnecessary suffering. It has a huge healthcare cost, with readmissions to hospital, prolonged lengths of stay and an overuse of services.

In this chapter, I will focus on loss of health and depression.

Why is depression important in sick old people?

Depression that warrants intervention occurs in 10% of people over the age of 60. Nearly a third of older people admitted to hospital for acute care experience depression. The lifetime experience of depression is 15–20%. Unipolar depression is the fourth leading cause of temporary and permanent disability worldwide.[4]

Physical illness can cause or be the result of depression. Depression worsens the prognosis of many medical disorders. Those with depression have a two-fold increase in cardiac mortality. It is a risk factor for non-suicidal mortality. Suicide in old age is associated with multiple physical illnesses and a history of hospital-treated depression.[6] Yet many people do not receive therapies that are of proven effectiveness – even up to eight years after the onset of their condition.

The relationship between depression and physical illness
The hospital and care home environment

Most hospitals were not designed with the welfare of older patients in mind. Hospital routines are not always conducive to well-being and few older patients after discharge wished that they had spent more time in hospital. Interviews of hospitalised patients in Australia revealed that all of them felt depressed. They were demoralised, feeling unable to cope. They disliked having to rely on others and felt that they were a burden. They perceived themselves as being helpless and hopeless, with a low sense of self-esteem.[7]

Many residents in residential and nursing homes are depressed. The diagnosis is underestimated and few residents are referred for specialist psychiatric care.

A high prevalence of suicidal ideation occurs in medically ill nursing home residents – particularly those with severe depression, medical comorbidity and little social support.[8]

Cardiovascular disease

There is a semantic association between grief and a broken heart. In some cases, depression precedes the clinical manifestations of cardiovascular disease. Major depression can predict first cardiac events.[9]

Depression is independently associated with coronary heart disease (as are social isolation and lack of social support).[10] The increased mortality seems to be related to the *severity* rather than the *presence* of depression – in a study of 763 patients who had sustained a myocardial infarction, depression *per se* was not an indicator of death. There was a higher death rate on those with more marked depression who had non-Q wave myocardial infarction.[11]

In heart failure, depression is related not only to the degree of physical impairment but also to how the individual copes with the impairment.[12] Koenig *et al.*[13] found that less than 50% of patients with heart failure who had major depression had it treated and few had psychiatric consultations.

Conversely, cardiovascular disease is a risk factor for late-onset depression. The mechanisms whereby depression and heart disease affect each other are uncertain. Part of the reason may be that depressed subjects tend to have poor concordance with their drug therapy – not surprisingly, health status is worse if people do not take their drugs.[14] Altered autonomic function may also explain the relationship between depression and cardiac mortality.[15] In depression, heart rate recovery after exercise is slower. Heart rate variability (a measure of autonomic function) is less in those with major depression than controls. An acutely depressed mood can trigger life-threatening cardiac events. It is speculated that biological responses involving inflammatory cytokines and platelet activation may be contributory.[16]

Chronic obstructive airways disease (COPD)

Thirty per cent of people with COPD are depressed. Depression is also a factor in the frequency of hospital readmissions for acute exacerbations.[17] Risk factors for depression in COPD include disease severity, lack of carer support, inadequate pulmonary rehabilitation, being underweight, use of psychotropic drugs and being a smoker. In COPD, depression and anxiety are significantly related to negative quality of life outcomes.

Their depressive symptoms improve if inpatient rehabilitation results in symptom relief and reduced disability.[18]

Depression is also common during recovery from acute respiratory failure.

Stroke

Stroke is the major cause of serious disability and its incidence increases exponentially with age. Depression is common, with about 50% of survivors being depressed at six months – especially those with poor mobility or limitations in activities of daily living. A history of depression is also associated with low mood after stroke. In a pan-European study of 626 non-disabled older people,[19] depressive symptoms were associated with white matter ischaemia on CT scan. The presence of lacunes (small, deep infarcts) was not associated with the development of depression.

After stroke, there is usually a reduction in social interaction over time.[20] Not surprisingly, the GDS score rises between the third and six month post-stroke.

Some stroke patients have difficulty controlling the expression of their emotions (emotionalism). They may have a low threshold for crying or laughing. The usual triggers are sadness, sentimentality and discussion of this symptom. Some people cry for no obvious reason. Emotionalism can distress the patient, who may feel that they are losing control. It can also be disturbing for the family, who might worry that their loved one is being badly treated in the hospital or care home. It is therefore wise to explain emotionalism to the patient and the family. Antidepressants can considerably reduce the frequency of crying or laughing episodes.[21] The improvement is not specific to a particular type of drug.[22]

Communication difficulties as a result of stroke are the strongest predictor of the severity of depression and its prognosis. The presence of depression can impede stroke rehabilitation.[23]

Depression in stroke is often undiagnosed and inadequately treated. A study of seven trials with 780 participants[22] found that antidepressants are associated with a reduction in scores on mood-rating scales. However, there was no reduction in the frequency of clinically diagnosable depression. Treating non-depressed stroke patients with sertraline in the first two weeks does not reduce the incidence of depression at 24 weeks.[24] Two small trials of psychotherapy showed no benefit. Physical exercise may improve post-stroke depression: a three-month programme was associated with less depression and an improved quality of life.[25]

There have been no studies of ECT in patients with stroke.

Cancer

People will be understandably depressed on being told that they have cancer. Depression can be the presenting feature of occult cancers – especially pancreatic cancer. Breast cancer and gastrointestinal malignancies are particularly likely to be associated with depression. Depression is also a manifestation of non-metastatic malignancy.[26] Patients with cancer who are also depressed have a significantly increased risk of death.[27] Some cancer patients date their depressive symptoms to the onset of treatment with chemotherapy or deep X-ray treatment.

Bone and joint disease

Antidepressants double the risk of falls and people who are depressed are more likely to break their hips. Almost a half of patients with a range of traumatic orthopaedic conditions are depressed. Open fractures can increase the rate of depression.[28] Patients with rheumatoid arthritis may be depressed because of the physical impact of the disease (pain, disability) or such psychological factors as low self-esteem and perceived impact of the disease.[29]

Neurodegenerative disease

Old people who are depressed are more likely to develop Alzheimer's disease, vascular dementia and Parkinson's disease. Depression may also be associated with mild cognitive impairment: this is independent of underlying cerebrovascular disease.[30]

Dementia may be accompanied by depression but it is not known whether drug treatment is effective or whether the balance of benefits versus adverse effects is favourable. The clinician should therefore be cautious in prescribing antidepressants to patients who are demented.[31]

Recurrent depression is a particular risk factor for dementia. Depression can mimic dementia, but depressive pseudo-dementia is not so common nowadays. Depression may be secondary to dementia – particularly in the early stages, when the patient has insight into their cognitive decline. Of course, depression and dementia may coexist – they are both common conditions.

Depression is also common in Parkinson's disease. Apathy may be a core feature of this illness and may occur in the absence of depression. Because of symptom overlap, there may be diagnostic difficulties.[32] There are no studies of ECT or behavioural therapy in Parkinson's disease. There are insufficient data from the few trials to help us make informed choices on whether, when or with which drug to treat depression in Parkinsonism.[33]

Endocrine disorders

Depression in diabetes mellitus is three times more common than in the general population. Those with diabetes may forget to log their blood glucose measurements, not manage their disease well and not attend for clinic appointments. Only a third of those with diabetes mellitus have their major depression identified and treated, partly because some of the somatic symptoms of depression (sleep disturbances, weight gain or loss, fatigue) may be attributed solely to the diabetes.

Depression occurs in most people with Cushing's disease. It also should be considered in hypothyroidism and hyper-parathyroidism.

Sensory impairment

Depression is likely in old people who are deaf or visually impaired. In age-related macular degeneration (the commonest cause of blindness in old people in Western countries, where it affects 30% of those over 75) is associated with depression – especially in those with impaired physical function.[34]

Other disorders

Depression can occur in a range of clinical disorders. Depression is common in old people with genito-urinary diseases and injuries that require admission to hospital.[6] Elderly Chinese men with moderate-to-severe lower urinary tract symptoms are at increased risk of having clinically relevant depression.[35] Depression is associated with impaired immune activity and altered inflammatory response. Depression can therefore be instrumental in causing physical illness or result from it. It should be considered in any older person, but especially those with disability, pain, chronic disease as well as those who do not take their drugs regularly or fail to attend for clinic appointments.

Why is depression under-recognised in medically ill old people?

Patients

Old people tend to under-report or deny depression. This may be a cohort effect of a generation of stoical individuals who often minimise their symptoms. The old person may attribute constipation, weight loss and chronic aches and pains to normal ageing. The dominant symptoms might be anxiety or irritability and they may not feel particularly sad. There may be inadequate privacy on the ward or at the clinic consultation. The patient may fear the stigma that still accompanies psychiatric disease. Or they simply may be unaware that they are depressed. The diagnosis may be difficult if the patient is deaf, dysarthric or dysphasic, or if their first language is not English. The general public has a poor understanding of antidepressant drugs, confusing them with tranquillisers and regarding them as addictive.

The family

Relatives may be unaware that their loved one is depressed. If the depression is associated with memory impairment, they may fear that the person is becoming demented. Depression may also be overlooked in informal caregivers, especially those who are under strain. Common causes of caregiver stress include sleep disturbance, faecal soiling and behavioural disorders.

How to improve the recognition of depression in medically ill patients

We should consider the possibility of depression in the following circumstances:

+ sadness – this is the commonest presentation
+ poor physical health
+ weight loss
+ alcohol abuse
+ not eating properly or refusal to eat

> + living in squalor
> + poverty
> + isolation
> + poor concordance with medication
> + not exercising
> + not rehabilitating successfully
> + living in a care home
> + living at home with chronic illness or bereavement
> + not attending for medical appointments.

Conversely, frequent attendances at the general practitioner's surgery (after controlling for physical illness, depression was found in those who attended the primary care physician more than once a month for the past six months).[36]

Not attending for influenza vaccination – this has been seen in depressed caregivers who are looking after an elderly person with dementia.[37]

Physical signs that should raise the possibility of depression include:
1 a slowed-up patient
2 flattening of affect
3 lack of eye contact
4 taciturnity
5 unkempt clothing or poor personal hygiene
6 an aura of heaviness or gloom.

Behavioural features that should alert the physician to the diagnosis include:
> + agoraphobia
> + anhedonia – little relish for life, not enjoying things that once gave pleasure
> + anxiety or being worried for no obvious reason
> + bad moods
> + dark thoughts
> + crying
> + importuning
> + being argumentative
> + being suspicious about others, including friends and family
> + complaining of feeling tired all the time
> + expressing repeated concerns about death and dying
> + feeling worthless or hopeless
> + fearing that they have an incurable disease.

We should also consider depression if the patient has several volumes of case notes. Some patients have somatisation, or their symptoms may not be readily diagnosable and these patients can present to different specialists. They may have undergone numerous investigations before the possibility of depressive illness is considered.

As depression is so common and may present in so many ways, it is wise to administer screening tests as a routine part of the assessment of old people.

Which tests for depression?

There is a bewildering array of tests, reflecting the fact that there is no ideal instrument for measuring depression. Some screen for the presence, others assess the degree of depression. The busy physician wants assessment tools which are easy and quick to administer, do not upset the patient and are valid.

The Geriatric Depression Scale (GDS) is probably the most useful in older patients. In patients referred to a specialist geriatric outpatient memory clinic, an abbreviated form consisting of five questions has been found to rapidly identify those with depression (positive predictive value of 97%).[38]

The questions are as follows.
 » Do you often feel downhearted or sad (blue)?
 » Do you often feel helpless?
 » Do you feel that your life is empty?
 » Do you feel happy most of the time?
 » Are you basically satisfied with your life?

The key questions to pose to all elderly patients are therefore on mood and loss of interest or pleasure in activities.

Investigating depression

It is important to consider underlying medical conditions which are associated with depression as the treatment may improve the patient's affect. Examples include the following.
1 Vitamin B12 and folate deficiency – there is a two-fold increase in depression in people with these deficiencies.
2 Subclinical hypothyroidism (in which the T4 level is normal but the TSH is elevated) is associated with a four-fold increase in depression – more common than in established overt hypothyroidism.[39]

We should also be aware that many drugs can cause depression. The older antihypertensive drugs such as reserpine and methyldopa are rarely used now, but beta-blockers and nifedipine can cause depression. Steroids are another recognised cause. Centrally acting drugs which might be incriminated include barbiturates, benzodiazepines and phenothiazines.

The management of depression in physically ill old people

To the non-specialist, the treatment of depression can be vexing. There are so many drugs as well as physical and herbal remedies. In recent years, there have been a number of clinical trials and literature reviews which have made management decisions a little easier for the physician.

The fact that there are so many therapies tells us that no single treatment is uniformly effective. The decision on whether to treat, with what treatment and for how long must be based on the individual's wishes, degree of depression, suicide risk, previous response to antidepressants, other drugs taken and concomitant medical problems.

Antidepressant drugs

About two-thirds of those with severe depression will respond to drug therapy (compared with a third who will respond to placebos). In recent years, there has been a big increase in the number and type of drugs available. We will briefly consider those that might be considered by the physician treating older patients and review the evidence for effectiveness and safety.

There are several classes of drugs for depression. All of them make various neurotransmitters more available in the brain but their precise mode of action is still not fully understood.

Tricyclic antidepressants (TCAs)

These were the first group of antidepressants to be developed and have been in use for over 50 years. They have effects on serotonin as well as noradrenaline (and perhaps on other neurotransmitters). Examples include amitriptyline, clomipramine, dosulepin (dothiepin), trazodone and trimipramine (which have sedative effects) and imipramine, nortriptyline and lofepramine (which are less sedating). Amitriptyline and dosulepin are dangerous in overdose. Lofepramine is safer but can cause hepatic toxicity. These drugs should be used with caution in patients with epilepsy. Older people are prone to syncope and falls when taking these drugs, which also cause hyponatraemia in some elderly users.

Tricyclics should be started with low dosage, which is then gradually increased. They usually begin to work within a few weeks. Patients taking these drugs should be advised to avoid alcohol, as the combination can result in drowsiness.

They are particularly useful in severely ill depressed patients. They improve sleep patterns. They are generally given once each evening (they usually have a long half-life). These often cause anti-cholinergic side-effects (dry mouth, constipation, confusion, urinary hesitancy and dribbling). They can also cause orthostatic hypotension and falls. They are best avoided in subjects with ischaemic heart disease or cardiac rhythm disturbances.

Newer drugs in this class have fewer side-effects than earlier compounds. Because they are much cheaper than SSRIs, they should be considered as first line treatment – unless there are medical contraindications (which is often the case in geriatric patients).

Physicians have been criticised for administering sub-optimal doses of TCAs. A systematic review of 39 studies found that doses between 75 and 100 mg per day (and even lower doses) resulted in a better response than placebo. Interestingly, one study found there to be no evidence that standard doses of TCAs were more effective than lower dose schedules.[40]

Selective serotonin reuptake inhibitors (SSRIs)

SSRIs are front line therapy in patients at risk of overdose, patients with diabetes mellitus and cardiac problems. In general, they have low toxicity and good tolerability. Which SSRI should be prescribed? There are claims made for the advantages of individual drugs but we have no good large trials to inform us when to prescribe individual SSRIs.[41]

This group of drugs includes citalopram, escitalopram, paroxetine, sertraline and fluoxetine. Fluoxetine has been shown in a well-conducted placebo-controlled study to be efficacious in minor depression. However, is less used now because of its long half-life and potential for drug–drug interactions.[42] It can also occasionally reduce blood glucose levels and make it difficult for people to sit still. Escitalopram is a new SSRI, being the S-enantiomer of citalopram. It has been promoted as being superior to citalopram. However, there is no compelling evidence that this drug is more effective or has a faster onset of action than its parent compound.[43] Tachycardia is a side-effect of citalopram. SIADH also occurs in patients on this drug and untoward effects with the two drugs are similar. Paroxetine is associated with tiredness. It has a short half-life and patients should be advised not to stop taking it suddenly. Sertraline can cause diarrhoea.

These drugs should be introduced gradually and the dose slowly increased. There is a risk of increased anxiety in the early days of treatment. Soon after starting these drugs, patients may become nauseated or anxious. If the drugs are stopped suddenly, there is a risk of a withdrawl syndrome. These unpleasant symptoms occur in the first five days of discontinuation of the drug. Patients may experience stomach upsets, anxiety, flu-like symptoms, vivid dreams and sensations of electric shocks. They are more likely with paroxetine, which has a short half-life.

Other adverse effects of SSRIs are falls and fractures, gastrointestinal bleeding and hyponatraemia. Hyponatraemia is three times more common in patients taking SSRIs than in those taking other antidepressants.[44] Hyponatraemia is potentially life-threatening. It should be suspected in all patients who become drowsy, delirious or who have seizures while taking an anticonvulsant. It usually occurs in the first few weeks of treatment and is probably secondary to inappropriate antidiuretic hormone (ADH) secretion. The syndrome of inappropriate ADH is characterised by a low serum sodium (<135 mmol /L), a high urinary osmolality (>200 mOsm/kg), a urinary sodium of over 20 mmol per litre and a serum osmolality of less than 280 milliOsmoles per kilogram.[44] It is commoner in older people, women, those of low body weight and those with a low baseline sodium concentration. It is also more common if diuretics are used concomitantly. Patients receiving multiple medications may also be at increased risk. Treatment is with fluid restriction, severe cases requiring a loop diuretic and isotonic saline.[45]

Despite a large catalogue of possible adverse effects, few users get serious side-effects with SSRIs.

If a patient cannot tolerate a specific SSRI, or there is no remission of symptoms after about three months' therapy, one in four will respond to a second step choice.[46]

Serotonin and noradrenalin reuptake inhibitors (SNRIs)

These include venlafaxine (and duloxetine) which is used for both anxiety and depression and there is some evidence that venlafaxine might be more effective than SSRIs for major depression. Two thirds of patients with anxiety respond to this drug. It should be avoided in patients with renal impairment, uncontrolled hypertension, or cardiac disease. The treatment effect can be delayed. This drug can cause tremor, raised cholesterol, increased blood pressure (which may be sustained with the slow-release preparation) as well as gastrointestinal disturbances and tiredness. Patients on this drug should have their blood pressure monitored. There is a risk of overdose especially in patients with conduction disturbances or ventricular dysrhythmias. Up to a third of users who stop taking these drugs experience withdrawal symptoms (the same proportion as in those who stop SSRIs). They should therefore be tapered rather than stopped suddenly. The SNRIs are second line drugs best prescribed and monitored by an old age psychiatrist.

Lithium

This drug is efficacious in both the treatment and prevention of bipolar depression. Lithium reduces the suicide risk in bipolar disorder.[47] It is also used in acute mania. This drug is inexpensive and can be used as a second line drug for maintenance treatment of depression. It has a narrow therapeutic window and it is therefore important to monitor serum levels 12 hours after the last dose taken the previous evening. In older patients, the recommended level for prophylaxis is 0.4–0.6 mmol/L and for treatment of an acute episode 0.8–1.0 mmol/L. Before starting the drug, it is wise to measure renal and thyroid function (the drug can induce hypothyroidism). Lithium levels are decreased by acetazolamide and theophylline and increased by some antibiotics, anti-hypertensives and several diuretics (e.g. thiazides, spironolactone and metolazone).

Mono-amine oxidase inhibitors (MAOIs)

These drugs are rarely used now because they are less effective than TCAs and SSRIs. There is a risk of hypertension with foods containing tyramine and therefore the need for observing strict dietary limitations.

Noradrenergic and specific serotoninergic antidepressants (NaSSAs)

Mirtazapine, a pre-symptomatic alpha antagonist, causes initial sedation and can cause oedema, dizziness, weight gain and GI disturbances. It is used for major depression and is best prescribed by experts.

Tryptophan

Hydroxytryptophan and tryptophan are so-called 'natural' alternatives to conventional antidepressants. They are recommended for dysthymia and unipolar depression. Only two clinical trials are good enough to be reliable: they suggest that these drugs are better than placebo at relieving depression, but more studies are needed on their safety and efficacy.[48] A rare but serious complication is eosinophilic-myalgia syndrome, characterised by myalgia, arthralgia, dyspnoea, neuropathy and an increased eosinophil count.

A Cochrane review of 17 studies involving TCAs, SSRIs and MAOIs administered to 2000 patients showed that they were effective in the treatment of older community patients as well as inpatients.[49]

Another Cochrane review scrutinised 32 studies of different classes of drugs used in the treatment of depression in old people.[50] Tricyclics (TCAs) and selective serotonin reuptake inhibitors (SSRIs) were equally efficacious. However, TCAs are less well tolerated, with a higher withdrawal rate because of side-effects. There appear to be no differences between discontinuation rates (either because of adverse reactions or lack of efficacy) between the SSRIs and other second-generation antidepressants (e.g. venlafaxine, mirtazapine, bupropion) in patients with major depression. The number needed to treat with paroxetine to prevent one recurrence of depression is four.

The Royal College of Psychiatrists[51] recommends that antidepressants should be taken for six to nine months after the depressive symptoms have abated. The British National Formulary suggests 12 months' continuance after remission for elderly people, with five years' (or even lifelong) therapy for recurrent depression. Certainly, depression is less likely to recur if the drug is given for two years.[46] In practice, 50% of GPs discontinue these drugs after six months.[42]

A more detailed discussion of antidepressant use in older people can be found in Chapter 4.

Herbal and other remedies

Many people do not wish to take powerful synthetic antidepressants, fearing habituation and side-effects. Eighty-two per cent of Americans over the age of 65 use complementary or alternative therapies in the course of a year. Those with self-reported depression or anxiety are more likely to use natural remedies, relaxation techniques or spiritual practices.[52]

St John's wort (*Hypericum perforatum*) has long been used for depression in Germany where it is also licensed for anxiety and sleep disorders. Extracts of the herb contain many different chemical classes, so the active agent is uncertain. Evidence of effectiveness is inconsistent (perhaps in part because of the differing formulations of the drug) but a Cochrane review of 37 trials[53] suggested that *Hypericum* may be as effective as standard antidepressants in treating mild to moderate – but not severe – symptoms (but other studies suggest it may have only limited benefit (*see* Chapter 4). Moreover, this preparation seems to have fewer side-effects than conventional drugs. However, it should not be taken in conjunction with antidepressant drugs. It can induce drug metabolising enzymes. Drug interactions include warfarin, digoxin, and anticonvulsants.

Long-chain omega-3 fatty acids might help relieve depression when given in addition to existing antidepressant medication but there is no good evidence justifying treating depression with these drugs alone.[54]

Physical activity

In a literature review of randomised controlled trials of exercise in depression, one study[55] found that it produced short-term gains in both major and minor depression. Another[25] found that exercise was helpful in treating post-stroke depression.

Psychological therapy

Historically, there was a bias against psychotherapy – largely because Freud believed that older people were too rigid to benefit from this form of treatment. Nowadays, most lay people consider that counselling therapy is the best way to treat depression. It helps people review how they see themselves, the world and other people.[51] GPs are more likely to offer counselling or psychotherapy than physicians.[1] Cognitive behavioural therapy is as effective as antidepressants for moderate (but not for severe) depression but takes longer to begin to work. There is an argument for using both concurrently but access to trained staff may make this unrealistic. Psychotherapy does not seem to be effective as maintenance treatment for major depression.[46]

Other approaches include behavioural activation (with scheduled restructured daily activities recorded in a diary), anxiety-management and problem-solving strategies (learning how to deal with retirement, bereavement or relocation). Family therapy is also helpful in helping people face up to unresolved intergenerational conflict, or deal with guilt or unrealistic expectations.

Support groups can be helpful, especially in dissipating the fears of dementia or inevitable institutionalisation.

Electroconvulsive therapy (ECT)

A recent Cochrane review[56] found only three trials which compared real ECT to simulated ECT and to antidepressants. Each study had serious methodological flaws. Despite the fact that this treatment has been in use for decades, it is not yet possible to say whether ECT is more effective than antidepressant medication. NICE[57] recommends that this treatment is used when the depression might be life-threatening or to achieve rapid and short-term improvement when other options have been ineffective.

A more detailed discussion of ECT use in older people with an affective disorder can be found in Chapter 6.

When to prescribe antidepressants

For most people who are depressed in the context of an acute physical illness, it is perhaps best to treat the physical illness first and review the patient in two to three weeks to see if the depression has resolved (watchful waiting). Once the pain has been controlled or the heart failure treated, the patient's spirits will often lift. Similarly, the patient is likely to be less depressed if their physical independence improves. If the depression persists but is mild, there is no need to prescribe an SSRI – this group of drugs is no better than placebo in the management of mild depression. In severe depression, antidepressants are more effective than placebo.

Given the paucity of studies and the poor quality of the published trials of antidepressant therapy, it is difficult to make many firm recommendations about the optimum treatment for depression. The older TCAs are best avoided in many old people, as these drugs often have unacceptable side-effects. Whether to prescribe a newer TCA or an SSRI as first line therapy will be a decision made on cost, potential drug interactions and patient preference.

The patient should be asked if they would like to consider medication. They should be reassured about the low risk of habituation. It is important to treat depression – if not, there is a two-fold increase in overall mortality. If in doubt, it is wise to treat the depression: better to treat the potentially reversible than to deny effective therapy.

When to refer to an old age psychiatrist

If a first line drug is not working, it is prudent to ask for specialist help. Decisions about whether to increase the dose to higher levels than physicians are comfortable with, to switch to another agent in the same class (e.g. another SSRI), to switch to another class of drugs ('out of class switch'), to use a dual agent (e.g. a drug which also inhibits the uptake of 5-hydroxytryptamine *and* noradrenaline) or to augment therapy with a different class of drug (such as lithium) are best made by consultants in old age psychiatry. Referral should also be considered if the patient is refusing to eat or drink – in severe cases, ECT may be considered.

Where do we go from here?

The priority is to do large high quality randomised controlled trials in older populations – it is unfortunate that studies still focus on younger subjects. These should be based in primary care as well as including hospital patients. They should include economic evaluations. We also need to find ways of improving the recognition of depression in old people by the patients themselves, their informal caregivers, nurses, therapists and physicians.

KEY POINTS

▶ Depression is common in old people but often unrecognised and untreated.
▶ It occurs in many medical conditions, particularly if there is pain, disability or prolonged or serious illness.
▶ It should always be considered in those who are bereaved and residents of nursing and residential homes.
▶ In mild depression, counselling is useful but drugs are not usually indicated.
▶ In moderate to severe depression, antidepressants should be considered.
▶ There is little difference in effectiveness between tricyclics and SSRIs.
▶ The newer tricyclics are sometimes suitable but should not generally be prescribed for old people with heart disease, constipation, glaucoma or those who fall.
▶ SSRIs are less cardiotoxic and safer in overdose and are generally well tolerated, but are more expensive and can cause unpleasant effects if they are suddenly withdrawn.
▶ When prescribing SSRIs, always check the blood urea and electrolytes after two weeks.
▶ The drugs should be taken for at least six to nine months after the depressive symptoms after the depression has resolved (some advocate a two-year course).
▶ In recurrent depression, lifelong treatment may be necessary.

REFERENCES

1 Harman JS, Veazie PJ, Lyness JM. Primary care physician office visits for depression by older Americans. *J Gen Intern Med.* 2006; **21**: 926–30.
2 Cullum S, Tucker S, Todd C, *et al.* Screening for depression in older medical inpatients. *Int J Geriatr Psychiatr.* 2006; **21**: 469–76.
3 Copeland JR, Beekman AT, Braam AW, *et al.* Depression among older people in Europe: the EURODEP studies. *World Psychiatry.* 2004; **3**: 45–9.
4 Rubinow DR. Treatment strategies after SSRI failure: good news and bad news. *NEJM.* 2006; **354**: 1305–6.
5 Pepersack T, De Breucker S, Mekongo YP, *et al.* Correlates of unrecognised depression among hospitalised geriatric patients. *J Psychiatr Pract.* 2006; **12**: 160–7.
6 Koponen HJ, Viilo K, Hakko H, *et al.* Rates and previous disease history in old age suicide. *Int J Geriatr Psychiatr.* 2007; **22**: 38–46.
7 Clarke DM, Cook KE, Coleman KJ, *et al.* A qualitative examination of the experiences of 'depression' in hospitalized medically ill patients. *Psychopathology.* 2006; **39**: 303–12.
8 Raue PJ, Meyers BS, Rowe JL, *et al.* Suicidal ideation among elderly homecare patients. *Int J Geriatr Psychiatr.* 2007; **22**: 32–7.
9 Bremmer MA, Hoogendijk WJ, Deeg DJ, *et al.* Depression in older age is a risk factor for first ischemic cardiac events. *Am J Geriatr Psychiatr.* 2006; **14**: 523–30.

10 Arthur HM. Depression, isolation, social support, and cardiovascular disease in older adults. *J Cardiovasc Nurs.* 2006; **21**(5 Suppl. 1): S2–7.

11 Sorensen C, Brandes A, Hendricks O, *et al.* Depression assessed over 1-year survival in patients with myocardial infarction. *Acta Psychiatr Scand.* 2006; **113**: 241–4.

12 Turvey CL, Klein DM, Pies CJ. Depression, physical impairment, and treatment of depression in chronic heart failure. *J Cardiovasc Nurs.* 2005; **21**: 178–85.

13 Koenig HG, Vandermeer J, Chambers A, *et al.* Comparison of major and minor depression in older medical inpatients with chronic heart and pulmonary disease. *Psychosom.* 2006; **47**: 296–303.

14 Morgan AL, Masoudi FA, Havranek EP, *et al.* Difficulty taking medications, depression, and health status in heart failure patients. *J Card Fail.* 2006; **12**: 54–60.

15 Hughes JW, Casey E, Luyster F, *et al.* Depression symptoms predict heart rate recovery after treadmill stress testing. *Am Heart J.* 2006; **151**: 1122.el–6.

16 Steptoe A, Strike PC, Perkins-Porras L, *et al.* Acute depressed mood as a trigger of acute coronary syndromes. *Biol Psychiatr.* 2006; **15**: 837–42.

17 Cao Z, Ong KC, Eng P, *et al.* Frequent hospital readmissions for acute exacerbation of COPD and their associated factors. *Respirology.* 2006; **11**: 188–95.

18 Alexopoulos GS, Sirey JA, Raue PJ, *et al.* Outcomes of depressed patients undergoing inpatient pulmonary rehabilitation. *Am J Geriatr Psychiatr.* 2006; **14**: 466–75.

19 O'Brien JT, Firbank MR, Krishnan MS, *et al.* White matter hyperdensities rather than lacunar infarcts are associated with depressive symptoms in older people: the LADIS study. *Am J Geriatr Psychiatr.* 2006; **14**: 824–41.

20 Kwok T, Lo RS, Wong E, *et al.* Quality of life of stroke survivors: a 1-year follow-up study. *Arch Phys Med Rehabil.* 2006; **87**: 1177–82.

21 House AO, Hackett ML, Anderson CS, *et al.* Pharmaceutical interventions for emotionalism after stroke. *The Cochrane Database of Systematic Reviews.* 2004; **2**. Available from: http://www.cochrane.org/reviews/en/ab003690.html

22 Hackett ML, Anderson CS, House AO. Interventions for treating depression after stroke. *The Cochrane Database of Systematic Reviews.* 2004; **3**. Available from: http://www.cochrane.org/reviews/en/ab003437.html

23 Thomas SA, Lincoln NB. Factors relating to depression after stroke. *Br J Clin Psychol.* 2006; **45**: 49–61.

24 Almeida OP, Waterreus A, Hankey GJ. Preventing depression after stroke: results from a randomised placebo-controlled trial. *J Clin Psychiatr.* 2006; **67**: 1104–9.

25 Lai SM, Studenski S, Richards L, *et al.* Therapeutic exercise and depressive symptoms after stroke. *J Am Geriatr Soc.* 2006; **54**: 240–7.

26 Katona CE. *Depression in Old Age.* Chichester: John Wiley and Sons; 1994.

27 Onitilo AA, Nietert PJ, Egede LE. Effect of depression on all-cause mortality in adults with cancer and differential effects of cancer site. *Gen Hosp Psychiatr.* 2006; **28**: 396–402.

28 Crichlow RJ, Andres PL, Morrison SM, *et al.* Depression in orthopaedic trauma patients: prevalence and severity. *J Bone Joint Surg Am.* 2006; **88**: 1927–33.

29 Covic T, Tyson G, Spencer D, *et al.* Depression in rheumatoid arthritis patients: demographic, clinical, and psychological predictors. *J Psychosom Res.* 2006; **60**: 469–76.

30 Barnes DE, Alexopoulos GS, Lopez OL, *et al.* Depressive symptoms, vascular disease, and mild cognitive impairment: findings from the Cardiovascular Health Study. *Arch Gen Psychiatr.* 2006; **63**: 273–9.

31 Bains J, Birks JS, Dening TD. Antidepressants for treating depression in dementia. *The Cochrane Database of Systemic Reviews.* 2002; **4**. Available from: http://www.cochrane.org/reviews/en/ab003944.html

32 Kirsch-Darrow L, Fernandez HH, Marsiske M, *et al.* Dissociating apathy and depression in Parkinson's disease. *Neurology.* 2006; **67**: 33–8.

33 Ghazi-Noori S, Chung TH, Deane K, *et al.* Therapies for depression in Parkinson's disease. *The Cochrane Database of Systematic Reviews.* 2003; **3**. Available from: http://www.cochrane.org/reviews/en/ab003465.html

34 Berman K, Brodaty H. Psychological effects of age-related macular degeneration. *Int Psychogeriatr.* 2006; **18**: 415–28.

35 Wong SY, Hoing A, Leung J, *et al.* Lower urinary tract symptoms and depressive symptoms in elderly men. *J Affect Disord.* 2006; **96**: 83–8.

36 Menchetti M, Cevenini N, De Ronchi D, *et al.* Depression and frequent attendance in primary health care patients. *Gen Hosp Psychiatr.* 2006; **28**: 119–24.

37 Thorpe JM, Sleath BL, Thorpe CT, *et al.* Caregiver psychological distress as a barrier to influenza vaccination among community-dwelling elderly with dementia. *Med Care.* 2006; **44**: 713–21.

38 Molloy DW, Standish TI, Dubois S, *et al.* A short screen for depression: the AB Clinician Depression Screen (ABCD). *Int Psychogeriatr.* 2006; **18**: 481–92.

39 Chueire VB, Romaldini JH, Ward LS. Subclinical hypothyroidism increases the risk for depression in the elderly. *Arch Gerontol Geriatr.* 2007; **44**: 21–8.

40 Furukawa T, McGuire H, Barbui C. Low dosage tricyclic antidepressants for depression. *The Cochrane Database of Systematic Reviews.* 2003; **3**. Available from: http://www.cochrane.org/reviews/en/ab003197.html

41 Cipriani A, Brambilla P, Furukawa T, *et al.* Fluoxetine versus other types of pharmacotherapy for depression. *The Cochrane Database of Systematic Reviews.* 2005; **4**. Available from: http://cochrane.org/reviews/en/ab004185.html

42 Fitch K, Molnar FJ, Power B, *et al.* Antidepressant use in older people: family physicians' knowledge, attitudes, and practices. *Can Fam Physician.* 2005; **51**: 80–1.

43 Drug and Therapeutics Bulletin. New drugs from old. *DTB.* 2006; **44**: 73–7.

44 Covyeou JA, Jackson CJ. Hyponatraemia associated with Escitalopram. *NEJM.* 2007; **356**: 94–5.

45 Jacob S, Spinler SA. Hyponatraemia associated with selective serotonin-reuptake inhibitors in older adults. *Ann Pharmacother.* 2006; **40**: 1618–22.

46 Reynolds CF III, Dew MA, Pollock BG. Maintenance treatment of major depression in old age. *NEJM.* 2006; **354**: 1130–8.

47 Freeman MP, Freeman SA. Lithium: clinical considerations in internal medicine. *Am J Med.* 2006; **119**: 478–81.

48 Shaw K, Turner J, Del Mar C. Tryptophan and 5-Hydroxytryptophan for depression. *The Cochrane Database of Systematic Reviews.* 2001; **3**. Available from: http://www.cochrane.org/reviews/en/ab003198.html

49 Wilson K, Mottram P, Sivanranthran A, *et al.* Antidepressants versus placebo for the depressed elderly. *The Cochrane Database of Systematic Reviews.* 2001; **3**. Available from: http://www.cochrane.org/reviews/en/ab000561.html

50 Mottram P, Wilson K, Strobl J. Antidepressants for depressed elderly. *The Cochrane Database of Systematic Reviews.* 2006; **1**. Available from: http://www.cochrane.org/reviews/en/ab003491.html

51 Royal College of Psychiatrists. *Antidepressants.* Available from: http://www.rcpsych.ac.uk/mentalhealthinformation/mentalhealthproblems/depression/antidepressants.asp (accessed 2007).

52 Grzywacz JG, Suerken CK, Quandt SA, *et al.* Older adults' use of complementary and alternative medicine for mental health: findings from the 2002 National Health Interview Survey. *J Altern Complement Med.* 2006; **12**: 467–73.

53 Linde K, Mulrow CD, Berner M, *et al.* St John's wort for depression. *The Cochrane Database of Systematic Reviews.* 2005; **4**. Available from: http://www.cochrane.org/reviews/en/ab000448.html

54 Drug and Therapeutics Bulletin. Do omega-3 fatty acids help in depression? *DTB.* 2007; **45**: 9–12.

55 Sjosten N, Kivela SL. The effects of physical exercise on depressive symptoms among the aged: a systematic review. *Int J Geriatr Psychiatr.* 2006; **21**: 410–18.

56 Stek M, Van der Wurff FB, Hoogendijk W, *et al.* Electroconvulsive therapy for the depressed elderly. *The Cochrane Database of Systematic Reviews.* 2003; **2**. Available from: http://www.cochrane.org/reviews/en/ab003593.html

57 National Institute for Clinical Excellence. Technology Appraisal: electro-convulsive therapy. In: *Compilation: summary of guidance issued to the NHS in England and Wales.* London: National Institute for Clinical Excellence; 2003. pp. 133–4.

CHAPTER 9

Relationship between physical illness and affective disorders

RICHARD MARRIOTT

Introduction

The relationship between physical illness and affective disorders, particularly depression, is a complex and fascinating one. In the earlier chapters we have seen that depression is common in older people, with an increasing prevalence in medical inpatient and outpatient populations. We have also seen that the diagnosis is often missed. This may be because of a lack of effective strategies to screen for depression. However, in patients with physical illness there is perhaps the tendency for professionals to view a patient's mental state as 'as one would expect' given the difficulties they have to struggle with.

Research[1] into 'life satisfaction' suggests that health (along with social relationships) is a much more important factor for older people as compared with their younger counterparts. However, it has been noted that older people tend to deal with objectively worse conditions than the young.[1,2] This may relate to findings that older people feel satisfied if they consider their situation to be what they deserve[3] and that they are no worse off than fair comparators.[4]

In this chapter I hope to focus on a number of related topics, as follows.

- Associations between depression and the incidence of physical ill health, particularly ischaemic heart disease.
- Assessment of affective disorders in patients with physical illnesses.
  This includes differentiation from adjustment disorders, dementia and delirium.
- Particular physical disorders where depression is a common association.
- The complex area of medically unexplained symptoms, exploring the

difficulties in this population of engagement and management. This has some interesting associations with anxiety disorders.

The impact of depression on physical health

While more extreme forms of depressive disorder obviously impact on general physical health through inactivity and self-neglect there is a growing body of evidence to suggest that depression may be bad for you in other ways.

Evidence from older general hospital populations, summarised by the Royal College of Psychiatrists in the document *Who Cares Wins*,[5] suggests that depression leads to:

» increased length of stay[6,7]
» increased rates of institutionalisation at six months[6,8]
» increased physical dependence at one year[9]
» poorer health[10,11]
» increased mortality.[6,8,10,11,12,13,14,15]

One of the most significant areas of research relates to the impact of depression on ischaemic heart disease. There is increasing evidence that psychosocial factors, particularly depression, are independent risk factors for myocardial infarction[16] and congestive heart failure.[17] It is not at present clear whether the main factors in the association are directly mediated by biological factors or whether their impact is more to do with behavioural change resulting in a less healthy life style[18] (*see* Chapter 3). Various biological mechanisms have been proposed to explain the association and it may well be multi-factorial. These include the following.

» Increased activity of the hypothalamic-pituitary axis,[19] with blunted reactivity and impaired recovery pattern.[20]
» Greater platelet activation.[21] We know that SSRI antidepressants inhibit platelet activation and are associated with an increased risk of bleeding. It is yet to be established whether SSRIs might have a direct impact on vascular outcomes because of this effect.
» Alterations in inflammatory markers associated with ischaemic heart disease have been found to be associated with depressed mood.[22]
» Decreased heart rate variability (HRV) is a risk factor for increased mortality following myocardial infarction. Rates of decreased HRV have been found to be higher in depressed patients.[23]

Despite these findings there is no clear evidence as yet that treatment of affective disorders improves cardiovascular outcomes and further research in this area would be welcomed. Nevertheless, this body of research shows that depression is common in these populations and is associated with significant morbidity and mortality. Clearly depression should still be treated effectively because of its impact on quality of life.

Assessment/identification

Having established that depression in the medically ill is a widespread and important problem the question is what should be done about it? Clearly one of the biggest challenges in assessment of the medically ill is establishing what symptoms are suggestive of a depressive disorder that may benefit from specific treatment. The differential diagnosis includes symptoms directly attributable to the physical illness, an adjustment disorder, mood changes associated with delirium and a dementing process.

A study by Clarke *et al.*[24] suggested, as might be expected, that psychological symptoms, such as guilt and hopelessness, differentiated better than somatic symptoms, between the depressed and non-depressed. However, they also found that somatic symptoms were more severe in depressed than non-depressed medical patients.

In considering the various possible causes of depressive symptoms in the physically ill it is important not only to focus on the cognitive symptoms but also the time course. In a delirium the symptoms are likely to have been of very recent onset and may fluctuate by the day and even the hour. Do the depressive symptoms pre-date the physical illness or is there a very close temporal relationship? If the onset is closely related this might suggest an adjustment disorder. In such cases the symptoms might be expected to improve if the physical condition does. The differentiation between an adjustment disorder and depression relies largely on the form, duration and severity of the symptoms. There may well still be a case for treatment of depressive symptoms that appear to have developed in response to physical illness, especially if the symptoms are especially severe or prolonged.

A cognitive assessment of the patient is important, particularly in older patients with depressive symptoms. A dementing illness may be associated with affective blunting, apathy and loss of interest in usual activities. While depression and dementia may coexist, in the absence of other symptoms of a depressive disorder it is unlikely that these features suggest a depressive disorder. Brief screening tools such as the Abbreviated Mental Test Score[25] or the Mini Mental Test Score[26] may flag up the possibility of delirium or dementia (although depression in itself can affect cognition and when it does this may be a prodromal sign of possible dementia – *see* Chapter 3).

A number of rating scales have been advocated for the detection of depression. These include the Geriatric Depression Scale (GDS),[27] the Hospital Anxiety and Depression Scale[28] (HADs), the Beck Depression Inventory[29] (BDI) and the General Health Questionnaire[30] (GHQ). Only the HADs was developed specifically for use with medically ill patients and unlike the others excludes somatic symptoms. However, a review by Creed (in Robertson and Katona,[31]) suggests that it may not have major advantages over other scales such as the GHQ in this population. The key message seems to be that if use of these scales leads to increased detection of depression they may be extremely useful but they cannot be a replacement for a detailed clinical interview.[32]

Specific medical conditions

Parkinson's disease

The typical neurological features of Parkinson's disease are well known and include a resting tremor, muscle rigidity and bradykinesia. However, psychiatric complications are common, particularly depression. Aarsland[33] reports rates of 38% and 20% for depression and anxiety respectively, which is broadly in line with reviews that suggest an average prevalence of 31% for depression (range 7–70%), depending on the populations studied, the rating scales used and the diagnostic criteria.[34]

These findings raise the intriguing question: is the high incidence of depression in Parkinson's disease a function of the biochemical changes associated with Parkinson's disease itself or related to the psychological processes common to many chronic disabling conditions? Mindham[35] showed a close relationship between degree of disability secondary to Parkinson's disease and depressive symptoms, whereas Celesia and Wanamaker[36] and Horn[37] suggested that severity of depression was independent of duration or severity of disease. Gotham et al.[38] related depression to impairment in activities of daily living, but with less self-blame and worthlessness and more hopelessness. Functional impairment, however, did not account for all the variability and they suggest that individual coping styles and availability of support are also important factors. More recently Aarsland et al.[33] and Tandeberg et al.[39] suggest that the highest correlations with depression are with impaired cognitive function. The review by Slaughter et al.[34] notes that any association between the degree of depression and degree of disability may be mediated by the underlying neurochemical abnormalities rather than a reaction to the physical limitations. They also report that the incidence of depression in Parkinson's disease is higher than for other comparable chronic medical conditions.

The key issue in assessment, as in many other chronic medical conditions, is having a high index of suspicion for depression in patients with Parkinson's disease. However, clinicians need to be particularly wary as a number of features of Parkinson's disease such as the mask-like face and slowed thinking add to diagnostic difficulty and may distract assessors from other features more suggestive of depression.

Another diagnostic complication is the high incidence of apathy in Parkinson's disease. Pluck and Brown[40] compared patients with Parkinson's disease with other patients with a chronic disabling condition (osteoarthritis). They showed significantly higher levels of both apathy and depression in the Parkinson's group. However, they found that apathy in patients with Parkinson's disease is not specifically correlated with depression. They replicated previous findings suggesting that apathy is probably more likely to be related to impaired cognitive (executive) function. This was despite having a relatively small proportion of patients with possible dementia in their sample. All of these were defined as apathetic, 'consistent with the classical description of fronto-subcortical dementia'.

Given this finding and those of Aarsland *et al.*[33] and Tandeberg *et al.*[39] noted above it is clear that an assessment of cognitive function should form part of the initial assessment of any patient with Parkinson's disease and any symptoms suggestive of depression. While depression can interfere with performance on cognitive testing, the patient may also benefit from separate treatment of their cognitive symptoms.

Having identified a probable case of depression in Parkinson's disease, treatment needs to consider biological, psychological and social factors.

Biological factors

1 Psychotropic medication: Despite the incidence of Parkinson's disease, Slaughter *et al.*[34] found few studies examining the effectiveness of antidepressants. They note that while tricyclics (TCAs) have previously been commonly used that they may induce delirium and memory impairment, because of the anti-cholinergic effects; and postural hypotension, because of alpha-adrenergic blockade. They cite Richard and Kurlan,[41] whose survey found that over 50% of physicians used SSRIs in preference to TCAs because of these concerns. This was despite reports of deteriorating motor function reported by some clinicians in certain cases. This may relate to CSM reports of extra-pyramidal symptoms, especially with paroxetine.[42] Sertraline and citalopram might be preferred because of this finding and the fact that they are also associated with fewer drug interactions during metabolism in the liver via cytochrome P450.

2 Electroconvulsive therapy (ECT): A review by Cummings[43] cites a number of studies that report that ECT can be an effective treatment for depression in Parkinson's disease and that there is often an improvement in the motor symptoms in the short term as well. However, the likelihood of subsequent delirium probably limits its use to more extreme or resistant cases.

3 Treatment for the motor symptoms of Parkinson's disease may also be beneficial, by improving independence and social opportunities.

4 Possible future developments: A number of trials have noted good results for cholinesterase inhibitors in the treatment of the neuropsychiatric complications of Parkinson's.[44,45,46] Given the associations noted above between cognitive impairment and both apathy and depression, it might be postulated that similar treatments might have a role in the treatment of a subgroup of Parkinson's patients with low mood.

Psychological factors

There appear to be few trials of psychological therapies specifically for depression in Parkinson's disease. However, both theoretically[47] and from anecdotal reports it seems likely that cognitive behaviour therapy would be an appropriate approach, although further research is necessary.

Social factors

Patients with Parkinson's disease and depression will obviously have many of the social difficulties common to many older people and assessments of their needs should include finances, housing, aids and adaptations required and opportunities for social interaction and availability of practical support and care.

Stroke

As with all disorders, estimates of incidence depend on the populations studied and the assessments used.[48] Two large Scandinavian studies suggest that the incidence of affective disorders after stroke is high with up to a quarter of patients suffering from major depression and many more with significant depressive symptoms.[49,50] An Australian study looking just at patients in the community (i.e. excluding inpatient and rehabilitation unit populations) showed a somewhat lower incidence (15% major depression, 8% minor depression).[51] They also found high levels of anxiety disorders in both men and women post stroke (26% and 39% respectively). There is also evidence that most of those that were found to be depressed three months after a stroke were still depressed at one year.[49]

There has been ongoing controversy as to whether lesion location affects the risk of depression. However, this view is not supported by a systematic review by Carson et al.[52]

Looking at prognosis there is evidence that major depression at three months is correlated with both depression and also poor functional recovery at 15 months.[53] There is also evidence that depressive symptoms are associated with increased mortality at 12 and 24 months, after adjusting for stroke severity.[54]

Andersen et al.[55] found that a previous stroke, a previous history of depression, female gender, living alone and social distress were the main risk factors for post-stroke depression.

Clearly, the most important issue having identified a patient with depression post stroke is what treatments may be beneficial? A Cochrane review looking at this issue was disappointing.[56,57] They found nine trials that were eligible for inclusion in the review. Both the seven trials examining the use of antidepressants and the two looking at psychotherapy showed a trend for improvements on depression rating scales but no strong evidence that either demonstrated clear benefit with regards to remission of depression. Nor did a study of cognitive therapy for depression post stroke show any benefit.[58] Hackett et al.[56] suggest that there is insufficient evidence to support the routine use of antidepressants to prevent depression or improve recovery from stroke and they call for more research to define the role of antidepressants post stroke. Similarly, a further review of non-drug strategies aimed at resolving psychosocial difficulties after stroke[59] failed to find convincing evidence of their effectiveness. However, a study comparing areas of Finland with and those without community follow-up and intervention programmes did demonstrate lower levels of depression at three months in the areas with these arrangements.[49]

Another associated problem commonly encountered after a stroke is emotionalism, characterised by persistent crying following minor provocation. Calvert *et al.*[60] found that 21.5% of stroke survivors had emotionalism (38% of whom also had depression). Andersen[61] states that the mechanism may be partial destruction of the serotonergic raphe nuclei in the brainstem or their ascending projection to the hemispheres. This might explain the positive results of trials of antidepressants (tricyclics and SSRIs) in the treatment of emotionalism.

Depression and hypochondriasis/somatoform disorders/ chronic pain

There is a significant overlap between affective disorders and medically unexplained symptoms, with approximately 50% of patients with medically unexplained symptoms having comorbid anxiety, depression or severe sleep disturbance.[62] There is little research into medically unexplained symptoms in older people, but the prevalence is probably similar to that in younger people.[63] GPs in a study by Sheehan *et al.*[64] suggested that over 35% of older patients had physical symptoms at least equally of psychological origin.

The terminology used to describe physical symptoms without a medically explained, organic cause is unsatisfactory. Terms such as hypochondriasis and somatisation have been used both to describe psychiatric syndromes with prominent somatic symptoms and to describe the mechanisms whereby these symptoms may be generated. However, they are also included within the DSM-IV[65] and ICD-10[66] classifications of categories of somatoform disorders.

DSM IV[65] states that

> the common feature of the somatoform disorders is the presence of physical symptoms that suggest a general medical condition (hence the term somatoform) and are not fully explained by a general medical condition, by the direct effects of a substance, or by another mental disorder (e.g. panic disorder). The symptoms must cause clinically significant distress or impairment in social, occupational or other areas of functioning.

Somatoform disorders do not include ones where physical symptoms are intentionally induced, nor do they include psychological factors affecting a medical condition, as the symptoms cannot be accounted for by any medical disorder.

ICD-10[66] (section F45.4) describes persistent somatoform pain disorder.

> The predominant complaint is of persistent, severe and distressing pain, which cannot be explained fully by a physiological process or physical disorder, and which occurs in association with emotional conflict or psychosocial problems that are sufficient to allow the conclusion that they are the main causative influences. The result is usually a marked increase in support and attention, either personal or medical.

In DSM-IV[65] it states that 'psychological factors are judged to have an important role in its (the pain's) onset, severity, exacerbation or maintenance'. This definition perhaps changes the focus slightly by not *requiring* the psychological factors to have a role in causation. As we will see later, cognitive therapists working in this area have drawn heavily on work from the field of the anxiety disorders to develop maintenance models for these disorders.

Approximately 20% of new consultations in primary care relate to somatic symptoms for which no cause can be found and it appears that pain is a common presenting symptom of emotional disorder.[67] While most of these unexplained symptoms are transient, 20% of them are distressing and persistent with a resultant resource issue.[68] Many hospital specialists will see patients with medically unexplained symptoms: e.g. atypical chest pain presenting to cardiologists, headache to neurologists and irritable bowel syndrome to gastroenterologists.

Katon *et al.*[69] report a case series of distressed, high utilisers of primary care services. The DSM-IV[65] criteria for somatisation disorder require more than 12 medically unexplained symptoms from various body systems. Katon *et al.*[69] found that patients with fewer medically unexplained symptoms still have significant clinical and behavioural features of somatisation. Furthermore, an increasing number of medically unexplained symptoms was associated with higher lifetime rates of panic disorder and major depression. They suggest that somatisation should be viewed as a continuum.

Chronic pain is a common symptom in older people presenting to health services in both primary and secondary care. The *Oxford Concise Medical Dictionary*[70] defines pain as 'an unpleasant sensation ranging from mild discomfort to agonising distress, associated with real or potential tissue damage. Pain is a response to impulses from peripheral nerves in damaged tissue'. However, despite advances in medical technology the evidence for a link between pain and tissue damage is often limited. Jensen *et al.*[71] report that many people with abnormalities on magnetic resonance imaging (MRI) do not report pain. On the other hand, Spitzer *et al.*[72] report that many people who report back pain have no identifiable pathology. Indeed Fordyce[73] suggests that 'fewer than 15% of persons with back pain can be assigned to one of the categories of specific low back pain'.

It has also long been recognised that physical pathology does not perfectly predict pain severity and that different people respond in a variety of ways to chronic pain.[74] Banks and Kerns[75] found that rates of depression in patients with persistent pain were high (30–54%) and it appears that this association is mediated by psychosocial variables such as perceived life control.[76]

So it would certainly appear that medically unexplained symptoms, especially pain, are common and disabling. The introduction of the Gate Control Theory of pain[77] opened the way for the use of words such as 'emotional experience' as a description of pain, acknowledging the influence of psychological variables. It proposed that rather than a simple mechanism of receptors that transmit noxious stimuli via afferent nerve fibres from the periphery to the spinal cord, the gate control mechanism receives a balance of afferent fibres of different types in addition to efferent fibres that can modulate the subject's experience. This complex theory allows an explanation of situations where the subject denies pain despite obvious tissue damage as well as situations where pain is experienced despite transection of pain pathways at numerous levels.

There is a vast amount written on the subject of pain and this chapter can only look at a small proportion of published studies. Evidence from the cognitive literature suggests that a number of factors are important in the maintenance of mood disorder, functional impairment and pain in such patients. I have tried to pick out a few studies that look at the concepts important in the model presented later.

Rosenstiel and Keefe[78] found that cognitive and behavioural coping strategies are commonly used but not particularly effective in giving patients a sense of control over their pain or reducing the pain. They found that catastrophising (e.g. 'I worry all the time about whether it will end') was related to poorer emotional adjustment in terms of anxiety and depression ratings, but not pain ratings. Geisser et al.[79] went on to suggest that 'catastrophising may be more important than depression in terms of how chronic pain patients ultimately evaluate their pain experience and may impact on how they cope with chronic pain.'

Two studies by Williams[80,81] examined beliefs about pain and found that patients who believed strongly that their pain would persist were poorly compliant with both physical and behavioural interventions. Patients who believed their pain to be mysterious exhibited more psychological distress, more somatisation and poorer compliance.

Eccleston[82] looked at the importance of attention. He suggests that any task pitted in competition with pain must be one that demands higher controlled attention, as pain seems designed to gain access to consciousness by interrupting all other current processing. Intensity (as shown in this study) and quality of the pain are also likely to be important in the pain's success in capturing attention. Eccleston[82] therefore goes on to ask, not whether distraction works, but under what conditions does it work? He raises concerns about patients with chronic pain being encouraged to use distractional coping strategies. A task that is sufficiently demanding of attention may be effortful and tiring. Once used repeatedly a task will require less central resource, thereby allowing pain to enter consciousness. Avoidant strategies may not only be ineffective but may have 'adverse and maladaptive effects'. Indeed Rosenstiel and Keefe[78] showed that patients who diverted attention or prayed had more pain and functional impairment. Eccleston[82] suggests that focusing on the pain and redefining its meaning may be a more effective way forward.

Asmundson et al.[83,84] examined fear of pain and found that it appeared to predict functional impairment. Vlaeyen et al.[85] examined how fear of movement/(re)injury relates to behavioural performance and various other variables in chronic low back pain patients. Included in the study were 103 patients with chronic low back pain who either had minimal organic findings or symptoms disproportionate to the demonstrable organic findings. When gender, pain intensity and compensation status were controlled for, the authors found a correlation between catastrophising and to a lesser extent depression and fear of movement/(re)injury. They moved on to examine whether fear of movement/(re)injury is related to behavioural performance. With a smaller number of patients they went on to expose subjects to a simple motor activity and found that indeed the patients with the higher fear of injury avoided motor activity more.

Sharp[86] proposes a cognitive-behavioural model (*see* Figure 9.1), which suggests that the problems a patient experiences in association with pain originate in the way the patient reacts to the pain. Reactions are defined as all forms of cognition, including imagery (not just observable behaviours). Thus distress or disability are determined more by appraisal and interpretation rather than sensory activity.

As indicated in Figure 9.1, there are a number of feedback loops that can lead to maintenance of the distress, disability and autonomic arousal, even in the absence of the original sensory stimulus. The model builds on the work of Salkovskis[87] in suggesting that safety behaviours may prevent disconfirmation of beliefs regarding pain and disability. Meanwhile anxiety and distress may maintain autonomic arousal, potentially confirming more negative interpretations. Sharp[86] suggests that affective disorders may lead to cognitive errors and negative appraisals being more likely, thus further maintaining the problem. Sharp[86] also alludes to the possible relevance of meta-cognitions, worries a patient has regarding pain,[88] and the possibility that cognitive coping strategies to suppress these worries may themselves be safety behaviours.

The model includes iatrogenic factors. These may be relevant because of side-effects or physiological responses to medication or investigations. The meaning of these symptoms for the patient may further confirm negative appraisals. These factors are thus added to the patient's evaluation of the doctor's behaviour in recommending the tests or medication in the first place. Kouyanou *et al.*[89] and Pither and Nicholas[90] support the view that doctors may inadvertently reinforce patients' anxieties and reinforce disability and a passive approach by accepting requests for further investigations or treatments.

The model is a complicated one and this may affect its utility. It would certainly be hard to develop this with a patient. However, the model certainly addresses many of the issues raised by the evidence put forward earlier. Perhaps it would be helpful to see more emphasis placed on cognitive coping strategies, especially given the wealth of studies that have looked at this area. The cognitive aspects of the model are lumped together as appraisals and evaluation. It is clear how beliefs about pain are incorporated but perhaps less so with respect to coping strategies. However, the use of so many feedback loops helps to illustrate the complicated nature of the problem and, clinically, individual maintenance cycles may be drawn out and addressed in therapy. Obviously, the utility of the model depends on the response to treatment obtained by patients and trials are required to test this.

In developing a similar cognitive model for somatoform disorders, Looper and Kirmayer[91] suggest that the various diagnoses that make up the somatoform disorders 'involve common processes of bodily preoccupation and symptom

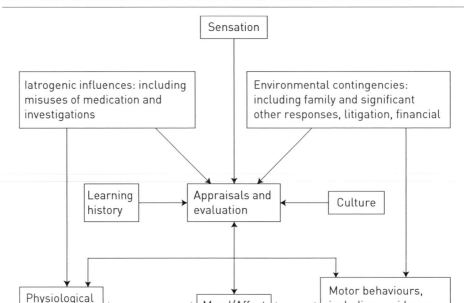

FIGURE 9.1 The reformulated cognitive-behavioural model of chronic pain.[86]

amplification', making it useful to conceptualise them together. They describe similar factors to Sharp[86] but perhaps stress more the interpersonal factors that may be important, as the reactions of others, particularly those in a caring role, may reinforce patterns of behaviour.

Approaches to engagement/management

One of the biggest issues in the treatment of patients with medically unexplained symptoms is the tendency of people, both professional and lay, to talk in terms of the mind/body split. If there is no demonstrable physical cause for symptoms then they must be 'all in the mind'. This creates a challenge for patients and professionals alike. Despite good evidence from systematic reviews that treatments work (CBT[92] and antidepressants[93]), there is also evidence that professionals are reluctant to refer.[64] Also, many patients are reluctant to consider engaging with mental health professionals. This tends to lead to a reliance on physical treatments that appear to have limited benefit, at least from the point of view of functioning. For example, 20% or fewer of lumbar surgery patients return to work.[94] Patients with chronic pain are often prescribed strong analgesics but there is emerging evidence that opioids rarely improve physical or emotional functioning (Turk, in press). There is now evidence that cognitive processes are important. CBT appears to lead to improvements in mood and daily activity by decreasing fear and avoidance. It appears that pain itself may be of limited importance in terms of functional recovery and a couple of studies have found that changes in pain or physical capacity accounted for relatively little or no variance in functional outcomes.[95,96] Furthermore, among patients referred to a pain clinic, the strongest predictors of satisfaction were: perceiving that the evaluation was complete, feeling they received an explanation for treatment and believing that treatment improved daily activity.[97]

So, one of the main issues seems to be developing a formulation with the patient, using the concepts described above, to shift their focus away from unhelpful medical investigations and treatments, towards an alternative perspective that looks more at functional outcomes than merely symptoms. Clearly, this can be a difficult process for many patients and doctors. It is obviously important that the patient feels that their symptoms are assessed and investigated appropriately. However, it is also important that this process is logical and has an appropriate end-point. A succession of normal investigations or unsuccessful symptomatic treatments gives the message that a definite diagnosis and/or cure are around the corner if only they are patient enough. This tends to shift the patient's focus more towards physical symptoms and in turn is likely to lead to further functional impairment and deterioration in affective symptoms. To reverse this trend it is important to engage not only the patient but also carers and doctors in agreeing a more helpful approach. (Although in older people inter-current health problems very frequently complicate this process.)

Even if there is no medical explanation for the symptom, the symptom is still there and distressing for the patient. This needs to be acknowledged as many patients will have had the experience of not feeling believed. Once the patient feels that they have been understood and that they have an understanding of how these various factors impact on their experience there is a greater chance of breaking the cycle of unhelpful medical interventions. It may then be possible to engage the patient in eliciting goals that are in keeping with their values and this in turn helps to focus work on areas of functional impairment rather than constantly focusing on symptom levels.

It seems likely that the concepts discussed here in relation to medically unexplained symptoms may still be useful in the management of patients with medically explained symptoms. Just because we are unable to discover a cause for a symptom it does not mean that the level of functional impairment experienced is not amenable to change.

KEY POINTS

▶ Depression is common in physically ill older people, particularly in Parkinson's disease and after stroke.

▶ Depression is associated with poor physical outcomes; in particular depression is an independent risk factor for myocardial infarction.

▶ One should have a high index of suspicion when assessing physically ill older people in whom psychological symptoms, such as guilt and hopelessness, appear to differentiate better than somatic symptoms, between the depressed and non-depressed.

▶ In chronic pain, beliefs in a mind/body split among both patients and professionals lead to a reliance on physical treatments that appear to have limited benefit, at least from the point of view of functioning.

▶ Even if there is no medical explanation for a symptom, the symptom is still there, is distressing for the patient and needs to be acknowledged. Once the patient feels that they have been understood and that they have an understanding of how these various factors impact on their experience there is a greater chance of breaking the cycle of unhelpful medical interventions.

REFERENCES

1 George LK, Okun MA, Landerman R. Age as a moderator of the determinants of life satisfaction. *Res Aging.* 1985; **7**: 209–33.

2 Herzog AR, Rodgers WL. Age and satisfaction: data from several large surveys. *Res Aging.* 1981; **3**: 142–65.

3 Carp FM, Carp A. Test of a model of domain satisfactions and well-being: equity considerations. *Res Aging.* 1982; **4**: 503–22.

4 Hagerty MR. Social comparisons of income in one's community: evidence from national surveys of income and happiness. *J Pers Soc Psychol.* 2000; **78**: 764–71.

5 The Royal College of Psychiatrists. *Who Cares Wins.* 2005. Available from: http://www. rcpsych.ac.uk/PDF/WhoCaresWins.pdf

6 Holmes J, House A. Psychiatric illness predicts poor outcome after surgery for hip fracture: a prospective cohort study. *Psychol Med.* 2000; **30**: 921–9.

7 Ingold BB, Yersin B, Weitlisbach V, *et al.* Characteristics associated with inappropriate hospital use in elderly patients admitted to a general medicine service. *Aging-Clin Exper Res.* 2000; **12**: 430–8.

8 Nightingale S, Holmes J, Mason J, *et al.* Psychiatric illness and mortality after hip fracture. *Lancet.* 2001; **357**: 1264–5.

9 Magaziner J, Simonsick EM, Kashner TM, *et al.* Predictors of functional recovery one year following hospital discharge for hip fracture: a prospective study. *J Gerontol.* 1990; **45**: M101–7.

10 Covinsky KE, Kahana E, Chin MH, *et al.* Depressive symptoms and 3 year mortality in older hospitalised medical patients. *Ann Int Med.* 1999; **130**: 563–9.

11 Covinsky KE, Firtinsky RH, Palmer RM, *et al.* Relation between symptoms of depression and Health Status Outcomes in acutely ill hospitalised older persons. *Ann Int Med.* 1997; **126**: 417–25.

12 Afken CL, Lichtenberg PA, Tancer ME. Cognitive impairment and depression predict mortality in medically ill older adults. *J Geront Series A-Bio Sci Med Sci.* 1999; **54**: M152–6.

13 Bula CJ, Weitlisbach V, Burnand B, *et al.* Depressive symptoms as a predictor of 6 month outcomes and service utilisation in elderly medical inpatients. *Arch Int Med.* 2001; **161**: 2609–15.

14 Inouye SK, Peduzzi PN, Robison JT, *et al.* Importance of functional measures in predicting mortality among older hospitalised patients. *JAMA.* 1998; **279**: 1187–93.

15 Ganzini L, Smith DM, Fenn DS, *et al.* Depression and mortality in medically ill older adults. *J Am Geriatr Soc.* 1997; **45**: 307–12.

16 Yusuf S, Hawken S, Ounpuu S, *et al.* Effect of potentially modifiable risk factors associated with myocardial infarction in 52 countries (the INTERHEART Study): case-control study. *Lancet.* 2004; **364**: 937–52.

17 Abramson J, Berger A, Krumholz HM, *et al.* Depression and risk of heart failure among older persons with isolated systolic hypertension. *Arch Int Med.* 2001; **161**: 1725–30.

18 Bonnet F, Irving K, Terra JL, *et al.* Anxiety and depression are associated with unhealthy lifestyle in patients at risk of cardiovascular disease. *Atherosclerosis.* 2005; **178**: 339–44.

19 Otte C, Marmar CR, Pipkin SS, *et al.* Depression and 24-hour urinary cortisol in medical out-patients with coronary heart disease: The Heart and Soul Study. *Biol Psychiatr.* 2004; **56**(4): 241–7.

20 Burke HM, Davis MC, Otte C, *et al.* Depression and cortisol responses to psychological stress: a meta-analysis. *Psychoneuroendocrinol.* 2005; **30**(9): 846–56.

21 Serebruany VL, Glassman AH, Malinin AI, *et al.* Enhanced platelet/endothelial activation in depressed patients with acute coronary syndromes: evidence from recent clinical trials. *Blood Coagul Fibrinolysis.* 2003; **14**(6): 563–7.

22 Empana JP, Sykes DH, Luc G, *et al.* Contributions of depressive mood and circulating inflammatory markers to coronary heart disease in healthy European men: the Prospective Epidemiological Study of Myocardial Infarction (PRIME). *Circulation.* 2005; **111**(18): 2299–305.

23 Carney RM, Blumenthal JA, Stein PK, *et al.* Depression, heart rate variability, and acute myocardial infarction. *Circulation.* 2001; **104**(17): 2024–8.

24 Clarke DC, Cavanaugh SVA, Gibbons RD. The core symptoms of depression in medical and psychiatric patients. *J Nerv and Ment Disord.* 1983; **171**: 705–13.

25 Hodkinson HM. Evaluation of a mental test score for assessment of mental impairment in the elderly. *Age Ageing.* 1972; **1**: 233–8.

26 Folstein MF, Folstein SE, Hugh PR. 'Mini-Mental State': a practical method for grading the cognitive state of patients for the clinician. *J Psychiatr Res.* 1975; **12**: 189–98.

27 Yesavage JA, Brink TL, Rose TL, *et al.* Development and evaluation of a geriatric depression screening scale: a preliminary report. *J Psychiatr Res.* 1983; **17**: 37–9.

28 Zigmund AS, Snaith RP. The Hospital Anxiety and Depression Scale. *Acta Psychiatr Scand.* 1983; **67**: 361–7.

29 Beck AT, Ward CH, Mendelson M, *et al.* An inventory for measuring depression. *Arch Gen Psychiatr.* 1961; **31**: 319–25.

30 Goldberg DP, Blackwell B. Psychiatric illness in general practice: a detailed study of a new method of case identification. *BMJ.* 1970; **1**(5707): 439–43.

31 Robertson MM, Katona CLE. *Depression and Physical Illness.* Perspectives in Psychiatry Volume 6. Chichester: Wiley; 1997. pp. 10–11.

32 Goldberg D. Use of the General Health Questionnaire in clinical work. *BMJ.* 1986; **293**: 1188–9.

33 Aarsland D, Larsen JP, Lim NG, *et al.* Range of neuropsychiatric disturbances in patients with Parkinson's disease. *J Neurol Neurosurg Psychiatr.* 1999; **67**(4): 492–6.

34 Slaughter JR, Slaughter KA, Nichols D, *et al.* Prevalence, clinical manifestations, aetiology and treatment of depression in Parkinson's disease. *J Neuropsychiatr Clin Neurosci.* 2001; **13**: 187–96.

35 Mindham R. Psychiatric aspects of Parkinson's disease. *Br J Hosp Med.* 1974; **11**: 411–4.

36 Celesia G, Wanamaker W. Psychiatric disturbances in Parkinson's disease. *Dis Nerv Syst.* 1972; **33**: 577–83.

37 Horn S. Some psychological factors in Parkinsonism. *J Neurol Neurosurg Psychiatr.* 1974; **37**: 27–31.

38 Gotham A, Brown R, Marsden C. Depression in Parkinson's disease: a quantitative and qualitative analysis. *J Neurol Neurosurg Psychiatr.* 1986; **49**: 381–9.

39 Tandeberg E, Larsen JP, Aarsland D, *et al.* Risk factors for depression in Parkinson's disease. *Arch Neurol.* 1997; **54**(5): 625–30.

40 Pluck GC, Brown RG. Apathy in Parkinson's disease. *J Neurol Neurosurg Psychiatr.* 2002; **73**: 636–42.

41 Richard IH, Kurlan R. A survey of antidepressant use in Parkinson's disease. *Neurology.* 1997; **49**: 1168–70.

42 Royal Pharmaceutical Society. *British National Formulary (52: 4.3.4).* London: BMJ Publishing/RPS Publishing; 2006.

43 Cummings JL. Depression and Parkinson's disease: a review. *Am J Psychiatr.* 1992; **149**(4): 443–54.

44 Emre M, Aarsland D, Albanese A, *et al.* Rivastigmine for dementia associated with Parkinson's disease. *NEJM.* 2004; **351**(24): 2509–18.

45 Fabbrini G, Barbanti P, Aurilia C, *et al.* Donepezil in the treatment of hallucinations and delusions in Parkinson's disease. *Neurol Sci.* 2002; **23**(1): 41–3.

46 Pakrasi S, Mukaetova-Ladinska EB, McKeith IG, *et al.* Clinical predictors of response to acetyl cholinesterase inhibitors: experience from routine clinical use in Newcastle. *Int J Geriatr Psychiatr.* 2003; **18**(10): 879–86.

47 Cole K, Vaughan FL. The feasibility of using cognitive therapy for depression associated with Parkinson's disease: a literature review. *Parkinsonism Relat Disord.* 2005; **11**(5): 269–76.

48 Knapp P, House A. Depression after stroke. In: Copeland J, Abou-Saleh M, Blazer D, editors. *Principles and Practice of Geriatric Psychiatry.* 2nd ed. John Wiley and Sons; 2002.

49 Kotila M, Numminen H, Waltimo O, *et al.* Depression after stroke: results of the FINSTROKE Study. *Stroke.* 1998; **29**: 368–72.

50 Pohjasvaara T, Leppavuori A, Siira I, *et al.* Frequency and clinical determinants of poststroke depression. *Stroke.* 1998; **29**: 2311–17.

51 Burvill PW, Johnson GA, Jamrozik KD, *et al.* Prevalence of depression after stroke: the Perth Community Stroke Study. *Br J Psychiatr.* 1995; **166**(3): 320–7.

52 Carson AJ, MacHale S, Allen K, *et al.* Depression after stroke and lesion location: a systematic review. *Lancet.* 2000; **356**(9224): 122–6.

53 Pohjasvaara T, Vataja R, Leppavuori A, *et al.* Depression is an independent predictor of poor long-term functional outcome post-stroke. *Eur J Neurol.* 2001; **8**(4): 315–9.

54 House A, Knapp P, Bamford J, *et al.* Mortality at 12 and 24 months after stroke may be associated with depressive symptoms at 1 month. *Stroke.* 2001; **32**(3): 696–701.

55 Andersen G, Vestergaard K, Ingemann-Nielsen M, *et al.* Risk factors for post-stroke depression. *Acta Psychiatr Scand.* 1995; **92**(3): 193–8.

56 Hackett ML, Anderson CS, House AO. Interventions for treating depression after stroke. *Cochrane Database of Systematic Reviews.* 2004; **3**. Available from: http://www.cochrane.org/reviews/en/ab003437.html

57 Hackett ML, Anderson CS, House AO. Management of depression after stroke: a systematic review of pharmacological therapies. *Stroke.* 2005; **36**(5): 1098–103.

58 Lincoln NB, Flannaghan T. Cognitive behavioural therapy for depression following stroke: a randomised controlled trial. *Stroke.* 2003; **34**(1): 111–15.

59 Knapp P, Young J, House A, *et al.* Non-drug strategies to resolve psycho-social difficulties after stroke. *Age Ageing.* 2000; **29**: 23–30.

60 Calvert T, Knapp P, House A. Psychological associations with emotionalism after stroke. *J Neurol Neurosurg Psychiatr.* 1998; **65**(6): 928–9.

61 Andersen G. Treatment of uncontrolled crying after stroke. *Drugs Aging.* 1995; **6**(2): 105–11.

62 Nimnuan C, Hotopf M, Wessely S. Medically unexplained symptoms: an epidemiological study in seven specialities. *J Psychosom Res.* 2001; **51**(1): 361–7.

63 Sheehan B, Bass C, Briggs R, *et al.* Somatization among older primary care attenders. *Psychol Med.* 2003; **33**(5): 867–77.

64 Sheehan B, Bass C, Briggs R, *et al.* Do general practitioners believe that their older patients' physical symptoms are somatized? *J Psychosom Res.* 2004; **56**(3): 313–6.

65 American Psychiatric Association. *Diagnostic and Statistical Manual of Mental Disorders (DSM-IV).* 4th ed. Washington, DC: American Psychiatric Association; 1994.

66 World Health Organization. *International Classification of Diseases 10: classification of mental and behavioural disorders.* Geneva: World Health Organization; 1994.

67 Bridges KW, Goldberg DP. Somatic presentations of DSM III psychiatric disorders in primary care. *J Psychosom Res.* 1985; **29**: 563–9.

68 Kroenke K, Mangelsdorff D. Common symptoms in ambulatory care: incidence, evaluation, therapy and outcome. *Am J Med.* 1989; **86**: 262–6.

69 Katon W, Lin E, Von Korff M, *et al.* Somatization: a spectrum of severity. *Am J Psychiatr.* 1991; **148**: 1: 34–40.

70 Martin EA. *Oxford Concise Medical Dictionary.* Oxford: Oxford University Press; 2003. p. 503.

71 Jensen M, Brant-Zawadzki M, Obuchowski N, *et al.* Magnetic resonance imaging of the lumbar spine in people without back pain. *NEJM.* 1994; **331**: 69–73.

72 Spitzer W, LeBlanc F, *et al.* Scientific approach to the assessment and management of activity-related spinal disorders: report of the Quebec Task Force on Spinal Disorders. *Spine.* 1987; **12**: 7S (European ed. Suppl. 1), S1–59.

73 Fordyce W. *Back Pain in the Workplace: management of disability in non-specific conditions.* Seattle: IASP Press; 1995.

74 Turk D. Biopsychosocial perspective on chronic pain. In: Gatchel R, Turk D, editors. *Psychological Approaches to Pain Management: a practitioner's handbook.* New York: Guilford Press; 1996.

75 Banks S, Kerns R. Explaining high rates of depression in chronic pain: a diathesis-stress framework. *Psychol Bull.* 1996; **119**: 95–110.

76 Rudy T, Kerns R, Turk D. Chronic pain and depression: toward a cognitive-behavioural mediation model. *Pain.* 1988; **35**: 129–40.

77 Melzack R, Wall P. Pain mechanisms: a new theory. *Science.* 1965; **50**: 971–9.

78 Rosenstiel AK, Keefe FJ. The use of coping strategies in chronic low back pain patients: relationship to patient characteristics and current adjustment. *Pain.* 1983; **17**: 33–44.

79 Geisser ME, Robinson ME, Keefe FJ, *et al.* Catastrophising, depression and the sensory, affective and evaluative aspects of chronic pain. *Pain.* 1994; **59**: 79–83.

80 Williams DA, Keefe FJ. Pain beliefs and the use of cognitive-behavioural coping strategies. *Pain.* 1991; **46**: 185–90.

81 Williams DA, Thorn BE. An empirical assessment of pain beliefs. *Pain.* 1989; **36**: 351–8.

82 Eccleston C. Chronic pain and distraction: an experimental investigation into the role of sustained and shifting attention in the processing of chronic persistent pain. *Behav Res Ther.* 1995; **33**: 4, 391–405.

83 Asmundson GJG, Kuperos JL, Norton GR. Do patients with chronic pain selectively attend to pain-related information?: preliminary evidence for the mediating role of fear. *Pain.* 1997; **72**: 27–32.

84 Asmundson GJG, Norton GR, Allerdings MD. Fear and avoidance in dysfunctional chronic back pain patients. *Pain.* 1997; **69**: 231–36.

85 Vlaeyen JWS, Kole-Snijders AMJ, Boeren RGB, *et al.* Fear of movement/(re)injury in chronic low back pain and its relation to behavioural performance. *Pain.* 1995; **62**: 363–72.

86 Sharp TJ. Chronic pain: a reformulation of the cognitive-behavioural model. *Behav Res Ther.* 2001; **39**: 787–800.

87 Salkovskis P. The importance of behaviour in the maintenance of anxiety and panic: a cognitive account. *Behav Psychother.* 1991; **19**: 6–19.

88 Wells A. Meta-cognition and worry: a cognitive model of generalised anxiety disorder. *Behav Cog Psychother.* 1995; **23**: 265–80.

89 Kouyanou K, Pither CE, Rabe-Hesketh S, *et al.* A comparative study of iatrogenesis, medication abuse, and psychiatric morbidity in chronic pain patients with and without medically explained symptoms. *Pain.* 1998; **76**: 417–26.

90 Pither C, Nicholas M. The identification of iatrogenic factors in the development of chronic pain syndromes: abnormal treatment behaviour? In: Bond MR, Charlton JE, Woolf CJ, editors. *Proceedings of the Fifth World Congress on Pain.* Amsterdam: Elsevier Science Publishers; 1991.

91 Looper K, Kirmayer L. Behavioural medicine approaches to somatoform disorders. *J Consult Clin Psychol.* 2002; **70**(3): 810–27.

92 Kroenke K, Swindle R. Cognitive behavioural therapy for somatisation and symptom syndromes: a critical review of controlled clinical trials. *Psychother Psychosomat.* 2000; **69**(4): 205–15.

93 O'Malley PG, Jackson JL, Santoro J, *et al.* Antidepressant therapy for unexplained symptoms and symptom syndromes. *J Fam Prac.* 1999; **48**(12): 980–90.

94 Franklin GM, Haug J, Heyer NJ, *et al.* Outcome of lumbar fusion in Washington State workers' compensation. *Spine.* 1994; **19**(17): 1897–903.

95 McCracken LM, Faber SD, Janeck AS. Pain-related anxiety predicts non-specific physical complaints in persons with chronic pain. *Behav Res Ther.* 1998; **36**: 621–30.

96 McCracken LM, Gross RT, Eccleston C. Multimethod assessment of treatment process in chronic low back pain: comparison of reported pain-related anxiety with directly measured physical capacity. *Behav Res Ther.* 2002; **40**(5): 585–94.

97 McCracken LM, Evon D, Karapas-Eleftheria T. Satisfaction with treatment for chronic pain in a specialty service: preliminary prospective results. *Eur J Pain.* 2002; **6**(5): 387–93.

CHAPTER 10

Depression in primary care

STEPHEN ILIFFE

Introduction

Depression appears pervasive, being the most common mental health problem of later life, affecting approximately 15% of older people (when defined broadly), but fortunately only 2% (about the same prevalence as diabetes or schizophrenia) when considered in its most severe form. Every general practitioner or practice nurse will be encountering depressed older patients on a daily basis, either because they seek help for symptoms related to their depression, or because their depression is an aspect of long-term conditions monitored and managed in primary care.[1,2,5] Tiredness, sleep disturbance, low energy and demotivation are commonplace problems brought to general practitioners by depressed older people, but often as a second layer of symptoms behind the painful joints, shortness of breath or gastrointestinal complaints that dominate their daily life. This ubiquity is problematic for primary care, because it can make us expert in the recognition of and response to depression, as we gain clinical experience over thousands of encounters, or render depressed mood so usual that it comes to be seen as normal, particularly when associated with age.

The housebound are twice as likely to experience depression as more mobile older people,[5] a fact that needs to be remembered at every home visit, while those living in sheltered accommodation may have a prevalence of depression closer to one in four.[6] High rates of depression are found among users of home care services,[7] and older people who have just moved into a care home are particularly at risk of developing depression.[8] Both these associations should be part of the tacit knowledge of social care managers and providers, as well as the community and care home nursing staff that are the main clinical support for depressed older people. There is also some evidence that mistreatment and neglect in older people, including self-neglect, are associated with depression,[10] a factor that can be overlooked in the need to protect vulnerable individuals from harm.

Poverty and depression go together[10] and although poorer and less educated older people have no monopoly of depression, they are less likely to seek help or treatment for it.[11] The first wave of the English Longitudinal Study of Ageing (ELSA),[12] found that depression was widely associated with the key dimensions of social exclusion. In each of the dimensions of social exclusion (age itself, living alone, being in poor health, being from an ethnic minority and having a low income – but not limited possession of material goods) being depressed was strongly related to the likelihood of having a poor quality of life. Finally, depression particularly affects those older people caring for others, making carers an important group to identify in primary care.

Untreated, depression shortens life and increases healthcare costs, as well adding to disability from medical illnesses.[13] It seems to increase mortality from all causes,[14] and is the leading cause of suicide among older people.[15] Suicide is associated with physical illness in older age groups, rather than with the substance abuse and personality disorder that characterise younger cohorts.[16] High and rising rates of suicide among older adults – particularly men – are a worldwide phenomenon,[17,18] and the increasing incidence of depression in recent cohorts portends ominously for future generations of older adults. Late-life depression is also associated with higher than expected morbidity, disability and mortality from a wide range of natural causes.[19] One large-scale community study has shown that the relative risks of both all-cause mortality and cardiovascular mortality are highest in depressed individuals with established heart disease, but are also elevated in those with no evidence of cardiovascular pathology at entry to the study.[20] Depression is one of the main risk factors for sudden death up to one year after myocardial infarction, after adjustment for other risk factors,[21] and also predicts a poorer outcome after life-threatening illness like subarachnoid haemorrhage, pulmonary embolism or bleeding peptic ulcer, even allowing for illness severity.[21]

Depression in later life is associated with high use of both medical and social services,[23] making it an important issue for commissioners hoping to contain expenditure, and depressed older people are more likely to be treated for anxiety (or physical symptoms like pain) than with antidepressants or psychological therapies. Depression is pervasive in many senses, being connected to physical illness, poverty, disability and living circumstances, as well as being widespread in the older population. The impact of depression, and its associations with illness and disability, are now recognised in the NHS contract with general practice. Within the Quality Outcomes Framework (QOF) depression is not only identified as a disorder that needs to be identified, treated and monitored in its own right, but also in its relationship to heart disease, COPD and diabetes. This pervasiveness also gives us some clues about why responding to depression in later life can be difficult, but first we must think about the course of this disorder.

Prognosis

Depression in later life has a poor prognosis, with a chronic relapsing course.[24] A study from the Netherlands showed that among depressed older people attending general practice a third remitted without relapse after one year, a quarter remitted but relapsed and 40% remained chronically depressed.[25] However, this poor prognosis does not mean that recognition and response to depression in older people is pointless, because when depression is treated in older people, their quality of life improves.[26] The relapsing nature of depression in later life is a problem only if we see it as a homogeneous and curable disease; once we accept it as a spectrum of potentially long-term conditions, each with a variable course – variable enough to be experienced as remissions and relapses – then working with depressed older people gets easier.

Most depression is treated entirely in primary care,[27] but there is evidence of poor detection[28,29,30] and less than optimal treatment[31] among older adults. For example, community studies show consistent under-documenting of depression in medical records when compared with depression prevalence,[32] and 'physical' symptoms of depression may simply not be recognised for what they are.[33] Only a small minority of depressed older individuals with significant symptoms receive treatment or referral, even though their general practitioners frequently recognise their depressed state.[34] The severity of the depression and high levels of anxiety seem to be triggers for referral,[35] but as a whole it seems true to say that depression in later life is underestimated, under-diagnosed and probably under-treated. Both general practitioners and hospital doctors have been criticised for their tendency to miss depression in their patients,[36] but as we shall see the presentation and pattern of depression in older people in the community are so complex, and the uncertainties about the effectiveness of intervention so great, that under-diagnosis is almost assured. That is not to say that we cannot do better, and become more adept at seeing the depressive symptoms woven into a dense pattern of problems.

Most older patients with depression consult their general practitioner with a combination of physical and psychological symptoms, and more often than not depression is intertwined with other aspects of everyday life. The older woman disabled with arthritis of the lower spine, whose life has become restricted by pain and immobility, may also be struggling with events like the acrimonious divorce of one of her children, while also caring for a spouse with disabilities worse than her own. Her tiredness, pain, sleep disturbance and irritability seem to her to be the common ground for the different losses in her life, holding together her difficulties in an understandable pattern, rather than being an entity worth attending to in its own right. The older widower who finds himself increasingly alone as his friends die, and whose heart failure limits his ability to get about, may

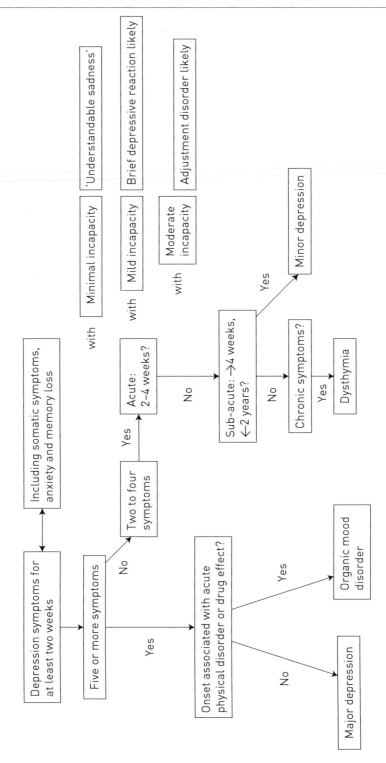

FIGURE 10.1 A map of late-life depression.

think that his low mood and loss of enthusiasm for life are entirely understandable and even appropriate, saying: 'What can I expect at my age?' These perspectives are important, and no general practitioner or practice nurse will get away with contradicting them, for they are the explanatory models that facilitate or impede self-care and the self-management of persistent problems, including depression. Equally, no primary care professional should accept them as the only explanatory model, and leave them unchallenged. At the very least an open discussion is needed about where depression – if it can be accepted as a distinct problem at all – fits into the everyday experience of the individual. To have that discussion clinicians need to have their own explanatory model, detailed and complex enough to match their patient's reality. This chapter is an attempt to outline such a model, both for primary care professionals and for specialists who are expected to provide guidance, education and training in the management of common disorders like depression,[37] knowing that collaboration between general practitioners and specialists is associated with better treatment outcomes for depression.[38,39]

The challenge for general practice

Let us start from first principles. The continuity of care that general practice still offers permits long-term care and commitment, and treatment can be given in a more familiar environment without stigmatising the patient.[40] Recognition and management of depression in older people do seem appropriate tasks for general practice, especially given the scale and pervasive impact of depression. However, four things get in the way of identifying depressed older people and initiating treatment: recognition can be difficult, acceptance of the diagnosis or any treatment may be contested, resources for any therapy other than medication may be limited, and awareness of the poor prognosis may inhibit action.

Recognition of depression in later life can be a problem in the community because the typical features of depressed mood or sadness may not be evident,[41] or may be masked by anxiety, cognitive disturbance or somatic complaints.[42] Sleep disturbance, failure to care for oneself, withdrawal from social life, appetite disturbance and 'joylessness',[43] unexplainable somatic symptoms or hopelessness about a coexisting physical disorder may be the clues to depression, which might be best understood by both patient and practitioner as a physical disorder with emotional symptoms and an unclear biochemical basis.[44,45]

Most older people with depression symptoms fall into the 'dysphoria' or 'demoralisation syndrome' group where the appropriateness of the clinical label of depression may be contested by patients and their families, often because the depression is associated with other problems, and where the effectiveness of treatments is less clear than in major depression, which is clearly amenable to treatment. It may be useful to consider late-life depression as a spectrum rather than a series of discrete diagnostic categories. For example, many so-called 'sub-threshold' (minor) depressions (*see* later) appear to be cases of incompletely resolved depressive episodes.[46] This spectrum can be visualised as a map, as shown in Figure 10.1, in which chronicity and severity (both in numbers of symptoms and their impact) are used to distinguish between subtypes of late-life depression.

Organic mood disorder is particularly important in general practice, given the salience of the disorders and medications that cause it. It is diagnosed when there is a direct link between the onset of depression and either a systemic or neurological condition or an ingested substance or drug. There are a large number of conditions which may act in this way, the most common being cancer, stroke, Parkinson's disease, hip fracture, myocardial infarction, heart failure, chronic obstructive pulmonary disease and asthma.[46] The prevalence of organic depressive disorder caused or aggravated by medication is not known, but it has been estimated that beta-blockers alone could account for 1–10% of depressive disorders in older people.[48] Alcohol can precipitate or prolong major depression or depressive symptoms.

Components of good practice

Placing an individual at a point on the map does help the practitioner to consider the best approach to treatment, assuming that common ground can be found between the perspectives of the patient and those of the professional. Although the evidence base is limited compared with that for depression in younger people, recent guidelines suggest the following statements can be made with some confidence.

1 Antidepressant drugs are effective in older patients with depressive episodes.
2 There is evidence for the efficacy of antidepressants in dysthymia and minor depressive disorder of at least four weeks' duration.[49]
3 Antidepressants are effective in depressed patients with a range of physical comorbid conditions, although tolerability varies.
4 There are no important differences in speed of onset of antidepressants, although in general older people take longer to recover than younger adults.[50]
5 Age should not be a barrier to receiving a psychological therapy.[51] With increased knowledge about their efficacy demand for psychological treatments by older people is likely to increase, with more opting for a psychological approach over drug treatment.
6 Psychological treatments such as those recommended by the English National Service Framework for Older People include cognitive behaviour therapy (CBT), interpersonal therapy (IPT) and brief focal analytic psychotherapy. These are effective treatments for depressive disorder in older people but are under-used. Other effective interventions include life review and problem-solving therapy.[52,53]
7 For moderate to severe (non-psychotic) depressive episode treatment which combines antidepressant medication with a psychological intervention such as CBT or IPT is associated with better outcomes than either intervention alone.

8 For adjustment disorder and minor depression (and possibly mild depressive episodes) offering structured support to the patient and caregiver may be effective. The structure involves active listening, weighing options, considering actions and reframing perceptions, and borders on the techniques used in cognitive behaviour therapy. Offering support is not doing nothing, nor is it 'having a chat'. In therapeutic trials quite high rates of symptomatic recovery have been observed in controls groups comprising 'attention' or 'support'.[54]

9 Psychological treatment delivered alongside physical treatment has been shown to be an effective preventive treatment for patients at high risk of relapse. Structured support, delivered by general practitioners and practice nurses, is one (albeit limited) form of such psychological treatment.

The messages for primary care are clear. General practitioners, practice nurses managing chronic diseases, and community nurses seeing the most disabled and dependent older people can and should offer ongoing therapeutic support. General practitioners can offer antidepressant treatment when appropriate, and practice counsellors can offer brief psychological interventions. There is no more rationale for nihilism in the treatment of late-life depression than there is for ignoring osteoarthritis, established heart disease or benign prostatic hypertrophy.

The management of late-life depression

Depression is manageable within everyday routine care, provided that encounters with the depressed older person occur often enough for these general management principles to be implemented.[55]

→ Educating the patient (and caregivers) about depression and involving him/her in treatment decisions.

→ Treating the whole person, including any coexisting physical disorders. This entails: paying attention to sensory deficits and other handicaps; signposting the patient to appropriate social care agencies; and reviewing medication with a view to withdrawing those unnecessary.

→ Treating depressive symptoms with the aim of complete remission (as residual symptoms are a risk factor for chronic depression).

→ Monitoring the risk of self-harm and promptly referring patients who should receive immediate specialist treatment.

Choosing an antidepressant

There is little evidence that one antidepressant is more effective than another. The choice is determined by patient characteristics (such as severity of depression – perhaps favouring tricyclics; safety – favouring newer antidepressants; prior response to a particular agent; tolerability; anticipated side-effects; drug interactions; compliance; and frailty) and by local protocols. In primary care, newer drugs such as the SSRIs have replaced tricyclics as the drugs of first choice. Newer antidepressants are better tolerated than older drugs but the difference is not great. In frail patients it is advisable to commence treatment with a low dose and titrate gradually to the therapeutic dosage range.

Collaborative care

We need to capitalise on and improve the capacity of the existing services used by older people to recognise and respond to late-life depression. Neither education of primary care professionals nor screening of older populations is likely to be effective as stand-alone strategies for enhancing capacity. We have an example from British general practice where use of a validated screening instrument for detecting depression did yield more cases than clinical judgement revealed, but better identification did not seem to lead to more treatment.[56] In a similar American study[57] feedback to primary care physicians about missed depression improved their recognition, but did not alter management. The general practitioners in these studies may have been categorising their patients by perceived treatability, and not initiating any form of therapy or referral for those with 'minor depression' for whom they felt they had no obvious treatment. Despite this evidence some specialist opinion continues to advocate screening of primary care populations.[58]

The most productive approach may be to emphasise the benefits of tailored treatment packages, and to demonstrate their usefulness. From studies of younger people with depression, strategies which have been associated with improved outcomes include the identification of a case manager (for example, a practice nurse) and integrating primary care services with those of specialist mental health services. Some other elements of these models of care have involved telephone support (a relatively low-cost intervention) and improved access to psychiatrists, which is more costly and may be impractical in many places.

Three studies have reported positive outcomes for community dwelling older people. A Community Psychiatric Nurse (CPN) from a specialist mental health team was more effective in the primary care management of depression in older people than usual (general practitioner) treatment[59] and a research psychiatrist implementing a management plan in frail older depressed patients (defined by the amount of home care they received) living at home was more effective than general practitioner treatment alone.[60] In a large randomised multi-centred trial involving 1800 patients aged 60 years or above with either a depressive episode, dysthymia or both, an intervention involving a depression care manager with the deployment of either an antidepressant or problem-solving treatment was significantly more effective than usual GP care.[39]

Conclusions

From the primary care perspective depression is a common relapsing syndrome with a variable pattern of symptoms that can have a disabling effect on older people. Late-life depression should be viewed in the same light as other chronic conditions and care delivered accordingly.[38] Inclusion of depression in relationship to chronic disease in the Quality Outcomes Framework in general practice will be a useful incentive to enhancing the quality of care for depressed older people, if it helps change clinical practice. While late-life depression cannot necessarily be 'cured', it can be reduced, ameliorated and contained, so that the individual's quality of life improves. All treatment approaches start from the provision of psychological support, and can include specific therapies, both pharmacological and psychological. General practitioners and practice and community nurses are pivotal to this process, providing continuity of care, exploring the patient's understanding and perceptions of their problems, providing structured support and engaging other services as necessary. Specialists in community mental health nursing and old age psychiatry can assist with making sense of symptoms and coming to conclusions about the depth and severity of depression, and can advise about the best combinations of therapies. Close working relationships with old age psychiatrists are worth developing and sustaining.

REFERENCES

1 Beekman ATF, Copeland JRM, Prince MJ. Review of community prevalence of depression in later life. *Br J Psychiatr.* 1999; **174**: 307–11.

2 Watts SC, Bhutani GE, Stout IH, *et al.* Mental health in older recipients of primary care services: is depression the key issue? Identification, treatment and the general practitioner. *Int J Geriatr Psychiatr.* 2002; **17**(5): 427–37.

3 Olafsdottir M, Marcusson J, Skoog I. Mental disorders among elderly people in primary care: the Linkoping Study. *Acta Psychiatr Scand.* 2001; **104**(1): 12–18.

4 Lyness JM, Caine ED, King DA, *et al.* Psychiatric disorders in older primary care patients. *J Gen Int Med.* 1999; **14**(4): 249–54.

5 Bruce ML, McNamara R. Psychiatric status among the home bound elderly: an epidemiologic perspective. *J Am Geriatr Soc.* 1992; **40**(6): 61–6.

6 Field, EM, Walker MH, Orrell MW. Social networks and health of older people living in sheltered housing. *Aging Ment Health.* 2002; **6**(4): 372–86.

7 Patmeore C. Morale and quality of life among frail older users of community care: key issues for the success of community care. *Qual in Ageing.* 2002; **3**(2): 22–9.

8 Bagley H, Cordingley L, Burns A, *et al.* Recognition of depression by staff in nursing and residential homes. *J Clin Nurs.* 2000; **9**(3): 445–50.

9 Dyer C, Pavlik V, Murphy K, *et al.* The high prevalence of depression and dementia in elder abuse and neglect. *J Am Geriatr Soc.* 2000; **48**(2): 205–8.

10 Beekman A, Copeland J, Prince M. Review of community prevalence of depression in later life. *Br J Psychiatr.* 1999; **174**: 307–11.

11 Mills TL, Edwards CDA. *Ageing and Society.* Cambridge: Cambridge University Press; 2002.

12 Office of the Deputy Prime Minister. *Social Exclusion of Older People: evidence from the first wave of the English longitudinal study of Ageing (ELSA), New Horizons Research Summary no. 1.* London: Office of Deputy Prime Minister; 2006.

13 Penninx BW, Deeg DJ, van Eijk J, *et al.* Changes in depression and physical decline in older adults: a longitudinal perspective. *J Affect Disord.* 2000; **61**: 1–12.

14 Montano CB. Primary care issues related to the treatment of depression in elderly patients. *J Clin Psychiatr.* 1999; **60**: 45–51.

15 Lebowitz BD, Pearson JL, Schneider L, *et al.* Diagnosis and treatment of depression in late life. *JAMA.* 1997; **278**: 1186–90.

16 Szanto K, Gildengers A, Mulsant BH, *et al.* Identification of suicidal ideation and prevention of suicidal behavior in the elderly. *Drugs Aging.* 2002; **19**: 11–24.

17 La Vecchia C, Lucchini F, Levi F. Worldwide trends in suicide mortality 1955–1989. *Acta Psychiatr Scand.* 1994; **90**: 53–64.

18 McIntosh JL. Older adults: the next suicide epidemic? *Suicide Life Threat Behav.* 1992; **22**: 322–32.

19 Walker Z, Katona CLE. Depression in elderly people with physical illness. In: Robertson MM, Katona CLE, editors. *Depression and Physical Illness.* West Sussex: John Wiley; 1997.

20 Aromaa A, Raitasalo R, Reunanen A, *et al.* Depression and cardiovascular disease. *Acta Psychiatr Scand.* 1994; **377**: 77–82.

21 Ahern DK, Gorkin L, Anderson JL, *et al.* Biobehavioural variables and mortality or cardiac arrest. *Am Cardiol.* 1990; **66**: 59–62.

22 Silverstone PH. Depression increases mortality and morbidity in acute life-threatening medical illness. *J Psychosom Res.* 1990; **34**: 651–7.

23 Beekman ATF, Deeg DJH, Braam AW, *et al.* Consequences of major and minor depression in later life: a study of disability, well-being and service utilization. *Psychiatr Med.* 1997; **27**(6): 1397–409.

24 Cole MG, Bellavance F, Mansour A. Prognosis of depression in elderly community and primary care populations: a systematic review and meta-analysis. *Am J Psychiatr.* 1999; **156**(8): 1182–9.

25 Beekman ATF, Deeg DJH, Smit JH, *et al.* Predicting the course of depression in the older population: results from a community-based study in the Netherlands. *J Affect Disord.* 1995; **34**(1): 41–9.

26 Shmuely Y, Baumgarten M, Rovner B, *et al.* Predictors of improvement in health-related quality of life among elderly patients with depression. *Int Psychogeriatr.* 2001; **13**: 63–73.

27 Ustun TB. In: Jenkins R, Ustun TB, editors. *Preventing Mental Illness: mental health promotion in primary care.* West Sussex: John Wiley and Sons; 1998.

28 Marks J, Goldberg D, Hillier V. Determinants of the ability of general practitioners to detect psychiatric illness. *Psychol Med.* 1979; **9**: 337–53.

29 Briscoe M. Identification of emotional problems in postpartum women by health visitors. *BMJ.* 1986; **292**: 1245–7.

30 Plummer S, Ritter SAH, Leach RE, *et al.* A controlled comparison of the ability of practice nurses to detect psychological distress in patients who attend their clinics. *J Psychiatr Ment Health.* 1997; **4**: 221–3.

31 Iliffe S, Haines A, Gallivan S, *et al.* Assessment of elderly people in general practice. 1. Social circumstances and mental state. *Br J Gen Pract.* 1991; **41**(342): 9–12.

32 Garrard J, Rolnick SJ, Nitz NM, *et al.* Clinical detection of depression among community-based elderly people with self-reported symptoms of depression. *Geront.* 1998; **53**: M92–M101.

33 Watts S, Bhutani G, Stout I, *et al.* Mental health in older adult recipients of primary care services: is depression the key issue? Identification, treatment and the general practitioner. *Int J Geriatr Psychiatr.* 2002; **17**(5): 427–37.

34 MacDonald AJD. Do general practitioners miss depression in elderly patients? *BMJ.* 1986; **292**: 1365–7.

35 Eustace A, Denihan A, Bruce I, *et al.* Depression in the community dwelling elderly: do clinical and sociodemographic factors influence referral to psychiatry? *Int J Geriatr Psychiatr.* 2001; **16**(10): 975–9.

36 Audit Commission. *Forget Me Not.* London: The Audit Commission; 2000.

37 Department of Health. *National Service Framework for Older People.* London: Department of Health; 2001.

38 Von Korff M, Goldberg D. Improving outcomes in depression. *BMJ.* 2001; **323**: 948–9.

39 Unützer J, Katon W, Callahan C, *et al.* Collaborative care management of late-life depression in the primary care setting. *JAMA.* 2002; **288**: 2836–45.

40 Cooper B. Psychiatric illness, epidemiology and the general practitioner In: Cooper B, Eastwood R, editors. *Primary Health Care and Psychiatric Epidemiology.* New York: Tavistock/Routledge; 1992.

41 Gallo JJ, Rabins PV. Depression without sadness: alternative presentations of depression in late life. *Am Fam Physician.* 1999; **60**: 820–6.

42 Rabins PV. Barriers to diagnosis and treatment of depression in elderly patients. *Am J Geriatr Psychiatr.* 1996; **4**: S79–83.

43 Kockler M, Heun R. Gender differences of depressive symptoms in depressed and nondepressed elderly persons. *Int J Geriatr Psychiatr.* 2002; **17**: 65–72.

44 Fogel BS, Fretwell M. Reclassification of depression in the medically ill elderly. *J Am Geriatr Soc.* 1985; **33**: 446–8.

45 Milne A, Williams J. Meeting the mental health needs of older women: taking social inequality into account. *Ageing Society.* 2000; **20**: 725–44.

46 Judd LL, Akiskal HS, Maser JD, *et al.* A prospective 12-year study of subsyndromal and syndromal depressive symptoms in unipolar major depressive disorders. *Arch Gen Psychiatr.* 1998; **55**: 694–700.

47 Baldwin RC, Chiu E, Katona CLE, *et al. Guidelines for Depressive Disorder in Later Life: practising the evidence.* London: Martin Dunitz; 2002.

48 Dhondt ADF, Hooijer C. Iatrogenic origins of depression in the elderly. *Int J Geriatr Psychiatr.* 1995; **10**: 1–8.

49 Williams JW, Barrett J, Oxman T, *et al.* Treatment of dysthymia and minor depression in primary care: a randomised controlled trial in older adults. *JAMA.* 2000; **284**: 1519–26.

50 Mottram PG, Wilson KCM, Ashworth L, *et al.* The clinical profile of older patients' response to antidepressants: an open trial of sertraline. *Int J Geriatr Psychiatr.* 2002; **17**: 574–8.

51 Katona C, Freeling P, Hinchcliffe K, *et al.* Recognition and management of depression in late life in general practice: consensus statement. *Prim Care Psychiatr.* 1995; **1**: 107–13.

52 Gatz M, Fiske A, Fox LS, *et al.* Empirically validated psychological treatments for older adults. *J Ment Health Aging.* 1998; **4**: 9–46.

53 Pinquart M, Sorensen S. How effective are psychotherapeutic and other psychosocial interventions with older adults? A meta-analysis. *J Ment Health Aging.* 2001; **7**: 207–43.

54 McCusker J, Cole M, Keller E, *et al.* Effectiveness of treatments of depression in older ambulatory patients. *Arch Int Med.* 1998; **158**: 705–12.

55 World Psychiatric Association, WPA International Committee for Prevention and Treatment of Depression. *Depressive Disorders in Older Persons.* New York: NCM Publishers Inc; 1999. Available at: http://www.wpanet.org/sectorial/edu4.html

56 Iliffe S, Gould MM, Mitchley S, *et al.* Evaluation of brief screening instruments for depression, dementia and problem drinking in general practice. *Br J Gen Pract.* 1994; **44**: 503–7.

57 German PS, Shapiro S, Skinner EA, *et al.* Detection and management of mental health problems of older patients by primary care providers. *JAMA.* 1987; **257**: 489–93.

58 Arthur A, Jagger C, Lindesay J, *et al.* Using an annual over-75 health check to screen for depression: validation of the short Geriatric Depression Scale (GDS15) within general practice. *Int J Geriatr Psychiatr.* 1999; **14**: 431–9.

59 Waterreus A, Blanchard M, Mann A, *et al.* Community psychiatric nurses for the elderly: few side-effects and effective in the treatment of depression. *J Clinl Nurs.* 1994; **3**: 2 99–306.

60 Banerjee S, Shamash K, Macdonald AJD, *et al.* Randomised controlled trial of effect of intervention by psychogeriatric teams on depression in frail elderly people at home. *BMJ.* 1996; **313**: 1058–61.

The role of the nurse in the assessment, diagnosis and management of patients with affective disorders

RICHARD CLIBBENS AND PAULA RYLATT

Introduction

For many older people experiencing affective disorders such as depression, anxiety and psychosis, nurses are the health professionals they are most likely to have contact with. Whether a nurse working on an inpatient medical ward in a large acute hospital, a health promotion nurse or a community mental health nurse, most nurses will have a significant range of contact with older people and will need to have an understanding of the assessment, diagnosis and management of these conditions when experienced by older people. This chapter seeks to present an overview of common affective mental health problems experienced by older people, with guidance on appropriate nursing assessment and interventions, applicable to nurses working with older people in any setting. The second section of the chapter provides a more detailed approach to the development of a bio-psychosocial framework for the provision of nursing interventions in psychosis experienced by older people.

Nursing assessment, diagnosis and management of depression and anxiety in older people

As many as 10 to 15% of older people in the UK experience undiagnosed and untreated depression. This is recognised as resulting in significant distress and a negative impact on the quality of life and physical health for affected individuals.[1] Despite the large and reportedly growing numbers of older people affected, recent national reports and strategies consistently indicate that this remains an under-recognised (and under-diagnosed) problem, and even when identified does not always lead to appropriate intervention and treatment. In 2003, the National Statistics office of the UK identified that 10% of people aged 60 to 75 years living in private households in Great Britain had a common mental disorder such as anxiety, depression or phobias.[2] This report was based on a survey of psychiatric morbidity carried out in 2000 by the Office of National Statistics. These mental health problems were strongly associated with the presence of disability for older people in completion of common activities of daily living. At every level of physical ill health those with mental disorder were more likely to have problems with activities of daily living, than those without. This has significant implications across the whole spectrum of environments in which nurses provide care for older people. Physical and mental health are inextricably linked. Physical health and activity reduces depression and can prevent the occurrence of depression in the first place. Physical ill health and disability are the most consistent factors contributing to depression in later life. Promoting well-being and active ageing reduces mental health problems for older people who are usually motivated to remain active and involved in their community.[1,3]

Nurses provide healthcare to older people in a wide range of diverse settings, including: health screening in primary care, specialist disease-specific clinics, acute hospital care, teams working with people experiencing chronic illness and end of life care. This breadth of assessment contact with older people means that nurses across all specialities and settings caring for older people have a role in improving the detection and treatment of depression and anxiety. Nurses often have sustained contact with older people in care settings, which can enable the identification of possible mental health needs through this privileged knowledge of the individual over time.

Nurses are often the members of the multidisciplinary team with the greatest opportunity to develop a trusting therapeutic relationship with an older person in contact with health services. Such relationships can provide a safe and trusting atmosphere for an older person to disclose potentially upsetting or sensitive information regarding their thoughts, mood and feelings. Where the presence of depression or anxiety has been identified, nurses are often well placed to obtain crucial relevant assessment information, to enable discussion with the wider multidisciplinary team regarding the most appropriate intervention. The use of national guidelines or local protocols that are informed by national guidance can enable a systematic approach to the assessment of depression and anxiety and identification of appropriate interventions.

CASE HISTORY 11.1

Deirdre is 81 years of age, and lives alone in her home of 50 years. Over the past six months Deirdre has experienced increasing pain and difficulty when mobilising in the presence of her arthritis. She complains of feeling dizzy at times and is embarrassed about recent occasions where her clothes have been stained with urine. When Deirdre attends an annual health check appointment with her practice nurse at the health centre, the practice nurse is concerned that she may be depressed. Following a review of Deirdre's currently prescribed medication, her dizziness subsides, and she receives more effective pain control for her arthritis. Adaptations are made to Deirdre's home, which enable her to access the toilet more safely and quickly. Following assessment by the continence nurse specialist, Deirdre is using continence aids which have increased her confidence to leave her home to visit family, friends and a local social centre. These practical interventions have all promoted Deirdre's independence, increasing her ability to meet her social needs and need for stimulation and activity.

This example demonstrates the potential for general health and social interventions to directly impact on a person's mental health, improving activity, confidence and pleasure in life.

Promoting mental health

Age Concern and the Mental Health Foundation have identified the crucial importance of promoting mental health and well-being in later life: 'It is widely acknowledged that the mental health and well-being of older people has been neglected across the spectrum of promotion, prevention and treatment services.'[4] The negative effects of age discrimination in reducing opportunities for employment or effective participation in society and the absence of a 'sense of belonging' for many older people have been identified as key contributors to mental health problems in old age. Age Concern identify that one in seven people over the age of 65 experience 'major depression', which is severe and persistent and affects their day to day functioning. The benefits for older people in maintaining their mental health are clearly summarised in the following extract from the mental health and well-being report published by Age Concern and the Mental Health Foundation:

> With good mental health we can:
>
> - Develop emotionally, creatively, intellectually and spiritually
> - Initiate, develop and sustain mutually satisfying personal relationships
> - Face problems, resolve and learn from them
> - Be aware of others and empathise with them
> - Use and enjoy solitude
> - Enjoy life and have fun
> - Laugh, both at ourselves and the world.[4]

A wide range of factors clearly impact on a person's potential to sustain effective mental health in old age. Poverty can severely limit an older person's capacity to maintain a range of hobbies and interests or engage in travel and other activities. Where finances are very limited this may impact on the person's ability to enjoy a varied diet and the treats and luxuries that most of us expect to enjoy from time to time.

Mental illness in old age is common in all care settings and for older people living at home without provision of care services it is mostly unrecognised.[5,6] The Department of Health anticipates that the majority of mild and moderate severity mood disorders among older people will be managed in mainstream settings by staff without psychiatric training. Nurses who specialise in older people's mental health therefore have a key function in supporting colleagues in the

> development and implementation of guidance for the detection and initial management of mental illness in later life in mainstream settings, and assisting with the elucidation of referral pathways to specialist and generic support services for older people with mental illness.[6]

In 2006 the Healthcare Commission identified that little evidence had been found of communities developing systematic ways of tackling loneliness and social exclusion among older people in order to promote good mental health, since publication of the National Service Framework for Older People in 2001.[1,7] In 2002 the Audit Commission identified that there continued to be very limited provision for services which are acceptable and appropriate for people from black and minority ethnic communities.[8] Improving the appropriateness of older people's mental health services for people from black and minority ethnic communities remains a significant development need in the commissioning and provision of services. Many nurses have a lead role in local health and social care partnership projects designed to tackle social exclusion and exclusion related to ethnic and cultural identity. As nurses it is essential that we promote at every opportunity the importance of social inclusion for all older people and more specifically better access to assessment, diagnosis and treatment of mental health problems in old age for marginalised or excluded groups.

A range of accredited tools for use at overview assessment as part of the single assessment process (SAP) can be employed at initial assessment contact with older people.[9,10] Typically, these global assessment tools will include brief measures of mood state. The EASYcare tool, for example, includes a three item Geriatric Depression Rating scale.[11] It can be difficult for non mental health practitioners to know how to interpret the results from such brief scales, however, unless a clear pathway or protocol for more detailed mood assessment is in place.

Locally agreed protocols for the detection and treatment of depression have been introduced widely across the NHS, in part as a requirement of the NSF for Older People.[7] The National Institute for Health and Clinical Excellence guideline on depression[12] recommends using the ICD-10 criteria for diagnosing and assessing the severity of depression,[13] but identifies that one occasion of 'counting the number of symptoms' is not a realistic way to accurately identify the true severity of someone's depression. Assessment should also include the past history and family history of depression and the degree of disability experienced.[14]

What is depression?

Depression refers to a wide range of mental health problems characterised by a loss of interest and enjoyment in ordinary things and experiences, low mood and a range of associated emotional, cognitive and behavioural symptoms. Distinguishing between 'normal' mood changes and major depression can be problematic. The persistence and severity of the changed mood, presence of other symptoms and functional and social impairment form the basis of distinguishing between the two.[12,14]

Depression is more common in people with chronic medical conditions such as diabetes, chronic obstructive pulmonary disease and cardiovascular disease. At least two thirds of depressed people who see their general practitioner (GP) present with physical symptoms rather than psychological symptoms. Nurses working in primary care should ensure that screening for depression in high-risk groups of older people takes place, such as those with a history of depression, significant physical illness causing disability and people with other mental health problems such as dementia.[12,14]

Mental health nurses can lead in the identification of contact with and referral rates for older people experiencing depression, in light of the national statistics which reveal this as a common but hidden problem. Depression in older people has been reported as frequently under-detected and untreated in primary care.[8] Core to the treatment of depression is an explanation to the person of their diagnosis and of their symptoms. Mental health professionals should provide training and support for primary care teams, making particular effort to contact those who refer very few people.[5,6,12]

All nurses working with older people should ensure screening takes place for adverse drug effects as a cause of identified depression. Drugs that may be involved include centrally acting antihypertensives (e.g. methyldopa), lipid soluble beta-blockers (e.g. propranolol), benzodiazepines or other central nervous system depressants and opioid analgesics.[14]

Distinguishing grief from depression

Grief in the presence of bereavement or other significant loss is a normal psychological process of adjustment. This may be a necessary if distressing process for an individual and it is important that this normal and natural process is not misinterpreted as a formal mood disorder such as major depression. Where there is concern that the severity or extended duration of a grief reaction is presenting a risk of harm or excessive distress, specialist mental health assessment will be appropriate. For most individuals experiencing prolonged or significant grief, bereavement counselling may be offered as a helpful intervention.[15]

NICE recommend that when older adults are experiencing depression, their physical state, living conditions and risk of social isolation should be assessed.[12] This may clearly require a multi-agency approach to tackling the underlying causal factors or background to an older person's experienced depression.

Identifying depression

The clinical presentation of depression in older people is in many ways the same as for younger adults.[16] Standardised diagnostic criteria for the identification of depression are recommended for use in adults regardless of age, as outlined below:

Ask about the following key symptoms:
* persistent sadness or low mood
* loss of interest or pleasure
* fatigue or low energy.

If any of the above have been present most days, most of the time, for at least two weeks, ask about *associated* symptoms:
* disturbed sleep
* poor concentration or indecisiveness
* low self-confidence
* poor or increased appetite
* agitation or slowing of movements
* guilt or self-blame
* suicidal thoughts or acts.

Major depression is diagnosed if the person has experienced four or more of the above symptoms for at least two weeks. Major depression is classified according to severity, as follows.
* **Mild** depression: four symptoms, one key and three associated (usually able to carry out normal activities).
* **Moderate** depression: five or six symptoms (at least one a key symptom). Likely to have great difficulty continuing with normal activities.
* **Severe** depression: seven or more symptoms at least one a key symptom with or without psychotic features. Highly dysfunctional with prominent feelings of worthlessness and guilt, with suicidal thoughts. (Adapted from Prodigy.[14])

Always ask people with depression about suicidal ideas and intent directly or ask if they feel hopeless or that life is not worth living. Also ask if they have previously attempted suicide. If suicidal ideation is present it is essential to determine whether the person has a current suicide plan and the extent of their intent to carry it out. When assessing an older person with depression, direct questions should be asked about suicidal ideation and intent.[14,17,18] Professional carers, family and friends should all be advised to be vigilant for changes in mood, and increased expressions of negativity and hopelessness. Medication changes and periods of increased stress may increase the risk of suicidality for some individuals.[16]

Carer stress and depression

Many older people are carers providing support to partners, other family members, friends and neighbours. Those with significant caring responsibilities can be at risk of low mood, from the accumulation of stress due to the demands of caregiving. Where nurses encounter older people fulfilling the role of carer, an assessment of that person's needs may be appropriate to identify the degree to which they may be at risk of carer stress and associated health problems. Older carers have been identified as a particular group at higher risk of depression.[19]

What is anxiety?

Anxiety is often present in the presence of depression, when the diagnosis may be:

> depression
> anxiety, or
> mixed depression and anxiety.

The diagnosis is dependent on which features are most dominant in the clinical presentation. When depression and anxiety are both present, NICE recommends that the depression is treated first.[20] Older adults are identified as more likely to present with somatic symptoms of depression (physical sensations which may be of pain or discomfort), and less likely to complain of low mood.[12] Depression can exacerbate pain and distress in the presence of physical disease. The stigma associated with mental health problems and the negative public view of people experiencing depression may account for the reluctance of depressed people to seek help. All nurses working with older people need to be alert to the possible presence of a 'hidden' depression, or need to further explore possible psychological and emotional factors associated with the presence of complaints of physical symptoms.[12,20]

Anxiety is typified by feelings of worry, fearfulness, distress or panic that seem out of proportion or inexplicable.[21] Anxiety can be present in a range of forms, from generalised feelings of continued unease, to more specific forms such as phobic anxiety or panic attacks. Anxiety can be disabling, particularly where older people become socially isolated, through avoidance of situations that may increase anxious thoughts and feelings. Specific treatment of anxiety without the use of antidepressants is problematic, due to the potential for unwanted effects from medication such as anxiolytic benzodiazepines. Psychological interventions often reduce anxiety and antidepressant medication may also have a sedative and anxiolytic effect in reducing anxiety.[12,20] Psychological therapies such as cognitive behaviour therapy (CBT) may be particularly effective for anxiety and can be feasibly employed by nurses with appropriate training and supervision.[20]

Guidance produced by NICE on the management of anxiety contains a helpful algorithm for differentiating between anxiety and depression when considering which forms of interventions are most appropriate. For generalised anxiety disorder psychological therapy (CBT) is identified as having best evidence for the longest duration of effect.[20]

Nursing interventions for depression and anxiety

The Department of Health has clearly identified that nurses are key to the provision of psychological therapies, and should be part of a multidisciplinary provision with a range of available approaches for older people with mental health needs. These therapies should be seen as a routine treatment option. This includes access for older people in mainstream services, with physical disability, stroke, falls and challenging behaviours.

When (in a minority of cases) older people require admission to inpatient mental health services, this should only be in the presence of problems which require a level of intensive support or expertise unavailable in their home setting. This may additionally require their detention under the Mental Health Act in some cases. Due to the likely needs of people admitted under these circumstances, the Department of Health has identified that such inpatient units need to be staffed accordingly to ensure the safety and well-being of service users and staff.[6] Nurses working in environments where older people with mental health problems are experiencing acute episodes of mood disorder have opportunity to lead in the provision of an effective recovery-based model of multidisciplinary practice.[22]

Nurses have been identified as sometimes reluctant to use formalised psychosocial interventions with older people, either with individuals or in groups, because they can lack confidence in which therapies are appropriate for older people and how to implement these effectively.[23] Nurses may undertake specific specialist formal programmes of education and training for psychotherapeutic and/or psychosocial interventions, but this can be both time consuming and potentially expensive. It may be more practical within some mental health teams for nurses to receive case supervision from qualified and experienced therapists, which enables them to safely develop competence and knowledge in the implementation of psychologically based or formal psychosocial interventions.

CASE HISTORY 11.2

Within an older people's community mental health team in Wakefield, the community mental health nurses access planned case supervision with a consultant clinical psychologist, nurse specialist for psychosocial interventions with older people and old age consultant psychiatrist with a post-graduate qualification in cognitive behaviour therapy. Nurses are able to present and discuss live cases in a confidential and developmental environment, using case supervision to implement appropriate psychological and psychosocial approaches.

Registered nurses working with older people, and especially those trained in mental health, will usually have developed specific skills in the development and maintenance of therapeutic relationships.[24] An effective collaborative relationship between the older person and the nurse is in many ways the cornerstone and essential first step in the provision of any psychologically based therapy such as CBT. An empathic relationship, which promotes disclosure and a clear perception from both parties of working towards a shared goal, underpins effective therapeutic work for nurses with older people experiencing mental health problems.

A lack of resources in primary care has been identified for interventions to identify mild depression and set in place supportive interventions for older people.[25] Baldwin has identified a need for further evidence to explore the role of newer psychological interventions for the treatment of depression in older people, in primary care. Centres to provide talking therapies could be a way forward. In East Scotland, a network of tea shops and coffee bars with open access provides group therapy as part of a joint-funded service open to multi-professional and multi-agency referral.[26]

Psychotropic medication for depression and anxiety

Nurses working with older people have a responsibility to ensure that other non-pharmacological interventions are appropriately considered, either as an alternative to or in conjunction with any pharmacological treatments.[27] Recognition and respect for individual treatment preferences identified by older people requires timely appropriate information from nurses administering or prescribing medicines available to treat anxiety and depression. Nurses working with older people can promote choice and independence in the selection of treatment options and ensure that, where appropriate, prescribing, such as of antidepressants, follows good practice guidelines.[12]

The Mental Capacity Act 2005 enables people to plan ahead for any time when they may lack capacity and, where a person lacks capacity, identifies who can take decisions, in what situations and how they should go about this. The Mental Capacity Act Code of Practice provides guidance for anyone working with or caring for a person who lacks capacity.[28] It is essential that nurses ensure that their practice and that of colleagues meets the requirements of the Mental Capacity Act. The code of practice usefully clarifies capacity issues that may be present where an older person is experiencing a severe depression or other significant mental health problem. Nurses are well placed to promote advanced decision making and choice in considering treatment options for depression and anxiety.

Hypnotics and anxiolytics should be avoided where possible and when prescribed used for short courses of treatment only after causal factors have been identified and alternative, more appropriate initial interventions considered. These may include sleep hygiene advice that promotes independent preventative action by the older person to manage their experienced difficulties.[27,29]

Nurses have a vital role in ensuring a partnership approach with older people that empowers true choice in selecting treatment alternatives, based on the right information at the right time. Whether administering medicine prescribed by a doctor or acting as a nurse independent or supplementary prescriber,[30] every nurse working with older people should ensure they have appropriate knowledge regarding the prescribing of psychotropic medication. Nurses must take account of the physiology of ageing and the increased risk with age of altered distribution, metabolism and excretion of drugs.[31]

Alcohol misuse

Older people who drink alcohol excessively often experience higher levels of anxiety.[32] Older people with alcohol problems benefit from similar interventions to those offered to younger people and should have appropriate access to alcohol misuse advice, information and services regardless of age. Alcohol misuse in older people has been described as an evolving silent epidemic, where the incidence of problem drinking among older people is underestimated, including within national policy documents on reducing alcohol harm.[33] Physiological changes of ageing can make some older people more vulnerable to alcohol harm at lower levels than younger people. Memory loss, depression, anxiety, self-neglect and self-harm may be associated with alcohol misuse in older people.

The prevalence of problem drinking among older people in the UK has been estimated at between 2% and 15%, with significant reported variation depending on the populations studied.[34] Published literature often distinguishes between chronic drinking which extends into later life and 'late-onset drinking'. Depression, phobias and anxiety are associated with alcohol misuse in old age. Alcohol is also contraindicated with many prescribed medicines including psychotropic drugs which may be prescribed for older people. A key challenge identified by Alcohol Concern is in altering the mind set that older people with alcohol problems are unable to change or modify their drinking behaviour. In contrast to such views one London project to assist older drinkers reported a 72% improvement in participants' self-care, and psychological or social functioning.[35] Alcohol misuse in older people is a hidden issue.[33] While often not being diagnosed and treated, older people may be experiencing greater harm than younger people through alcohol misuse. Assessment tools need to be adapted for older people and attitudes need to change. Nurses in a wide range of care settings such as GP surgeries, day centres and fracture clinics, as well as in mental health services, need to be alert to the potential presence of alcohol misuse.

Psychosis and psychosocial interventions

Policy factors

In order to consider the role of the nurse in the assessment, diagnosis and management of affective disorders, it is essential to explore the core role of the contemporary mental health nurse. The Chief Nursing Officer's (CNO) review of mental health nursing[22] reports a need for 'positive human qualities, as well as a range of technical knowledge and skills', as identified by service users and carers. The review promotes a holistic approach to mental health nursing, requesting nursing practice to widen its skills in the pursuit of social inclusion and mental health recovery. These recommendations are further enhanced by the Department of Health's publications of the 10 essential shared capabilities framework for the mental health workforce,[36] and the best practice competencies and capabilities for pre-registration mental health nursing in England.[37]

Key roles in mental health nursing include expert assessment and intervention and the 'fundamentals of care': safety, privacy, dignity, hygiene, nutrition, hydration, continence and pressure area care.[38] In summary: 'Mental health nursing needs to move away from a traditional model of care towards a bio-psychosocial and values based approach'.[22] Nursing assessment, diagnosis and management of affective disorders should therefore operate within the above clinical guidance.

There is much consideration and discussion regarding the diagnostic classification of schizophrenia and psychosis and the relationship between psychosis and affect. In clinical nursing practice, however, working with the individual service user's experience and presenting difficulties is more significant than an applied diagnosis of schizophrenia, schizoaffective disorder or bipolar disorder, for example. Personal clinical experience suggests a significant relationship between affect and the development of psychosis, as suggested within psychological theories regarding the development of psychosis considering the role of self-evaluation and emotion.[39]

Psychosis-related problems affect 900 in a 45 000 population of adults over age 65.[6] The Department of Health reports that integrated specialist mental health services are required where people are experiencing complex mental health difficulties including psychosis, with specialist and mainstream services pivotal to integrated community mental health teams.[6] Additionally, with reference to older people with severe mental health difficulties associated with psychosis, the National Service Framework for Older People clearly states 'they will require the packages of care set out in the NSF for Mental Health and the same standards should apply for working age adults' (standard seven,[7] p. 19). Recommendations clearly promote flexibility within local mental health services and advocate person-centred, needs-led service provision.

Additionally, the National Institute for Health and Clinical Excellence guidelines for schizophrenia[40] report that five in 1000 individuals aged 16 to 74 experience psychotic disorder and recommend a range of psychosocial interventions including family work, cognitive behavioural therapy, counselling, medication management, psycho-education and assertive community treatment within integrated health and social services and a recovery model for service users with a diagnosis of schizophrenia before 60 years of age. The guidelines report additional guidance will be published regarding late-onset schizophrenia and complex factors associated with ageing, along with additional specialist recommendations regarding dual diagnosis, depressive psychosis, sensory impairment and psychosis. However, guidelines clearly recommend psychosocial interventions and integrated services for a specific population of older people experiencing psychosis. There is no exclusive evidence base regarding psychosocial interventions and older people. Therefore, ageless person centred clinical practice considering the idiosyncratic and political concept of age and the wealth of effectiveness research regarding working age adults and psychosocial interventions is a standard of best practice using the best available evidence.

Considering the above policy guidance, the nurses' role in the assessment, diagnosis and management of psychosis is an integrated role providing holistic, person-centred services. The Chief Nursing Officer's review of mental health nursing[37] (p. 15) reports desired outcomes for service users including psychological and psychosocial models that inform practice, and evidenced-based psychosocial assessment and interventions.

The therapeutic process

In clinical practice psychosocial assessment and interventions are considered within the context of the therapeutic process of engagement, assessment, formulation, intervention, evaluation and relapse prevention.[41] This process is continuous and evolving within clinical practice, and may not be undertaken in a linear approach. Furthermore, the recovery approach addressed by the CNO[22] as a guiding principle of mental health nurse practice was also pioneered in reference to psychosis care,[42] and is intrinsic to nursing practice with affective disorders and the concept of psychosocial interventions for psychosis. The nurse's role in the assessment, diagnosis and management of psychosis is perhaps more usefully considered as the nurse's role in engagement, assessment, formulation, interventions and relapse prevention in working with psychosis care.

Engagement

The process of engagement is recognised in the CNO's report on mental health nursing (p. 16): 'The relationship between the mental health nurse and service user needs to be positive, trusting, meaningful, therapeutic and collaborative, with the mental health nurses having sufficient clinical time in which to build, develop and sustain such relationships.'[22] While acknowledging difficulties with sincere engagement due to, for example, lack of time and human resources, the nurse's role in establishing and maintaining service user and carer engagement is paramount to all the therapeutic activity and a continuous and evolving relationship. We may ask whether, in the absence of adequate time and commitment to engagement, assessment, formulation, care planning and interventions can be accurate.

Barriers to engagement may be multidimensional, including service user barriers, issues for clinical staff and difficulties with service organisation and delivery. It is essential, however, that nursing and professional staff attempt to overcome such barriers by challenging negative attitudes towards mental health recovery and maintaining an optimistic, recovery-focused work ethic, supported by a motivation for continued professional development and training and supervision. Furthermore, staff involvement with service change and review is essential in order to promote the implementation of a flexible working approach and opportunities for creative engagement with service users, e.g. to meet with a service user in the local café, park or venue of choice, rather than in their home environment. Sincere engagement with service users experiencing psychosis is significant and a collaborative endeavour dependent upon an individual's level of insight into their experiences and associated distress and risks, and their willingness and ability to engage with professional services.

Assessment

Nursing staff have a key role in providing holistic assessment using statutory assessment procedures and global and specific symptom measurement tools in a range of formal and informal environmental settings. Nursing assessment is a continuous process requiring a range of observational, interpersonal and analytical skills and a bio-psychosocial knowledge base. Fowler *et al.*[43] suggest the core elements of assessment for psychosis include past and current holistic assessment, specific assessment of positive and negative symptoms of psychosis and beliefs about psychosis, existing coping skills and behaviour using a cognitive ABC analysis of activating events, beliefs about activating events and cognitive, behavioural, social, physiological and affective consequences of beliefs. The use of a time line is a practical and effective method of assessing the history and context of presenting difficulties. It enables the identification of personal stress and vulnerability factors in the course of psychotic relapse and experience, and possible symptom maintenance factors, e.g. habitual avoidance of feared stimuli resulting in lack of opportunity to test one's hypothesis.

A range of global and specific individual and family assessment tools for psychosis are available with differing licensing agreements including the KGV,[44] the Psychotic Symptoms Rating Scale,[45] the Social Functioning Scale,[46] the Maudsley Assessment of Delusions Scale,[47] the Belief about Voices Scale,[48] the LUNSERS medication scale[49] and the Knowledge about Schizophrenia Interview.[50] The use of assessment tools enables baseline and comparable measurement of change, and should be used as appropriate and agreeable with an individual and within local service or individual licence agreements. Relevant tools for depression are discussed elsewhere in this volume. Assessment tools are complementary to, and not a substitution for, clinical interview and discussion whereby using interpersonal skills an individual's beliefs about experiences can be elicited and discussed and one's assessment and initial formulation of events undertaken. In clinical practice, it is not always appropriate to introduce specific assessment tools and approaches and this may depend upon one's level of engagement with the service user and timing of an intervention.

Formulation

The nursing process has been described as a process of assessment, formulation of nursing diagnosis, identification of expected outcomes, identification of nursing objectives, implementation of interventions and evaluation.[51] Schultz and Videback describe the formulation of a nursing diagnosis as 'a statement of an actual or potential problem or situation amenable to nursing interventions . . . the nurse's perception of the factors related to the problem or contributing to its aetiology'.[51] In addition, the process of psychological case formulation has been described by Persons as 'a hypothesis about the nature of the psychological difficulty (or difficulties) underlying the problems'.[52] that, according to Haddock and Tarrier, 'takes place within the context of a generalised explanatory model of that particular disorder or problem category.'[53] With psychosis, cognitive theorists have focused on a developmental and symptom maintenance cognitive behavioural formulation, and case formulation is a core element of psychosocial interventions and the therapeutic process with psychosis care. Chadwick *et al.* state: 'Within the cognitive model formulation connects early experience, interpersonal style, significant life events, onset, and current analysis of problems. Formulations are tentative and speculative, and are likely to change as therapy progresses'.[54] In clinical practice this may translate as the development of a current or maintenance formulation, namely factors that maintain difficulties including the identification of the ABC: activating event (A), belief about A (B), and the consequences of B (C). The cognitive ABC approach when working with psychosis is developed from Ellis;[55] however, in formulation and psychosis the concept of B in the ABC analysis represents cognitions and not behaviour.[54] It is significant that psychological work with psychosis aims to support the beliefs about activating events, or experiences, rather than the events or experience itself. In addition to the identification of the ABC, in practice one may form a developmental or case-level formulation: identification of early experiences, key core beliefs, assumptions, trigger factors, critical incidents, and the ABC. A formulation may also identify potential obstacles to therapy.[52] There are several models of individual and family formulation which represent the above. However, in practice one may choose to simply map the ABC and assessment information on a note pad and begin to explore the case. The detail and complexity of an individual or family formulation will be determined by several factors, including the level of engagement and accuracy of assessment between a nurse or clinician and the service user, and the level of clinical skill and training. The introduction of a formulation-based approach to interventions aims to individualise care, accounting for the idiosyncratic and complex factors that may be involved in one's presentation. Formulation may be more collaborative and multidimensional than diagnosis-led or manualised treatment options, particularly where stress vulnerability models of schizophrenia[56,57] and psychosis are considered to underpin the psychosis care approach.

Interventions

Psychosocial interventions (PSI) are evidenced-based psychological, sociological and biological interventions applied in the assessment, management and support of individuals with schizophrenia and psychosis and their families. In practice, the same broad approaches are appropriate for severe depression and for bipolar disorder. Psychosocial interventions promote recovery and quality of life and reduce the incidence of relapse.[58] The stress vulnerability model of schizophrenia and psychosis[56,57] underpins psychosocial interventions, considering numerous factors in the onset and development of complex mental health problems.

A range of psychosocial interventions have reported clinical effectiveness, including: family work considering expressed emotion, problem solving, psycho-education;[59,60,61] case management;[62,63] cognitive behaviour therapy;[64,65] social functioning interventions;[66] social skills training;[67] symptom management strategies;[68] medication concordance therapy;[69] supportive counselling;[70] coping strategy enhancement[71] and relapse prevention.[72,73] The NHS Centre for Reviews and Dissemination[58] reports systematic evidence for effective psychosocial interventions for schizophrenia in working age adults, including: psycho-education and family interventions and reduced risk of relapse; cognitive behaviour therapy and decreased relapse and readmission rates; the effects of token economy upon negative symptoms of schizophrenia; assertive community treatment and engagement and reduced likelihood of hospitalisation; and the effective use of case management in maintaining service user contact. As discussed, the National Institute for Health and Clinical Excellence[40] also recommends a range of psychosocial interventions including family work, cognitive behavioural therapy, counselling, medication management, psycho-education and assertive community treatment within integrated health and social services and a recovery model for service users with a diagnosis of schizophrenia before 60 years of age.

The nurse's role in the management of psychosis is bio-psychosocial, involving an array of skills and extending practical roles. However, the complexity of an intervention or management plan will evidently differ depending on the case formulation, the level of practitioner skill and confidence, and service organisational issues. Implementation of the NICE[40] recommendations for schizophrenia and psychosis should, however, inform nursing practice.

Considering 'family work' for psychosis[40] several theoretical approaches may inform individual practice: behavioural family therapy,[74] cognitive behavioural family therapy[75] and integrated systemic and family management approaches.[76] In nursing practice, one's approach to supporting family members or carers is determined by the assessment and case formulation, and interventions may be multi-modal and less structured than formal family therapy. Common components of family interventions include education, communication training, goal setting, problem solving, cognitive-behavioural self-management and increasing family well-being and maintenance of skills[77] and psycho-education regarding symptom management strategies.[78] With appropriate training and supervision the above family interventions are integral to nursing care for psychosis and can be adapted for severe affective disorder.

Cognitive behavioural therapy, counselling, medication management and psycho-education recommended by the NICE guidelines for schizophrenia[40] can all be considered nursing interventions. The complexity of cognitive behavioural intervention and counselling interventions is determined by the level of professional training. However, the assimilation of varying therapeutic approaches is common to mental health nursing practice.

Medication management is a traditional and continued key role within mental health nursing and the extent of intervention may vary depending on extending nursing roles including non-medical prescribing. More common interventions, however, include the administration of medication and assessment of benefits and side-effects, including routine blood and physical investigations required with certain treatment regimes. Additionally, nursing practice involves interventions aimed to improve medication concordance where treatment adherence is minimal or erratic.

Psycho-educational interventions are essential within mental health nursing practice and although implemented routinely in terms of informal literature regarding common mental health problems and access to services, structured idiosyncratic psycho-educational interventions may be less routine. An individual experiencing a range of complex mental health difficulties may benefit from detailed discussion regarding aetiology, experiences and treatment choice, and in clinical experience psycho-education regarding stress vulnerability models[56,57] can be a beneficial premise to other psychosocial interventions for individuals and families. Psycho-education can be two-way as many service users and carers have a wealth of experience regarding experience and coping styles to share with clinical staff. If sensitively provided and supported psycho-education can reduce anxieties regarding blame, stigma and fear often associated with mental health.

The Department of Health has identified both the Care Programme Approach and Single Assessment Process arrangements relevant for older people experiencing psychoses.[7] Nursing staff who assume the role of the care coordinator for service users are required to coordinate care services within the above organisational or 'system management' approaches.[63] However, individual practitioners may also adopt a variety of practical case management styles to meet the needs of the service user group. Askey[79] defined various case management styles, but in personal experience a hybrid model of intensive and clinical case management features more prominently in community mental health services for older people. It may be supported by assertive community treatment or assertive outreach services recommended within the NICE guidelines for schizophrenia[40] where services are resourced and available. In the absence of a specialist outreach service, the implementation of designated clinical staff with the remit of assertive community treatment for psychosis care enables team organisation of clinical caseloads in a service providing multiple services including attending to acute and severe and enduring mental health needs. The following is a best practice example:

> Appointment of a specialist practitioner for psychosocial interventions in Wakefield Older People's Services, South West Yorkshire Mental Health Trust. The post created an opportunity for intensive and assertive case management with individuals and families experiencing severe and enduring mental health problems, specifically schizophrenia and psychosis.

In addition to the above interventions and recommendations, nurse management roles may include effective leadership and promotion of best practice, and the development of organisational partnerships. Best practice examples in psychosis care include the following.

> A staff questionnaire[80] exploring knowledge and skills regarding PSI undertaken in Wakefield Older People's Services, South West Yorkshire Mental Health Trust. The questionnaire and a small sample of service user interviews regarding service delivery and experience enabled the development of a local internal training and development workshop programme regarding psychosis care. The awareness workshops include various topics regarding psychosocial interventions and psychosis, stress vulnerability models, recovery, engagement, assessment, formulation, interventions and relapse prevention.

> The development of psychosis care standards in Wakefield Older People's Services, South West Yorkshire Mental Health Trust. The purpose of the tool is to enable a process of benchmarking and subsequent continuous training and service development to promote best practice in psychosis.[81]

Relapse prevention and evaluation

Relapse prevention is an essential process within psychosis care and aims 'to identify the earliest signs of impending relapse and to offer timely and effective intervention to arrest their progression towards frank psychosis'.[73] Birchwood et al.[73] report that early warning signs occur over a period of less than four weeks and suggest that the development of an individual 'relapse signature' may prevent an acute relapse by enabling professional services, family, carers and the service user to recognise deterioration and intervene. There are several generic and structured approaches to relapse prevention, and individual practice may be determined by local service arrangements. However, an idiosyncratic plan incorporating psycho-education, self-monitoring and collaboratively agreed coping strategies, shared by all involved personnel, can be clinically effective and support anticipatory anxieties about the future for individuals and their family members, thus enabling a sense of control and empowerment. Again, exactly the same principles can be applied to early detection of relapse in recurrent affective disorders.

REFERENCES

1 Commission for Health Care Audit and Inspection. *Living Well in Later Life: a review of progress against the National Service Framework for Older People.* London: Commission for Health Care Audit and Inspection; 2006.

2 National Statistics Office. *Mental Health of Older People.* London: National Statistics Office; 2006. Available from: http://www.statistics.gov.uk

3 Department of Health. *A New Ambition for Old Age: next steps in implementing the National Service Framework for Older People.* London: Department of Health; 2006.

4 Age Concern. *UK Inquiry into Mental Health and Well-Being in Later Life.* London: Age Concern and the Mental Health Foundation; 2006. Available from: http://www.mhilli.org/

5 Department of Health. *Securing Better Mental Health for Older Adults.* London: Department of Health; 2005.

6 Department of Health. *Everybody's Business: integrated mental health services for older adults; a service development guide.* London: Department of Health; 2005.

7 Department of Health. *National Service Framework for Older People.* London: Department of Health; 2001.

8 Audit Commission. *Forget Me Not: developing mental health services for older people.* London: Audit Commission; 2002.

9 Department of Health. *Single Assessment Process for Older People: assessment tools and accreditation.* London: Department of Health; 2004.

10 Department of Health. *The Single Assessment Process: assessment tools and scales.* London: Department of Health; 2002.

11 Sheffield Institute for Studies on Ageing. *EASY-Care Elderly Assessment System.* Sheffield Institute for Studies on Ageing, University of Sheffield; 1999.

12 National Institute for Clinical Excellence. *Depression: management of depression in primary and secondary care. Clinical Guideline 23.* London: National Institute for Clinical Excellence; 2004. http://www.nice.org.uk

13 World Health Organization. *The ICD–10 Classification of Mental and Behavioural Disorders: clinical descriptions and diagnostic guidelines.* Geneva: World Health Organization; 1992.

14 Prodigy. *What is Depression?* 2006. Available from: http://www.prodigy.nhs.uk

15 MIND. *Older People and Mental Health.* London: MIND; 2005. Available from: http://www.mind.org.uk

16 Hughes C. Depression in older people. In: Redfern S, Ross F, editors. *Nursing Older People: independence, autonomy and self fulfilment.* 4th ed. London: Churchill Livingstone; 2005.

17 Littlejohn C. Understanding the nurse's role in improving suicide prevention. *Nurs Times.* 2004; **100**(46): 28–9.

18 Manthorpe J, Iliffe S. Suicide among older people. *Nurs Older People.* 2006; **17**(10): 25–29.

19 Australian Psychological Society. *Understanding Late Life Depression.* 2006. Available from: http://www.psychology.aug.au/publications/tip-sheet/late_depression

20 National Institute for Clinical Excellence. *Guidelines for the Management of Anxiety (Panic Disorder, with or without Agoraphobia and Generalised Anxiety Disorder) in Adults in Primary Secondary and Community Care.* London: National Institute for Clinical Excellence; 2004.

21 Manthorpe J, Iliffe S. Anxiety and depression. *Nurs Older People.* 2006; **18**: 1.

22 Department of Health. *From Values to Action: the Chief Nursing Officer's review of mental health nursing.* London: Department of Health; 2006. p. 13.

23 Minardi H, Hayes N. Nursing older adults with mental health problems: therapeutic interventions, part 1. *Nurs Older People.* 2003; **15**: 6.

24 Brough C. Developing and maintaining a therapeutic relationship, part 1. *Nurs Older People.* 2004; **16**: 8.

25 Baldwin RC, Anderson D, Black S, *et al.* Guideline for the management of late-life depression in primary care. *Int J Geriatr Psychiatr.* **18**(9): 829–38.

26 Bright L. From loneliness to illness: Les Bright wonders when talking therapies will be widely available. *Nurs Older People.* 2006; **8**(5): 8.

27 Clibbens RJ. The role of the nurse in the assessment, diagnosis and treatment of older people with psychotropic drugs. In: Curran S, Bullock R, editors. *Practical Old Age Psychopharmacology: a multi-professional approach.* Oxford: Radcliffe Publishing; 2005.

28 Department for Constitutional Affairs. *Mental Capacity Act and Related Documents.* Department for Constitutional Affairs; 2007. http://www.dca.gov.uk/memincap/legis.htm

29 Prodigy. *Guidance: hypnotic or anxiolytic dependence.* 2007. http://www.prodigy.nhs.uk

30 Department of Health. *Medicines Matters.* London: Department of Health; 2006.

31 Trounce J. *Clinical Pharmacology for Nurses.* Edinburgh: Churchill-Livingstone; 2000.

32 Watts M. Incidences of excess alcohol consumption in the older person. *Nurs Older People.* 2007; **18**(12): 27–30.

33 Dyson J. Alcohol misuse and older people. *Nurs Older People.* 2006; **18**(7): 32.

34 Alcohol Concern. *Acquire: Alcohol Concern's Quarterly Information and Research Bulletin.* Autumn 2002.

35 Taber M. *Project Update: CASA Older Person's Service.* London: Alcohol Concern; 2001.

36 Department of Health. *The Ten Essential Shared Capabilities: a framework for the whole of the mental health workforce.* London: HMSO; 2004.

37 Department of Health. *Best Practice Competencies and Capabilities for Pre-Registration Mental Health Nurses in England: the Chief Nursing Officer's review of mental health nursing.* London: Department of Health; 2006.

38 Department of Health. *The NHS Plan: an action guide for nurses, midwives and health visitors.* London: Department of Health; 2001.

39 Freeman D, Garety PA, Kuipers E, *et al.* A cognitive model of persecutory delusions. *Br J Clin Psychol.* 2002; **41**: 331–47.

40 National Institute for Clinical Excellence. *Schizophrenia: core interventions in the treatment and management of schizophrenia in primary and secondary care.* London: National Institute for Clinical Excellence; 2002.

41 Haddock G, Morrison AP, Hopkins SL, *et al.* Individual cognitive-behavioural interventions in early psychosis. *Br J Psychiatr.* 1998; **172**(Suppl. 33): S101–6.

42 Anthony WA. Recovery from mental illness: the guiding vision of the Mental Health Service system in the 1990s. *Psychosoc Rehab J.* 1993; **16**(4): 11–23.

43 Fowler D, Garety P, Kuipers E. *Cognitive Behaviour Therapy for Psychosis: theory and practice.* Chichester: Wiley; 1995.

44 Krawiecka M, Goldberg D, Vaughan M. A standardised psychiatric assessment scale for rating chronic psychotic patients. *Acta Psychiatr Scand.* 1977. **55**: 299–308.

45 Haddock G, McCarron J, Tarrier N, *et al.* The psychotic symptom rating scales (PSYRATS). *Psychol Med.* 1999; **29**: 879–89.

46 Birchwood M, Smith J, Cochrane R, *et al.* Social Functioning Scale. *Br J Psychiatr.* 1990; **157**: 853–9.

47 Buchanan A, Reed A, Wesseley S, *et al.* Acting on delusions. 2. The phenomenological correlates of acting on delusions. *Br J Psychiatr.* 1993; **163**: 77–81.

48 Chadwick PDJ, Birchwood MJ. The omnipotence of voices. I. The beliefs about voices questionnaire. *Br J Psychiatr.* 1995; **166**: 11–19.

49 Day JC, Wood G, Dewey M, *et al.* A self-rating scale for measuring neuroleptic side-effects: validation in a group of schizophrenic patients. *Br J Psychiatr.* 1995; **166**: 650–3.

50 Barrowclough C, Tarrier N, Watts S, *et al.* Assessing the functional value of relatives' knowledge about schizophrenia: a preliminary report. *Br J Psychiatr.* 1987. **151**: 1–8.

51 Schultz JM, Videback SL. *Psychiatric Nursing Care Plans.* 7th edition. Philadelphia: Lippincott Williams and Wilkins; 2005. p. 29.

52 Persons J. *Cognitive Therapy in Practice: a case formulation approach.* New York: WW Norton; 1989. p. 37.

53 Haddock G, Tarrier N. Assessment and formulation in the cognitive behavioural treatment of psychosis. In: Tarrier N, Wells A, Haddock G, editors. *Treating Complex Cases: the cognitive behavioural therapy approach.* Chichester: John Wiley and Sons; 1998. p. 155.

54 Chadwick P, Birchwood M, Trower P. *Cognitive Therapy for Delusions, Voices and Paranoia.* Chichester: Wiley Press; 1996.

55 Ellis A. *Reason and Emotion in Psychotherapy.* New York: Lyle Stuart; 1962.

56 Zubin J, Spring B. Vulnerability: a new view of schizophrenia. *J Abnormal Psychol.* 1977; **86**(2): 103–26.

57 Neuchterlein KH, Dawson ME. A heuristic vulnerability-stress model of schizophrenic episodes. *Schizophr Bull.* 1984; **10**: 300–12.

58 NHS Centre for Reviews and Dissemination. Psychosocial interventions for schizophrenia. *Eff Health Care.* 2000; **6**(3).

59 Leff JP, Vaughn C. *Expressed Emotion in Families: its significance for mental illness.* New York: Guilford Press; 1985.

60 Zhang M, He Y, Gittelman M, *et al.* Group psycho-education of relatives of schizophrenic patients: two year experiences. *Psychiatr Clin Neurosci.* 1998; **52**(Suppl.): S344–7.

61 Tarrier N, Barrowclough C. *Families of Schizophrenic Patients: cognitive behavioural intervention.* Chichester: Wiley; 1998.

62 Stein LI, Test MA. Alternative to mental hospital treatment. *Arch Gen Psychiatr.* 1980; **37**.

63 Thornicroft G. The concept of case management for long-term mental illness. *Int Rev Psychiatr.* 1991; **3**: 125–32.

64 Bentall R, Haddock G, Slade P. Psychological treatment for auditory hallucination: from theory to therapy. *Behav Ther.* 1994; **25**: 51–66.

65 Kuipers E, Fowler D, Garety P, *et al.* London-East Anglia randomised trial of cognitive behavioural therapy for psychosis: effects of the treatment phase. *Br J Psychiatr.* 1997; **171**: 319–25.

66 Howard L, Leese M, Thornicroft G. Social networks and functional status in patients with psychosis. *Acta Psychiatr Scand.* 2000; **102**: 376–85.

67 Granholm E, McQuaid JR, McClure FS, *et al.* A randomised, controlled trial of cognitive behavioural social skills training for middle-aged and older outpatients with chronic schizophrenia. *Am J Psychiatr.* 2005; **162**(3): 520–9.

68 Nelson HE, Thrasher S, Barnes TR. Practical ways of alleviating auditory hallucinations. *BMJ.* 1991; **15**: 240–51.

69 Kemp R, Hayward P, David A. *Compliance Therapy Manual.* London: The Maudsley; 1997.

70 Tarrier N, Kinney C, McCarthy E, *et al.* Two year follow up of cognitive behavioural therapy and supportive counselling in the treatment of persistent symptoms in chronic schizophrenia. *J Consult and Clin Psychol.* 2000; **68**(5): 917–22.

71 Tarrier N, Beckett R, Harwood S, *et al.* A trial of two cognitive-behavioural methods of treating drug-resistant residual psychotic symptoms in schizophrenic patients: outcome. *Br J Psychiatr.* 1993; **162**: 524–32.

72 Birchwood M. Early detection in psychotic relapse: cognitive approaches to detection and management. *Behav Change.* 1995; **12**: 2–9.

73 Birchwood M, Spencer E, McGovern D. Schizophrenia: early warning signs. *Adv in Psychiatr Treat.* 2000; **6**: 93–101.

74 Falloon IRH, Boyd JL, McGill CW. Family management in the prevention of exacerbations of schizophrenia: a controlled study. *NEJM.* 1982; **306**: 1437–40.

75 Barrowclough C, Tarrier N. *Families of Schizophrenic Patients: cognitive behavioural intervention.* London: Chapman and Hall; 1992.

76 Burbach FR, Stanbridge RI. A family intervention in psychosis service integrating the systemic and family management approaches. *J Fam Ther.* 1998; **20**(3): 311.

77 Kavanagh D. Recent developments in expressed emotion and schizophrenia. *Br J Psychiatr.* 1992. **160**: 601–20.

78 Anderson CM, Reiss DJ, Hogarty GE. *Schizophrenia in the Family: a practitioner's guide to psychoeducation and management.* New York: Guilford Press; 1986.

79 Askey R. Case management: a critical review. *Ment Health Pract.* 2004; **7**(8).

80 Brewin A, Svanberg J. *Knowledge about Schizophrenia Questionnaire.* City Wide Specialist Psychology Therapies Department, Complex Psychological Problems and Psychosis Service/ Adult Mental Health Services: Continuing Treatment and Recovery Service. Leeds Mental Health Trust. (Unpublished); 2004.

81 Rylatt P. *Psychosis Care Standards for Older People.* South West Yorkshire Community Mental Health Trust. (Unpublished); 2006.

CHAPTER 12

Occupational therapy and affective disorders

MARY DUGGAN

Introduction

Occupational therapy is directly concerned with a person's ability to meet their personal needs for engagement in activity within the context of their physical and social environments. The role of the occupational therapist is to work with individuals who find that illness or disability impairs their ability to meet these needs.

The theory on which this chapter is based is that of the Model of Human Occupation[1] and explores:

- ageing and occupation
- the impact of affective disorders on a person's engagement with activity
- the assessment of occupational performance
- occupational therapy interventions
- mental health and well-being in later life.

Ageing and occupation

The Model of Human Occupation is founded on the belief that engagement in meaningful activity is central to our well-being, and that human occupation can best be understood as a dynamic system that involves:

- motivation
- roles and routines
- skills
- physical and social environments.

Motivation is the impulse that we experience to engage, or not to engage, in an activity. It is based on our previous experience of success in that activity, or similar activities, and is also influenced by our level of interest in the activity and the extent to which that activity fits with our personal values. As we grow older, the range of activities in which we can successfully engage may shift and even diminish. Our expectation of success may become more limited. In addition, the reduction in personal income that can accompany retirement may place real limits on the activities that we can afford to take part in. Our personal values may change. Values linked to work and achievement may become superseded by those linked to social relationships. Sadly, in a society that places high value on youth (or a youthful appearance) and on economic productivity, we may come to feel less valued by others as we grow older.

Each of us has a repertoire of life-roles, and this role-set plays a large part in our sense of personal identity and indeed in how others perceive us. These roles are related to family, friends, work (or productive activity), study, community involvement and leisure activity. Our role-set and its focus naturally change as we move through life. Ageing can sometimes represent a contraction of our overall role-set. Our children become independent adults. We reach retirement age, and lose what can be our most powerfully defining role. Increasing physical ill-health may limit the occupations that we are now able to take part in.

Our ability to engage in a satisfying and effective way with our chosen roles is supported by a range of routines. These are patterns of habitual or automatic behaviour that are acquired over time. Routines can be daily, or cyclical, taking place over longer periods of time. A degree of flexibility in routine behaviour is important to our well-being, but as we grow older our routines may become more rigid simply by their repetition over a very long time.

Occupational behaviour is enabled by physical, cognitive and interpersonal skills. Ageing may reduce our physical endurance but does not inevitably lead to an overall reduction in skills.

The physical environment consists of the natural world and the built environment, and of the objects that populate it. It encompasses areas over which we have greater control, such as our own homes and areas over which we have little or no control. In general, the wider physical environment may become less accessible for us as we age, as a result of decreasing energy and loss of physical fitness. Our more immediate physical environment may be populated by objects and influenced by occupational choices that were more relevant in earlier stages of our lives (for example, a home that was chosen with the needs of children in mind) and may therefore be less supportive of engagement in meaningful occupation as we grow older.

Our social environment is made up of a varied and complex network of family, friends, colleagues and acquaintances; the people who provide the interaction that we enjoy and value, and the services that we need. It forms the framework within which we act out our roles, and is an influencing factor on our choice of roles, the style with which we engage in them and the activities that support our role function. In earlier life, this network can be very flexible and fluid, and as we grow older is likely to become more static, and even eventually to become reduced as a result of bereavement. It may also be the case that the value set of an older network becomes more fixed, and may be seen to be less congruent with that of wider society. There is a risk, then, that the social environment becomes less enabling and more limiting for older people.

However, consider the following:

A 62 year old has become the oldest woman in Britain to have a baby. Benedict XVI had just celebrated his seventy-eighth birthday when he was elected as the Supreme Pontiff of the Catholic Church. The head of one of the world's largest media corporations is 75. Anna Mary Robertson Moses began painting in her seventies. Known as Grandma Moses, she became one of America's most renowned folk artists and by the time of her death had created over 1500 works of art. Mary Wesley, a highly successful author, published her first novel when she was 70, and was quoted as saying, 'Sixty should be the time to start something new, not to put your feet up.' Henri Matisse, one of the best known artists of the 20th century, completely changed his creative methods in his seventies after surgery for cancer left him physically weakened, in a way that enabled him not just to continue working but also to create some of his most memorable pieces. The state pension age is to rise to 68 by 2044.

The impact of affective disorders on engagement with activity
Motivation
The more powerfully an individual is motivated, the more likely they are to actually participate in an activity, and affective disorders can have a profound impact on an individual's motivation towards engagement in activity.

Even though someone may have experienced significant success in a wide range of activities or occupations, the loss of self-confidence and indeed the loss of hope that are both characteristic of depression tend to lead to an expectation of failure rather than success. One of the strongest influences on motivation is the degree to which a particular activity interests us. Anhedonia, where an individual loses the capacity to experience pleasure, effectively removes the interest value of any activity; an invitation to a party becomes as attractive as an invitation to do the dishes. In addition, the loss of energy that is often a part of low mood removes the initial impetus to do something rather than do nothing. Therefore, the individual who is experiencing depression is likely to disengage from activities that they would normally value and enjoy, because their motivation is significantly impaired.

Motivation can also be affected by the experience of hypomania. Although raised mood and over-activity may predispose an individual to activity, they may have unrealistic expectations of success that are not based on previous experience. This, accompanied by levels of disinhibition, risks engagement in activities at which the individual will fail, or which are not appropriate for him or her. This can have a serious impact on the individual's financial stability or relationships.

Routines and habits

The experience of affective disorder can have a serious effect on an individual's ability to maintain their normal routines, and consequently on their ability to carry out their roles.

The losses of energy and drive that are features of depression have an obvious impact on the maintenance of routines. If an individual feels tired and lacking in energy, they are less likely to keep up with daily routines. This is exacerbated by sleep disturbances and by the aches and pains that can also accompany low mood. Some people also experience agitation and restlessness as part of their depression. Although this may produce an increased level of motor activity, it is rarely a purposeful pattern of activity. It reduces an individual's ability to carry out routine tasks. In extreme circumstances, a person with severe depression may cease to carry out even the most basic of routines such as washing, changing their clothes and preparing food. An aspect of role-function that may be less often taken into account with older people is that of sexual expression. The impact of depression on libido and sexual function is well known, but may not be considered with older people. However, the cessation of sexual activity may have a profoundly destructive impact on a relationship, just at the time when that relationship needs to be at its most supportive.

In hypomania, over-activity can be equally disruptive to routines; it tends to take the form of disorganised engagement in activity. The individual may start an activity, but is not so likely to see it through to the end, or to be too concerned about the end result of the activity. Their routines become chaotic.

The loss of engagement in normal routines has an inevitable impact on the individual's ability to maintain their role-set. This can be further exacerbated by feelings of guilt and worthlessness, which can cause the person to question the value and validity of the roles themselves. A subset of motivation is particularly significant here: that of role incumbency. This is the extent to which an individual perceives that they have a right to a particular role, and this perception can be temporarily skewed by the experience of depression. Conversely, a person in a hypomanic state may have very unrealistic beliefs about their capacity to acquire or engage in particular roles.

Roles are not just a way of perceiving ourselves in relation to others – they are also part of how others perceive us. Disengagement from, or dysfunctional engagement in, existing roles has an impact on an individual's family and friends.

In addition to the impact of affective disorders on an individual's ability to engage in their role-set, it is important to acknowledge the profound effect of role loss on mental health. A healthy individual has a set of roles with which they can engage in a satisfying manner. Where a person's role-set is limited, the impact of the loss of a significant role can literally be disabling. The most obvious of these in relation to later life is the loss of the work role on retirement. Many people define themselves in terms of this role, and therefore suffer at least a partial loss of identity. Roles also provide the framework for our daily routines and so role disruption can also leave people without a meaningful structure to their lives. Conversely, roles or routines can be acquired that tend to perpetuate disability even after the depression or anxiety has resolved. For example, an individual experiencing anhedonia (impaired ability to experience pleasure) is likely to lose the habit of engaging in a range of leisure activities. An important part of rehabilitation is the re-establishment of normal and functional roles and routines that support mental well-being.

Skills

Affective disorders can temporarily affect cognitive, sensorimotor and interpersonal skills. Impaired concentration frequently occurs with both depression and hypomania. The individual can find it difficult to make decisions or may be vulnerable to making ill-advised decisions. Both psychomotor retardation and over-activity may have an impact on an individual's motor skills. Any of these will reduce a person's ability to engage in purposeful activity to the level or standard that they would normally expect. In addition, common side-effects of many types of medication include blurred vision, dizziness and muscle tremors, which may temporarily exacerbate the impact of illness on an individual's skills.

The most profoundly affected skill area is likely to be that of interpersonal skills. Where an individual is sunk in their own distress, they may lose awareness of the emotional needs of others. They find it harder to interact as they normally would, and also others find it harder to interact with them. An individual experiencing hypomania can be equally difficult to maintain relationships with. Disinhibition may also lead them to form relationships or to act on relationships in a way that they would not normally do. As mentioned in the previous section, the impact of affective disorders on sexual behaviour should not be ignored with older people.

Physical and social environments

The experience of affective disorder may have less impact on an individual's environment, except perhaps for their ability to maintain their immediate environment. However, both physical and social environments can be contributory factors to depression in particular, and both play a powerful role in mental health. *Everybody's Business*[8] cites estimates of mental ill health in older people which suggest a prevalence of perhaps 50% of general hospital inpatients and 60% of care home residents.

The assessment of occupational performance

The Model of Human Occupation[1] gives a framework for assessing the impact of illness or disability on an individual's occupational performance. The areas to be addressed include:

* the individual's ability to perform the activities that they need to do and those that they want to do within their normal physical and social environment
* the extent to which their environment supports or gets in the way of occupational performance
* the roles that the individual wishes or needs to engage in
* the ability of the individual to maintain the routines, both daily and cyclical, that support these roles
* the skills demanded by roles and routines, and the extent to which the individual possesses these skills, and
* the individual's motivation towards roles, routines and activities and their expectation of success within these.

There is no universal assessment tool, but it is possible to use a battery of tools and approaches that provide a comprehensive evaluation of a person's needs, capabilities and aspirations in terms of meaningful engagement in occupation. This could usefully include the following.

Occupational self-assessment[2]

This is a self-assessment that explores the person's performance, habits, roles, volition, interests and environment. It helps the individual to identify their personal values and to set priorities for change.

Occupational Performance History Interview II[3]

This assessment explores:

* the roles that a person engages in
* the ways that a person organises and uses their time
* critical life events that have shaped the individual's occupational history
* the person's occupational environments, including home, productive activity and leisure, and taking into account the physical and social aspects of those environments
* the factors that have influenced how that person makes choices about activity, and
* the individual's life story.

The assessment is summarised in three scales.

* *The Occupational Identity scale:* the extent to which that person has goals, values, interests and an expectation of success.
* *The Occupational Competence scale:* the extent to which the person is able to engage to their satisfaction in occupational behaviour.
* *The Occupational Behaviour Settings scale:* the extent to which the person's environment supports their choice of activity, and also the extent to which the activities that they engage in match their interests, abilities and personal resources.

Role checklist[4]

This checklist identifies the roles that an individual engages in on a regular basis, and the value that each of these roles has for that person. It is a useful indicator of changes in role-set, particularly of diminution of the role-set, and of the balance of roles that the individual engages in.

Interests checklist[5]

This leisure interest inventory, originally developed by Matsusuyu,[5] identifies an individual's range of interests, and their desire to engage with them in the future. It requires some adaptation to reflect British as opposed to American leisure interests, and would also require some adaptation for use with people from ethnic minority groups within Britain.

Occupational therapy interventions

Occupational therapy interventions traditionally involve:
> the use of specific, focused and graded activity as a treatment medium
> modification or adaptation of tasks
> modification or adaptation of the environment.

If, as the Model of Human Occupation describes, occupation is a dynamic system, it follows that alterations to one part of the system will have an effect not only on that part but on the whole system. This can be seen to be the case in the treatment of affective disorders, as will be outlined below. In addition, the subsystems that have been described above do not have a hierarchical relationship; in other words, none of them acts as a governing or overriding subsystem that controls the function of the others. Rather, different subsystems come to the fore in different contexts. Although, in the writer's own experience, it is often the motivational subsystem that appears to be most significantly affected, particularly by depression, this is not universally the case. Even if the motivational subsystem is the most impaired, the therapist and service user may decide together to work on a different subsystem to achieve the desired changes. In fact, Kielhofner[6] argues that 'the most effective therapeutic route is to attempt to address simultaneously as many parts of the human system as possible'. It may, therefore, be simplest to consider the types of intervention that might be used in the earlier and later stages of recovery.

Interventions in the early stages of recovery

These are often quite simple, and also often very powerful. The objectives for these interventions are likely to include the provision of immediate and tangible experiences of success (acting on motivation), to begin to restore regular engagement in activity (acting on habituation), to increase the individual's ability to focus on specific tasks for increasing lengths of time and to provide an opportunity for non-demanding social interaction (acting on skills). These interventions benefit from being delivered in an environment that encourages and supports engagement in activity. Here, the writer unashamedly champions the use of practical activity that has a tangible end result. This is precisely because of the real and observable nature of the individual's efforts. The type and nature of the activity is of less importance than the way that it is structured, although the activity needs to relate to the individual's values. However, in the early stages of recovery it may be important to avoid activities that are of particularly high value or importance to the individual, as failure in them would be likely to reinforce a sense of worthlessness. The individual is less likely to be able to un-favourably compare current performance to past performance in an unfamiliar activity. This is not always the case, though (*see* Case History 12.1)

CASE HISTORY 12.1

Lily was admitted to hospital suffering from a profound episode of depression. She had been neglecting herself to the point of becoming emaciated. She did not appear to be able to do anything spontaneously, and took much prompting to even carry out the most basic self-care activities. She was not responding to medication, and the team were becoming pessimistic about her future. Eventually, she agreed to a course of electroconvulsive treatment. After a few treatments, she required less prompting to carry out self-care, but still spent her day sitting silently in a chair. The occupational therapist invited her to come to the kitchen to make a cup of tea. She did so, but sighed as she gazed around the room. 'You know, I used to love cooking, and I even used to bake all my own bread. Look at me now.' The therapist suggested that there was no reason why she should not bake her own bread now, if she wanted. There was a flicker of interest in Lily's eyes. To simplify the activity, the therapist used a bread mix, rather than separate ingredients, and used a half quantity so that kneading would not be too arduous. The resulting bread was delicious.

Until that point, Lily had lost all hope of being able to care for herself, or do anything at all. The ECT began to lift her mood, but her inactivity gave her little opportunity to experience this. The experience of success in a valued activity gave her the initial impetus to begin to re-engage with her life.

In the early stages, activity benefits from being structured so that its execution is broken down into simple stages if need be. The completion of one stage is less daunting than the completion of the entire task. Decision making should be minimised at this point. The activity should not place too high a demand on skills – it should have a high probability of being successfully completed, without patronising the individuals concerned. The opportunity for interaction can be provided simply by virtue of carrying out the activity in a group, but the focus should be on the activity, not the interaction. In this way, individuals are able to interact without pressure and indeed can choose not to interact and still remain an active participant (*see* Case History 12.2).

CASE HISTORY 12.2

Rose had suffered a stroke that left her arm weakened. She could manage most activities of daily living, and had returned home. However, her speech remained slightly slurred. Embarrassed by this, she began to avoid the social activities that had been an important part of her life, and became increasingly low in mood.

The initial focus of therapy was to re-engage Rose to being with other people. An activity group was chosen that did not demand any interaction from her, and allowed her to work independently on a task. Building on this, she was then introduced to a group project, which required more discussion and decision making on the part of group members. Initially quiet, Rose became captivated by certain aspects of the activity, and soon developed some expertise in the techniques that were being used. Group members began to approach her for advice and assistance, and her self-consciousness began to recede.

It is important not to work at this level for too long, though of course progress is dictated by the individual. The demand of the activities can be increased by making them more complex, by introducing tasks that have to be completed over a longer period of time, by introducing more decision points and increasing the responsibility that the individual takes for planning and structuring the process. The activities should begin to involve more risk and a less rigid structure. There should be time to discuss the individual's experience of the activity, and its effect on them. Did they, for instance, anticipate that they would complete the activity successfully? As the individual begins to anticipate success, to be able to structure activity for him or herself, to make decisions and to take risks, the focus of therapy will begin to shift. Here, it can be seen that an approach that is also grounded in cognitive behavioural intervention can act powerfully on the individual's self-perception, combining challenge to self-limiting beliefs with actual experience of success.

Interventions in the later stages of recovery

Having re-engaged the individual in a more functional pattern of activity, it is important to then look at their overall occupational performance in the context of their physical and social environment. This will involve supporting them in the construction or restoration of patterns of behaviour that enable engagement in a satisfying set of roles, supported by manageable routines and enabled by the environment, that are reinforced by the experience of interest and enjoyment.

A range of approaches can be used. Individual or group-based lifestyle evaluation is often of great value. This should be linked to making actual changes in occupational behaviour (*see* Case History 12.3).

CASE HISTORY 12.3

When Olive reflected on her life, she felt that her happiest times were when her children were young. Now they were successful adults, and she often felt that they looked down on her modest range of interests. This had become worse once her husband retired. Now that he spent all day at home, he began to make disparaging remarks about how she spent her time. Predictably, her mood became low.

Olive was actually continuing to maintain her normal routine, but had lost all sense of pleasure. She felt less and less inclined to do the things that she had previously enjoyed. She joined a lifestyle re-evaluation group. Very soon, she realised that the activities that had made up her daily and weekly routine were entirely congruent with her own set of values. With individual coaching in assertiveness skills, she began to accept that she had a right to be guided by those values, rather than those of her husband or sons. She realised that she would benefit from time away from the house, and began to explore outside activities that would not only support her values, such as leisure classes and volunteering, but that would also be carried out in a social environment that shared her values.

Mental health and well-being in later life

The Joint Inquiry into Mental Health and Wellbeing in Later Life[7] cites research that suggests that maintaining involvement in productive activity and social networks has a significant impact on mental health. It also refers to the positive impact of volunteering and sustained social activities, and the significance of routine for mental health in later life. Further, *Everybody's Business*,[8] the recently published service development guide for older people's mental health, states that:

> Staying mentally and physically active gives a sense of purpose and personal worth to people, as well as enabling people to make an effective contribution to their communities. Participating in valued activities can also provide an opportunity for social contact. Hobbies and leisure activities, lifelong learning, as well as volunteering, employment, and engagement in the development or delivery of local services should all be supported.

The impact of occupation on well-being is increasingly being recognised, highlighting the importance of occupational therapy in re-establishing mental well-being.

However, a note of caution must be sounded: occupational function is not just about being able to cope independently with activities of daily living, nor is it about having a routine crammed with activity. It is about having a satisfying balance of roles and routines that arise from and enhance an individual's values and sense of self-worth.

KEY POINTS

▶ The experience of affective disorder is likely to impair the ability of the individual to engage in meaningful occupation.

▶ Occupational therapy assessment of the person with an affective disorder should encompass their motivation towards activities and occupations, their ability to maintain roles and routines, their ability to perform the activities required by their roles and environment, and the extent to which their physical and social environments support their engagement in activity.

▶ Therapeutic interventions in the early stages of recovery will tend to focus on increasing motivation towards activity, restoring more functional routines and improving sensorimotor skills linked to successful task performance.

▶ Therapeutic interventions in the later stages of recovery will tend to focus on restoring or constructing occupational performance in the context of the individual's whole environment.

▶ Satisfying engagement in purposeful and valued activity is an important contributor to mental well-being in later life.

REFERENCES

1 Kielhofner G. *A Model of Human Occupation: theory and application.* 2nd ed. Baltimore, MD: Williams and Wilkins; 1995.

2 Baron K, Kielhofner G, Tyenger A, *et al. Occupational Self Assessment.* Version 2.2. Model of Human Occupation Clearing House, University of Illinois at Chicago. Available from: http://www.moho.uic.edu/

3 Kielhofner G, Mallinson T, Crawford C, *et al. Occupational Performance History Interview II.* Model of Human Occupation Clearing House, University of Illinois at Chicago. 2004. Available from: http://www.moho.uic.edu/

4 Oakley F, Kielhofner G, Barris R, *et al.* The Role Checklist: development and empirical assessment of reliability. *Occup Ther J Res.* 1986; **6**: 157–70.

5 Matsusuyu J. The Interest Checklist. *Am J Occup Ther.* 1969; **23**: 323–8.

6 Kielhofner G. *A Model of Human Occupation: theory and application.* 2nd ed. Baltimore, MD: Williams and Wilkins; 1995. p. 258.

7 Seymour L, Gale E. *Literature and Policy Review for the Joint Inquiry into Mental Health and Well-being in Later Life.* London: Age Concern England and the Mental Health Foundation; 2004.

8 Care Services Improvement Partnership. *Everybody's Business: integrated mental health services for older adults: a service development guide.* CSIP: 2005.

CHAPTER 13

Social services for older people with depression

JILL MANTHORPE

Introduction

Everyone who works with older people in social services or social care will encounter people with depression. The impact of depression among older people and those supporting them is profound. The social work response to older people with depression is three-fold: to uphold the social model of disability in order to improve or maintain the quality of life of those affected by depression; to ensure timely and tailor-made support is available for people with depression and their carers; and to work collaboratively with other professionals at difficult times, crises or transitions. These aims reflect a social model of depression, greatly espoused in social work training and practice wisdom. This underscores social workers' responsibility to respect people's rights to self-determination, to promote participation, to treat each person as an individual, and to identify and develop strengths among individuals and communities. For people with depression of all ages, and particularly older people, social workers see the principles of social justice as equally important, because they often work in environments where the quality of care and quantity of support are poor. Many social workers will see it as their role to challenge negative discrimination, to recognise and to respond to diversity, to be culturally sensitive, to distribute resources equitably and to work towards an inclusive society. That is no small task and one that cannot be undertaken alone; it may also conflict with a narrowly constructed medical model of depression.

This chapter discusses social services' contribution to reducing the experience of depression among older people from individual support and casework to development of community well-being. The main focus is on the workings of local authority adult services in England but these are readily transferable to other parts of the United Kingdom and potentially to other developed countries.

In this chapter, the role of the professional social worker is discussed, as well as the workings of social care services. Many people working in social care are not qualified but they are the practitioners who have the most regular and sustained contact with individual older people (Chapter 14 discusses carers, so this chapter does not cover family and friends in detail). Social care services (such as home care and care homes) in the UK are largely now provided by the private sector. Many of these services but not all are paid for by local authority social services departments or adult services departments. Local government (local authorities, or Councils with Social Services Responsibilities to give them their correct, if long-winded, title) in what used to be termed social services departments is the main employer of social workers, many of whom work as care managers. Their roles include being an advocate, counsellor, caseworker, risk assessor, and agent of authority.[1]

The separation of children's and adults' services that occurred from 2005 onwards has led to a variety of new organisational structures and names for social services departments. For ease of reading the term *adult services* department will be used in this chapter, but readers are advised to look at their local context to see where adult services are located in their local government corporate structure. Similarly, in some areas, the organisational landscape is composed of integrated mental health services between local authorities and NHS Trusts. Lastly, while integration of health and social care is important, wider changes in community well-being, community safety and community cohesion are increasingly relevant. These are touched on below.

This chapter moves from discussion of the role of social work and social care's roles in assessment and care management to consider wider public agendas around mental health in later life. One overarching theme is that social workers and social care staff are pivotal in providing support for many older people with depression, but that practice is variable and practitioners often lack confidence, resources and support for themselves. These are ingredients that other professionals may be in a position to share.

Depression: a problem in common

Social care services are *'concerned with managing or reducing the effect of impairment of people's daily lives'*.[2] These services may lie in the areas of food and nutrition; personal care; social participation and involvement; safety; and control over daily life. These are basic but essential supports that can easily be overlooked and many social workers' efforts will centre on achieving outcomes that relate to these areas. They include providing help with everyday activities to regain independence, such as getting up or getting dressed, or providing company to foster social participation. Strategies to reduce depression fit well into these domains, as this chapter discusses below. In effect they are trying to close the gap between environmental demands and personal capacity to meet these demands.

The aim of this chapter is to relate the tasks and roles of social workers and social care workers with those of others working in professional roles, in the English context. If you work with social workers or with social care practitioners and with older people with depression then you will have many service users and carers in common. Local circumstances affect our roles, the systems in which we work and their rules. These are often taken for granted, but social workers and those providing social care to older people with depression have at their core the task of listening to the individual, empowering them to seek and accept support, and to developing support that will enhance their quality of life. These are shared with other professionals, of course, who also see the benefits of encouraging personal agency and promoting family involvement in the support of older people who may be in distress. This may involve interventions at times of crisis, or long-term care management, or it may involve work to develop communities' capacity to support their vulnerable members.

Working together?

This is a time of gradual but great changes for mental health services for older people, particularly around integration of health and social care services for adults. The review of the National Service Framework for Older People (NSFOP)[3] examined the rate and extent of change in 10 local authorities in England. It considered one standard 7 of the NSFOP: 'Older people who have mental health problems have access to integrated mental health services, provided by the NHS and local authorities to ensure effective diagnosis, treatment and support for them and their carers.'[4]

The Healthcare Commission[3] found that there was limited progress in providing an integrated service to older people with mental health needs. Only four of the 10 inspected areas had integrated community mental health teams for older people. In its opinion, the range of services available to older people with mental health needs was generally inferior to that available to working age adults and it concluded that age discrimination was a significant explanatory factor. For example, mental health services for older people were less well resourced than mental health services for adults of working age. They found little evidence of opportunities and activities to tackle loneliness and social exclusion among older people in order to promote good mental health. It has also been argued that the current public health and social care policy framework does not offer any coherent overarching approach to mental health in later life.[5] Such criticisms have spurred local services to develop strategies for older people with mental health problems, in the context of government initiatives to improve the lives of older people more generally (for example, *Opportunity Age*[6]).

A Social Services Inspectorate summary of inspections concluded: 'Older people with mental health difficulties were often poorly served'.[7] Underlying reasons for difficulties in planning and provision at local level reflect national policy neglect and historically poor coordination between mental health and older people's services. This is symbolised by the presence of one National Service Framework for Mental Health and another for Older People.[5]

Entitlement to social care services

Targeting of social care and other services (help to those most in need or with the potential to benefit from it) is often considered to be inadequate for older people with mental health problems, and many have noted the extent of unmet need and the lack of preventive focus. The Audit Commission[8,9] reports on mental health services for older people, *Forget Me Not*, followed up two years later, located few specialist teams for older people with mental health problems. Shortages of respite care, the service most often wanted by carers, were common. Nearly a quarter of all areas surveyed had no clear service goals or plans.[6,10] Strategies for mental health services in later life often tend to concentrate on dementia.[11]

Targeting of social care services has been widely recognised as highly successful, in that older people with greatest needs do receive the largest amount of support and funding (illustrations of this are discussed below). Social care assessments of older people are carried out under the National Health Service and Community Care Act 1990 and the raft of later policies to modernise social and other public services. The Department of Health required English local authorities to standardise eligibility criteria for adult social care services under Fair Access to Care Services (FACS). In essence, adult services departments all have eligibility criteria or thresholds for access to their services, whether provided or funded by their departments. Within FACS, four eligibility bands (low, moderate, substantial and critical) were established. This was in response to criticism that local variations were unfair,[12] inconsistent and inequitable.[13] In most areas, social care services funded and arranged by the local authority are only provided to people whose needs or risks are categorised as substantial or critical.

These high thresholds are set because local authorities must take into account their budget when determining the amount of services that they provide to meet social care needs. Care managers (those who undertake assessments for social care and who may have a role in planning the 'package' of care and its review and monitoring) have commonly reported their frustration at the raising of the threshold for eligibility to social care services.[14] On behalf of their department they have to consider whether an individual older person meets the criteria or threshold for social care support. If they do not, the person will likely be referred back to the NHS or to the voluntary or community sector for support; for example, to an Age Concern group.

This makes the task of assessment a key activity in social services, for it enables the social worker or care manager to establish a person's needs but also if a person meets the criteria or threshold for support. Case Study 13.1 sets out an example of *substantial* need applied to a fictional service user, Mrs K. It also illustrates one form of working that is common in UK settings; that is, joint working around a particular case or client.

CASE STUDY 13.1

Mrs K has lived alone since her husband died 30 years ago, but had a strong social network of friends who used to speak with her every day by phone, and visitors who called once or twice a week. She used to be house proud, despite her failing eyesight (she has Age-related Macular Degeneration (AMD)). Five months ago her cat was killed on the busy road outside her home, and she has not been sleeping well since, often waking in the night and finding it difficult to return to sleep. She has visited her GP asking for sleeping tablets. She agrees to take an antidepressant at night. After a month she is sleeping better but remains depressed with a poor appetite, is not undertaking personal care to the same extent as she used to, and has fallen after feeling dizzy. The GP makes a referral to social services to help Mrs K with her housework and personal care, since she tells him that her house is getting beyond her and she sometimes cannot be bothered to cook, eat or wash at times. He also asks a community mental health nurse to make calls on Mrs K to monitor her progress and to provide some listening and encouragement. The social worker carries out an assessment of Mrs K, taking into account what is happening and the changes in her life and what she might like to be able to do. He uses information passed on by the GP but goes into greater depth about her social circumstances and networks, including asking about her income and resources, the friends who used to visit and her extended family. Her case is regarded as falling into the substantial, not critical, band as Mrs K has some support and can do some things for herself. The ensuing care package is built up of an assessment for visual aids, a regular voluntary visitor to encourage her to get back in touch with her friends, a weekday meals on wheels service (with the hope that Mrs K might be persuaded to attend a local lunch club) and a weekly visit by a care worker (working for a private home care agency) to help, through encouragement, with personal care (a bath or strip wash) and the laundry. The community mental health nurse talks this plan through with the social worker, and agrees this is the best plan for the moment. This support is reassessed after a month, and the meals on wheels service is stopped, as Mrs K is feeling more able to prepare her own food. Six months later, the voluntary visitor is the only part of the care package in place but the social worker has left his contact details with the voluntary group coordinator and has asked to be informed if things are changing. He has also let the GP and nurse know that the social care package has now been withdrawn.

Case Study 13.2 presents the case of Mrs L, whose needs are assessed as *critical*.

CASE STUDY 13.2

Mrs L has long-standing depression and was admitted to hospital under the Mental Health Act 1983 a few years ago. She now has mobility problems that cause her considerable discomfort and finds taking medication very difficult. The Approved Social Worker (ASW) has been monitoring Mrs L over the last few years, as part of the local Community Mental Health Team (CMHT) and communicates with Mrs L's consultant psychiatrist and her general practitioner. Following the recent and sudden death of Mrs L's sister, who provided substantial practical help and emotional support to Mrs L, the social worker undertakes a fresh assessment, looking at the personal and home care needs of Mrs L, her social contacts and her need for safety and company. Her level of need is assessed as *critical* because her sister provided vital help, such as help with all meals, managing of household money, and very close monitoring of medication. A substantial package of care is commissioned with a private home care agency that can offer experienced workers who will be alert to the risks presented by Mrs L and her bereaved state. The social worker agrees the care plan with Mrs L (she says she does not want Direct Payments at this moment; *see* below) and the CMHT, and acts as key worker since she has a good relationship with Mrs L, regularly updating the GP.

There is, of course, a fine line in the formal FACS criteria between being in *substantial* need (Mrs K) and being at the higher level of *critical* need (Mrs L). To qualify for the lower level of *substantial* need, the person being assessed would have to show that 'there is, or will be, an inability to carry out the majority of personal care or domestic routines'. However, if 'there is, or will be, an inability to carry out vital personal care or domestic routines' those being assessed would qualify as being in *critical* need. For those working with social workers, knowledge of their criteria may be helpful in determining why judgements are being made and what information might be useful to them.

Such is the extent of depression among users of social care services that while it tends to be overlooked it may also taken for granted. A social worker assessing either Mrs K or Mrs L might focus on the accompanying physical health problems or disabilities, in the knowledge that their depression might worsen in response to loss or change. McCrae *et al.*[15] found that social care workers frequently expected depression among the older people they worked with. In their view, depression was common among older people in a deprived inner London area, and they attributed this largely to the adverse social circumstances of the locality. The services that they considered to be potentially effective, social groups, leisure and psychological therapies, were in particularly short supply, although secondary mental health services were regarded positively and considered available if matters were very serious.

Social workers' tasks include the assessment of risk, and this is evident in the examples of Mrs K and Mrs L. As Approved Social Workers (a post-qualification role specialising in mental health), some have particular roles in considering assessment, care and treatment in the context of the Mental Health Act 1983:

→ to observe the civil liberties of the patient and ensure that procedures are followed
→ to provide an independent professional opinion and ensure that there are sufficient grounds to warrant admission
→ advocacy to ensure the case is examined against the principle of least restriction
→ administrative functions 1) to coordinate the assessment, 2) to involve and consult close relatives, 3) to address the issues of dependants and property, and
→ responsibilities to be supportive to the patient and relatives during and after a Mental Health Act 1983 assessment.

While few older people are compulsorily assessed or treated under the Mental Health Act (MHA) 1983, or subject to its provisions for guardianship in the community, this is an important task, although the role may be revised to include professionals other than social workers. In a parallel process, proposals for clinical supervisors may enable experienced social workers to take on further case management responsibilities for people who have particularly serious mental health problems or present major risks to themselves or others.

While mental health services from the NHS, and those provided under the Mental Health Act 1983, are free, another distinctive feature with older people who have mental health problems, such as depression (unless the care is part of MHA provision), is that social care services are provided on a means-tested basis and service users will often pay for them. So, for example, Mrs K will have her finances assessed and will be charged for the meals on wheels and home care service, and possibly some of the low-vision aids supplied. The community care assessment will include efforts to consider if Mrs K is receiving all the welfare benefits she might be entitled to (such as Attendance Allowance and Pension Credit) but she will likely pay for the social care services she receives.

In this context, Direct Payments (payment for social care services that is given to the service user/carer to use to make direct arrangements) were introduced in England and Wales under the Community Care (Direct Payments) Act 1996, extended to older people in 2000. Direct Payments must now be offered to everyone assessed as needing social care, although take-up by older people and their carers has been slow. Case Study 13.3 illustrates the potential of Direct Payments and these are likely to be taken up more extensively.

CASE STUDY 13.3

Miss J looks after her mother, Mrs F, who has dementia and depression. She draws together a complex care package, using Direct Payments and her mother's disability benefits and savings (she has Lasting Power of Attorney under the Mental Capacity Act 2005), and the care manager has approved this. Miss J employs a team of three care workers who agree a rota between them and who know and understand her mother's needs and preferences. They have been told that Mrs F can be irritable and distressed at times. Miss J has asked them to gently encourage her mother in undertaking activities, such as baking, that she used to enjoy, but also to understand that she has difficulties in paying attention. The care workers also monitor medication and encourage Mrs F to go for walks if she feels so inclined. One of them brings her dog on her visits; the other plays the piano.

A previous day centre arrangement was disliked intensely by Mrs F, and caused Miss J more anxiety than it seemed worth. It also exacerbated friction between Mrs F and Miss J. Rather than meals on wheels; the care workers bring lunch to share with Mrs F and encourage her to eat. They also do housework when Mrs F is asleep or dozing. Miss J does all the paperwork and discusses any matters of concern at the review with the care manager; she says she much prefers this to coming back tired from work and having to do housework.

New developments in adult services include Individual Budgets where people will be more involved in their own assessment, decide upon the outcomes they want and how to achieve them, and will know what resources they will be given (*see* Case Study 13.4).

CASE STUDY 13.4

Mrs T, who has long-standing depression and mobility problems arising from her arthritis, has received a resource allocation of £3000 per year from social services after assessment. She chooses to spend this on a care worker who will take her shopping in the wheelchair at weekends, which is a time that feels heavy for her as her family cannot visit her then and she has no other contacts. She uses the other part of the money for servicing of her wheelchair and to buy other minor aids and adaptations. Each month she also hires a taxi to visit her sister. A local advice and support service helps her with the paperwork and she lets her care manager know how it is going at six-monthly intervals. In this way adult services fulfil their requirements of offering people more choice and control and they also see that this enhances Mrs T's well-being and promotes her independence.

Care homes

Most expenditure on long-term care in England is funded by local authority social services departments (38%), just over a third (35%) by individual service users or their families, and a minority (27%) is funded by the NHS.[16] The extent of depression among older care home residents is high, estimated to affect up to 40% of older people who live in care homes.[8] Moreover, the move to a care home can prompt feelings of great loss and sadness. A social worker will often try to listen to people's worries and distress, as well as making practical arrangements.

Despite increasing understanding of this risk, Bagley *et al.*[17] found low levels of recognition of depression among residents by care home staff and virtually no specific training on depression. Identification of depression, of course, is only the first step: care home staff need to know that there is some point in doing this and how to take effective action that will relieve the depression, otherwise they might become possibly avoidant of residents who acquire the label of 'being depressed'. Personalising the care plan for a resident may help to address this risk specifically and healthcare professionals may have a part in advising on this.

This returns us again to the key adult services' roles in assessment, care planning, monitoring and review. All these are part of the care management process and are being affected, slowly, by the Single Assessment Process (SAP) for older people, introduced in April 2004 (in Wales, Unified Assessment procedures). This again may move to become the Common Assessment Framework.

The Single Assessment Process has the potential to resolve many long-standing issues about duplication of information, although it will not overcome the problems of different computer systems between adult services and health services, different thresholds for access to services, or necessarily collect information about feelings, fears and perceptions.

Prevention

It is widely agreed that too few resources are targeted on prevention.[18] We are not short of ideas of how to improve mental health among older people, particularly around depression (*see*, for example, Better Government for Older People/Older People's Programme[19] and Mental Health Foundation/Age Concern[20]). But we are short of evidence of benefit; for example, who will benefit from befriending schemes and which type of schemes work for whom, and how to keep them well supplied with volunteers.

There are plans to improve preventative services; these have been welcomed by the UK Inquiry into Mental Health and Well Being in Later Life,[20] as potentially ways of reducing isolation and loneliness, especially around times of bereavement. The Inquiry recommended setting up healthy ageing programmes to involve local authorities and other local agencies in mental health promotion. Local authorities are also asked to support community-based activities that involve older people.

To some extent this is pushing at an open door; the Social Services Inspectorate[7] found that:

> A majority of councils included prevention in their plans to promote independence. These included developing day services, luncheon clubs and befriending services, as well as increasing low-level practical support such as care and repair, shopping and handy-persons' schemes.

However, it noted that most councils (local authorities) had made little investment in, and had no strategy for, developing low-level prevention and support services. Usually the voluntary sector was providing an uncoordinated patchwork of services.[7]

The white paper *Our Health, Our Care, Our Say*[21] portrays integrated working as something much more than the coming together of health and social care. This has special poignancy in relation to older people with depression as it acknowledges that housing, transport, lifelong learning, leisure, social contacts and many other supports must be considered alongside health and social care if practitioners are to make a reality of independence, well-being and choice; all of which are often seen as potentially helping to address the problems of older people with depression and to go some way towards prevention. Documents, such as *Opportunity Age*,[6] present further challenges to mental health services. This argues that when 40% of the population is aged 50 or more, as will soon be the case, the distinction between services for older people and services for everyone will lose significance. The same might be said of mental health services and wider community well-being. The Local Government Association[22] sees the imperative is to deliver 'community well-being':

> Integrated commissioning will include all out of hospital care and support – community health services, public health, adult social care, housing and primary care. This will develop to include a wider range of services from across all tiers of local government and local partners which impact on people's health and well-being such as leisure, recreation, community safety, benefits advice and access to work.

Local authority Directors of Adult Social Services (DASS) will play strategic roles. They are charged with the conduct of regular needs assessments of the local population, looking 10–15 years ahead, and are central to commissioning local services. Their relationships with NHS commissioning colleagues will be essential in reversing the neglect of older people's mental health services.

Connections between older people's services and mental health services for those in later life have sometimes been loose. Currently these are being tackled through building partnerships, such as Local Area Agreements (LAAs) in England. Working through Local Strategic Partnerships, these agreements are between government, the local authority, the primary care trust and other major services, community and commercial partners in an area. They bring together funding streams, simplify auditing and monitoring processes, and reduce bureaucracy to develop greater organisational flexibility to find local solutions. Within this framework, older people's concerns may continue to be separate in 'older people's departments' or they may become more diffuse in 'adult' services. The challenge for social workers, social care staff and others in multi-agency and multidisciplinary teams is that this may leave depression further marginalised, with the patchwork of resources in the voluntary and community sectors meeting a new patchwork of adult services and health sectors. Both may become threadbare by trying to meet high levels of demand and even greater expectations.

The skills that social workers develop in their professional training often focus on managing uncertain and changing circumstances. Many are motivated to work as social workers by a desire to work directly with service users, especially within a therapeutic relationship.[1] They are generally skilled in building relationships, in being able to access a wide range of helping resources, and in identifying and addressing some of the social causes of depression. Such skills are not theirs alone but there is rarely a time where there is an oversupply of such skills, especially those that are available over the long term.

KEY POINTS

▶ Many working in social services will be supporting older people who have depression or their carers who may be at risk of depression.
▶ Social workers' ability to set up social care services for an individual is constrained by the threshold for services set by their employing local authorities; they target their support on people in highest need.
▶ Approved social workers have particular powers under mental health legislation and work with older people at high risk: their roles need to be understood so they can complement other professionals' input.
▶ Social workers will increasingly be able to offer people who are eligible for social care services the power to organise their own care.
▶ Knowledge of community and faith groups and community-based organisations is likely to be high among social workers.

REFERENCES

1 Statham J, Cameron C, Mooney A. *The Tasks and Roles of Social Workers: a focused overview of research evidence.* London: Thomas Coram Research Unit; 2006.
2 Netten A, Ryan M, Smith P, *et al. Using a Discrete Choice Experiment to Develop OPUS: a preference-weighted measure of outcome of social care for older people.* [Discussion Paper]. Canterbury: PSSRU, University of Kent; 2002.
3 Healthcare Commission. *Living Well in Later Life.* London: Healthcare Commission; 2006.
4 Department of Health. *National Service Framework for Older People.* London: Department of Health; 2001.
5 Seymour L, Gale E. *Literature and Policy Review for the Joint Inquiry into Mental Health and Well-Being in Later Life.* Commissioned by Age Concern and The Mental Health Foundation. Unpublished report; 2004.

6 HM Government. *Opportunity Age: meeting the challenges of ageing in the 21st century.* London: HM Government; 2005.

7 Bainbridge I, Ricketts A. *Improving Older People's Services: an overview of performance.* London: Social Services Inspectorate; 2003.

8 Audit Commission. *Forget Me Not.* London: Audit Commission; 2000.

9 Audit Commission. *Forget Me Not.* London: Audit Commission; 2002.

10 Moriarty J, Webb S. *Part of their Lives.* Bristol: Policy Press; 2000.

11 Manthorpe J, Iliffe S. *Depression in Later Life.* London: Jessica Kingsley; 2005.

12 Audit Commission/Better Government for Older People. *Older People: independence and well-being: the challenge for public services.* London: Audit Commission; 2004.

13 Challis D, Hughes J. Frail old people at the margins of care: some recent research findings, *Br J Psychiatr.* 2002; **180**(2): 126–30.

14 Ware P, Matosevic T, Hardy B, *et al.* Commissioning care services for older people: the view from care managers, users and carers. *Ageing Soc.* 2003; **23**: 411–8.

15 McCrae N, Murray J, Banerjee S, *et al.* They're all depressed, aren't they? A qualitative study of social care workers and depression in older adults. *Aging Ment Health.* 2005; **9**(6): 508–16.

16 Comas-Herrera A, Pickard L, Wittenberg R. *Thirty years on: future demand for long-term care in England.* PSSRU Research Summary 25. Canterbury: PSSRU, University of Kent; 2003.

17 Bagley H, Cordingley L, Burns A, *et al.* Recognition of depression by staff in nursing and residential homes. *J Clin Nurs.* 2000; **9**(3): 445–50.

18 Godfrey M, Randall T. *Developing a Locality-based Approach to Prevention with Older People.* Leeds: Nuffield Institute for Health; 2003.

19 Better Government for Older People/Older People's Programme. *Moving Out of the Shadows.* Bournemouth: Help and Care Development Ltd; 2005.

20 Mental Health Foundation/Age Concern. *Promoting Mental Health and Well-being in Later Life: a first report from the UK Inquiry into Mental Health and Well-being in Later Life.* London: Age Concern and Mental Health Foundation; 2006.

21 Department of Health. *Our Health, Our Care, Our Say.* London: Department of Health; 2006.

22 Local Government Association. *The Future of Adult Social Care: a partnership approach for well-being.* London: LGA; 2006.

CHAPTER 14

Carer and service user perspectives of affective disorders in older adults

VIRGINIA MINOGUE

Introduction

This chapter explores affective disorders from the perspective of the service user and the carer. It examines the policy and practice guidance driving the broader agenda of public participation, service user and carer involvement in shaping health service delivery. It also examines the critical issues of choice and control in the care and treatment of older adults.

A raft of health and social care literature, and policy guidance, over the last 10 years has advocated service user and carer involvement in their care and in decisions about their treatment.[1,2,3,4,5,6,7,8] Yet, older adults often feel disenfranchised from making decisions about their own healthcare as professionals, and sometimes their own families, may believe they are not capable of a balanced judgement. This can be born out of some of the symptoms of affective disorders and dementia-related illnesses such as memory loss, confusion and loss of concentration. However, similar symptoms may be prevalent in mental illnesses found in working age adults but it is notable that the language used in discussing typologies of treatment and the intervention are different. It is routine to talk in terms of the use of the Recovery Model[9,10] or the Tidal Model,[11] both based on a central concept of person-centred care, in working with adults but relatively few areas have adopted and evaluated similar principles in treating older adults.[12,13] This belief that older adults have no need for creative and diverse services was highlighted by a report published in 2005 (Moving out of the Shadows (MOOTS)[8]) which described the difference between adult and older adults' mental health services as the 'Berlin Wall'. Although recognised as having value, psychotherapy is rarely

217

available for older adults. This point was also picked up by Oishi and Unutzer,[14] Collins *et al.*[15] and Gallo *et al.*[16] who found that antidepressant medication was the predominant treatment, with psychological interventions unlikely to be considered and, when they were, referrals were rarely made. The National Service Framework for Older People[17] attempted to redress this by stating that older adults with depression should be offered psychological therapies alongside medication.

Service user and carer experience of services for older adults

Depression, in itself, breeds a sense of hopelessness and helplessness and, often, isolation. Old age may also bring about similar emotions of loss of worth, power and no longer being part of the economic machine that defines our culture. The 'cycle of depression'[14] for carers or older adults may be linked to physical illness, mental illness or the onset of old age. Rates of depression are particularly high for some chronic illnesses such as Parkinson's or Huntington's disease. Older adults are more likely to experience key life events, such as bereavement, and age discrimination.[18] Those who are already experiencing exclusion, for example the mentally ill or physically disabled, may find this becomes more acute during older age. Levels of health and wealth may also reduce, resulting in lifestyle changes and a time of insecurity and uncertainty. Moreover, many older adults also become carers and have to adapt to that full-time role as well as cope with the ageing process. Any of these issues may trigger depression and with an increasing ageing population, the delivery of services that meet health, social care, leisure and activity needs become even more important.

The symptoms of depression, i.e. apathy, loss of concentration, memory loss, melancholy, may be seen as part of the ageing process and therefore not necessitating treatment with 'talking therapies'. The root causes of depression, physical illness, effect of long-term pain, social isolation, stress of caring for a partner, poverty, are not always examined nor is there recognition that the illness may be the result of a range of different health and social factors. Older adults need holistic joined-up services meeting all health and social care needs and reflecting the need to retain their social inclusion. Quality of life is not seen as predominant for the older population who are viewed as needing care rather than being encouraged in techniques for self-care. The Joseph Rowntree Foundation[19] suggests that policy and practice in services for older adults is framed in the context of two models: deficit and heroic. The deficit model sees old age as an incurable illness where older adults are the passive recipients of care. Decisions about care and treatment are taken by professionals and when ill, older adults experience a loss of control and power. This is often accompanied by feelings of declining productivity, the lowering of sexual activity, decreasing mobility, and being regarded by society, and possibly family members, as a burden. The heroic model cites successful ageing as the ability to remain on a physical par with younger people. Neither of these models represents the reality for the majority of older adults who wish to play an active role in the community and retain a reasonable quality of life.

With the proportion of older adults in the population expected to continue to increase,[20,21] then, improving quality of life, mental health and well-being is crucial from both the perspective of the service user and carer, and the government, and agencies and organisations working with older adults. However, as indicated by the publication of the MOOTS report[8] this may require a change of culture in the way services are provided. Since the report, several initiatives have been launched to improve service delivery for older people. In 2006 the Department of Work and Pensions announced that it would be introducing 'Sure Start' for older adults aimed at improving their quality of life; the Department of Health also launched 'A New Ambition for Older People'[20] comprising 10 programmes for improving care and treatment. While both are welcome developments, without joined-up thinking between government departments to deliver on the stated aim to reduce social exclusion and empower older adults to participate in their local community, there is a danger of older adults once again becoming passive participants in their care and few really benefiting from the opportunities offered. Policy alone cannot change the underlying negative attitudes to older adults within our society which impact on health and care through a lack of respect and dignity being offered during treatment.

In accessing and using health and social care services, older adults feel disempowered, overlooked, a burden and a drain on health services in particular. They feel that because they are in general economically inactive, they are not seen as an individual so much as just an older person.[8,19] When old people seek help for a physical problem many doctors do not recognise the impact of physical illnesses, chronic pain and disability on mental health and do not make this part of their assessment of the service user. Substance misuse and domestic violence may also be issues faced by both service users and carers. Women are over-represented in studies of depression and the prevalence rate of depression among abused women is 47.6%.[22] It is known that almost 50% of women using mental health services have experienced violence and abuse and the effects of this may carry on into later life. This is such a high priority area that the Department of Health and NIMHE set up a violence and abuse programme on health and mental health in 2004. We also know that elder abuse is a major but generally unreported problem.[23]

Carers feel their needs are often not recognised at all as the focus is on the service user. Although not limited to services for older adults, to negotiate health and social care services requires a certain amount of knowledge about what is available, where to go, what is needed and who to ask. This can be particularly difficult for carers who do not know what is available for them or their entitlement to a carer's assessment. Of course, not all older adults are suffering from chronic or serious illness but they nonetheless have needs which, if met, can help them retain an independent lifestyle and social participation. However, these needs may be perceived as 'low level', e.g. help with shopping, gardening or household chores, and not be eligible for assistance. Yet to meet these very practical needs may make a significant difference to quality of life and social functioning, and reduce higher level uptake of services in the future. Understandably, services are usually concentrated on those with the greatest need or those in crisis, but focusing on prevention or early detection may in the longer term reduce pressure on more costly interventions.

What do older adults want?

Older adults are a diverse population with different characteristics of ageing, physical and mental health, lifestyles, economic power and ethnic diversity. However, the majority share the desire to be heard and valued for their contribution to society and to retain their independence. Mobility can be critical to retaining independence, friendships and a social life. Access to transport will mean that older adults can go to social and leisure activities, classes, or meet friends. Lack of these contacts will lead to isolation and increased risk of developing depression. Remaining in your own home, with adaptations and assistance in order to do so, is the key to retaining a reasonable quality of life and mental well-being for older adults. The importance of an environment that feels safe, secure and welcoming cannot be overstated in terms of its role in enhancing a person's well-being. To achieve physical and mental well-being, older adults want to be active and to have opportunities for involvement. This can have the key benefit of reducing the need for access to health and social care services. Health and social care services can provide some of these opportunities and these will be discussed later in this chapter, but it is also important to listen to the individual. They may simply want support to attend a weekly social event rather than be taken to a Day Centre or older adults group. In addition to the service user, it is essential that carers' needs are recognised as many remain hidden and the full-time nature of their role means they may not be able to take up opportunities for engagement. It is important to recognise that the needs of older and younger carers may differ and to understand that there may be practical and financial implications arising from long-term care giving. Carers may also need assistance in helping the person they care for develop self-management strategies. We cannot assume that carers are able to access knowledge or have the skills to help this happen.

In common with most consumers, older adults want choice when accessing the services they require. This ideal underpins much of recent public sector reform, particularly in the NHS.[24,6,4] The evidence is that increased choice of care and treatment and involvement in care planning increases satisfaction with services and encourages self-management, but this is a complex area as it depends on the availability of a range of services, the ability and capacity to make relevant choices, and the willingness of clinicians and professionals to accept the choices of service users and carers.[5,25,26] Organisational culture may also need to shift to facilitate a greater level of involvement or co-production in the planning and delivery of services,[27,28] but it is predicated on the understanding of the consumer's motives for involvement.[29] Moreover, service user involvement in mental health services is patchy with an emphasis on consultation rather than influence, partnership or control. The main barriers to involvement are lack of information, financial and time costs, professionals' concerns over the representativeness of service users and resistance to the idea of service users as experts. Many mental health service users and older adults lack information to facilitate choice or are excluded from involvement.[26,30,31] This can be particularly true for hard to reach groups, such as black and minority ethnic communities, and disabled groups, who may not know where to access information about available services.

Older adults and their carers want holistic and flexible services that respond to their practical, physical and psychological needs. They also want culturally relevant services which are based in the community and reflect local needs. The voluntary sector can play a key role in the provision of services, especially day services, particularly if they can work within local communities. Community groups, such as faith-based groups, could also play a key role in engaging members of the community and reducing social isolation. Older adults with depressive type illnesses welcome safe environments where they can receive psychological and emotional support. Local services increase social inclusion as those older adults with mobility issues, whether through physical or mental ill health, are unlikely to travel outside their community to access services. To achieve holistic service provision, services have to have routine screening tools that will assess an older person's physical, psychological and practical needs, and those of their carers. Primary, acute and secondary care professionals need to have knowledge of the impact of the ageing process, physical illness and chronic pain on mental heath and to undertake appropriate assessments. This means the workforce has to reflect the population's requirements and may even mean that older adults, and older adult's champions, are involved in the training of practitioners and clinicians. This would have the additional benefit of providing positive role models that disprove ageist myths about older adults being passive recipients of services, grumpy and inactive.

User involvement: power, choice and control

For older adults services to truly reflect their needs, older adults need to play a greater role in shaping policy and practice. People need to have a say and choice over what happens to them even if they are facing difficulties in their lives, e.g. life-limiting illnesses. Standard 2 of the National Service Framework for Older People[17] states that health and social care organisations must treat older adults as individuals and allow them to make choices about their care. A single assessment process, integrated commissioning and provision of services is the portal through which this should be achieved.

As stated at the beginning of this chapter, the last decade has heralded a raft of policies and guidance relating to public participation in the NHS. Two of the earlier papers espoused the view that the public should participate in decisions and policies that affect their health and shape health services.[32,33] *The NHS Plan*[1] and

Involving Patients and the Public in Healthcare[2] developed this further by giving patients and the public a greater say in the NHS and setting out proposals for implementing patient-centred care. The emphasis on patient-centred and patient-led services and public involvement remained central to government policy in subsequent moves to modernise services.[4,6] Similarly, public involvement in NHS research became more prevalent.[34,35] Despite the plethora of policy and guidance, Beresford[36] suggests service users are in danger of being overlooked in knowledge-based policy and practice. Service user and carer experience may not necessarily be seen as 'evidence' or 'knowledge' and a basis for policy and practice if regarded as intrinsically biased. This then undermines the concept of service user involvement in practice and service development.

'Health in Partnership'[5] stressed the importance of involving service users and carers in health decision making and research. Twelve studies examined involvement in service planning and delivery, decisions about treatment and care, and education and training. Findings echoed the themes identified in earlier sections: involvement in care and planning, quality information and good communication increase service users' satisfaction. However, in order to fully involve the public, health and social care organisations, and the community, need to develop a greater understanding of the mechanisms to achieve this goal. The public need information about opportunities for involvement and organisations need a culture of involvement led by boards and governing bodies. Staff are generally positive about involvement but require education and training, particularly on the importance of including all elements of the community. This is now reflected in the professional training of many health and social care workers.[37]

Creating a Patient Led NHS[6] based the future of the NHS on the creation of services which were patient led with people having greater choice and control. It advocated changes to systems including the introduction of Foundation Trusts, payment by results, and the measurement of the impact of services by their impact on patients. Nonetheless, despite modernisation of healthcare, participation by older adults is not common and to increase their involvement we have to recognise the specific barriers they face such as ageism, poverty, access to employment, societal perception and social exclusion. The Joseph Rowntree Foundation[19] identified two levels of involvement for older adults, individual and collective. Individual involvement at the level of taking part in decision making about the person's own care; collective involvement taking the form of membership of a service user or carer interest or support group, or representing the service user or carer view on a committee. Neither of these offers real choice or control to the service user. They fall within a managerialist/consumerist approach rather than a democratic approach to service delivery. It is questionable whether this can lead to participation and involvement at strategic level and at the level of organisational development, but in considering how to involve the public, it is of course important to consider whether public involvement is motivated by altruism, egoism, collectivism, or principlism.[29] These forms of motivation are not exclusive but are crucial to health and social care organisations' understanding and retention of public and community involvement. Meaningful involvement can exist on a range of levels from consultation through collaboration and partnership to service user-led services.

Meaningful involvement

Older adults, like other age groups, are a diverse group of people and while they share some experience they also have individual concerns and needs. These do not simply relate to healthcare as social and other needs are also crucial. Meaningful involvement starts from recognising the important role that older adults play in society, in families and as carers. Involvement may start at an individual (egoist) level with participation in care planning, decisions about treatment, choice, managing Direct Payments;[38,19] or may be more altruistic and take the form of participation in a support, advocacy or lobbying group or charitable foundation. Research into participation has tended to focus on the extent of involvement (using a model such as Arnstein's 'ladder of participation').[39] However, the level of involvement is not necessarily the issue if the principle of inclusion is based on responsiveness to needs and empowerment and choice for the service user and carer. Furthermore, to be effective, involvement on any level must have meaning in the person's life and lead to positive outcomes on a personal or more general level.

The Care Services Improvement Partnership[24] has published guidance for those involved in providing health or social care to older adults on how to involve service users and carers in decisions. Further examples of good practice and meaningful involvement are provided by the Joseph Rowntree Foundation[19] and MOOTS[8] under the key themes of: person-centred care, mental well-being, social inclusion, participation, choice and control. Both offer clear messages about starting with the person and service user and carer-defined ideas of what constitutes quality of life rather than basing policy and practice on assumptions. Participation, power, choice and control are facilitated by the provision of good quality information, consultation, engagement in decision making, and support. To increase social inclusion, it is important to recognise the need to work with local communities and integrate opportunities for older adults into provision. Ageing can lead to social isolation and this can be compounded by an affective disorder which might lead to the person withdrawing from social contact. One response to this has been to extend the Sure Start programme for families to older adults through Link-Age Plus,[40] which aims to reduce social exclusion and poverty.

Many different types of involvement currently exist within health and social care which offer opportunities for involvement, for example patient forums such as clinical governance councils, Patient and Public Involvement Forums, advocacy, service user development workers, volunteers, user researchers, education and training of healthcare professionals, to mention just a few. However, older adults are generally in the minority in these arenas and their views are not always considered. This lack of involvement may be through poor communication, social isolation, or lack of support to enable people to get involved. To address this issue, health and social care providers need to think carefully about the methods used to consult with older adults and the training they may need to support their involvement. Creative methods that have been utilised are life story interviews, video, and discussion groups.[41] Levels of involvement that are utilised can be categorised as: consultation, collaboration or partnership, and user led initiatives (*see* Table 14.1 for examples of each of these in practice). Consultation is the most frequently used as this is potentially the most straightforward means of engaging in a dialogue with service users and carers. Engaging in collaboration or partnership, providing adequate time is devoted to it, increases the empowerment of the service user and carer. Service user led initiatives allow the service user or carer to take full control. There are several examples of research led by service users and carers which has had an impact on participants and demonstrates the potential for influencing service development in a meaningful way.[42,43,44,45] Many older adults would like to see a move through the continuum of involvement from passive recipients of care or passive providers of opinions to active engagement in planning and delivery and the potential for user led or user controlled services being explored.

The main areas that user involvement can impact on are: providing feedback on services, evaluation and research, developing outcome measures, training and education for health and social care professionals and students, employees of social care and health services, and user led services, e.g. Social Enterprises. Training for involvement needs to recognise the learning styles of people who experienced a different educational system. Most older adults will have strong opinions on their care and treatment but may not be used to a discursive style of learning and will not communicate in medical jargon. Older adults can also play an important role in teaching others or in community groups. Many have time and would like to take up an opportunity to learn new skills or use old ones. They are usually committed, conscientious and reliable members of any voluntary or community groups they become involved with. Service users who become involved in such activities need to feel valued and listened to and this can be crucial in retaining commitment and interest.

Meaningful involvement must have at its centre the older person who is the expert at defining 'quality of life'. As the model on p. 226 illustrates (*see* Figure 14.1), person-centred services must be based on participatory principles of choice, inclusion, respect, dignity, independence and involvement in decision making. Services must be holistic and recognise the need for integrated community-based care from health, social care, housing and other services. Access to good quality information, self-help and self-care techniques, or programmes to reduce anxiety, stress and depression, alongside leisure and social activities, enable increased self-management and self-care. However, to engage with marginalised groups, clinicians and professionals need to go into their communities or environments and use activities that will foster involvement and that may need to utilise other means than meetings.

TABLE 14.1 Typologies of involvement with examples

Passive recipients	Consultation	Collaboration/ partnership	Service user led initiatives
Research participants as subjects Annual patient surveys	Consultation exercises, e.g. workshops, surveys PALS* Patient forum Inpatient unit meetings Audit, evaluation and research – seek views on project proposals Local Partnership Boards	PPI** Forum Service user or carer support groups Training and education of professionals and students Volunteers Experts by Experience Commissioning groups Membership of NHS Trust Boards or other governing bodies Service user and carer champions Service user and carer development workers Jointly led audit, evaluation or research	Service user and carer led support and activity groups Service user and carer led services Social enterprises Service user led audit, evaluation or research

*PALS – Patient Advice and Liaison Service

**PPI – Patient and Public Involvement

Conclusions

As the number of older adults in the population increases by up to 15% in the next 10 years, social policy and societal expectations will also shift. It is estimated that as many as 15% of those over 65 suffer from depression, more than the number suffering from long-term physical illness, thereby placing increasing pressure on mental health services.[24] As the older population grows, demand on services will also increase as will the cost to the economy. It is therefore crucial that health and social care services respond at an early stage and are responsive to people's needs in supporting independence and maintaining quality of life. Changes to the employment-related pension system and the age discrimination law introduced in October 2006[46] will lead to people retiring at a later age than the historical 65 years for men and 60 years for women. Inevitably, this will mean some older adults experiencing many of the symptoms of old age while in employment. Conversely, their economic power will be sustained for a longer period. Maintaining the social inclusion of older adults in the community will become even more important. The distinction between services for working age adults and older adults, i.e. those under and over 65 years may also be questioned as people work for longer. Will this mean older 'working' adults accessing services for the under sixty-fives

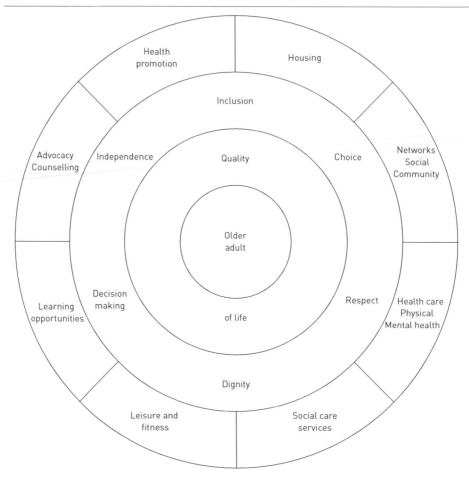

FIGURE 14.1 Person-centred care for older adults: a participatory model.

and those unemployed accessing older adults services thus introducing further inequities? (This distinction is not shared across government departments as the Social Exclusion Unit defines older adults as those aged over 50 years. Men over 65 years old and women over 60 are defined as 'pensioners'.)[47]

Although fewer older adults are now experiencing absolute poverty, according to the Social Exclusion Unit,[47] it is still anticipated that a substantial number will face social exclusion in later life. Recommendations for developing strategies for older adults' services have been well documented in the MOOTS and Joseph Rowntree Foundation reports[8,19] and stress the need for integrated strategies and investment plans. Person Centred Care, reflecting all needs including housing, leisure and mobility, is fundamental to any successful strategy as is provision of information. Service users and carers do not expect organisations and their staff to necessarily share their values but when involving consumers in service planning and delivery, it is vital to reach a shared understanding and to find a common language in order to communicate effectively. To have any real impact, older adults must be heard and be an integral part of service planning and service provision. Increasingly, we will require culturally relevant services to respond to an increasingly ethnically diverse older population.

KEY POINTS

▶ The active participation of older adults in the planning and delivery of services can have positive effects on their self-esteem, reduce social exclusion, and improve their quality of life.

▶ Involving older adults in the design of services, and decisions about their own care, leads to more appropriate and targeted service delivery which may result in individuals retaining a greater degree of independence and social participation.

▶ With a growth in the ageing population, there is an increased need to involve older adults in education and training of health and social care staff, service development and delivery to ensure relevant and properly planned services. Local and community-based groups can play a key role in facilitating the involvement of older adults and reduce social exclusion and increase empowerment.

▶ Carers have specific needs and need to be recognised as individuals distinct from the person they care for. Opportunities for influencing service delivery and access to support for their own health, social care, leisure and activity needs are crucial.

Acknowledgements

In writing this chapter, I would like to acknowledge the contribution of Rebecca Northern, and particularly John Girdlestone and Anne Haughie for sharing their experience with me.

REFERENCES

1 Department of Health. *The NHS Plan.* London: HMSO; 2000.

2 Department of Health. *Involving Patients and the Public in Healthcare.* London: HMSO; 2001.

3 Department of Health. *Health and Social Care Act: Section 11.* London: HMSO; 2001.

4 Department of Health. *NHS Improvement Plan.* London: HMSO; 2004.

5 Department of Health. *Patient and Public Involvement in Health: the evidence for policy implementation: a summary of the results of the Health in Partnership research programme.* London: HMSO; 2004.

6 Department of Health. *Creating a Patient Led NHS.* London: HMSO; 2005.

7 Care Services Improvement Partnership. *Our Choices in Mental Health.* London: Care Services Improvement Partnership; 2005.

8 Bowers H, Eastman M, Harris J, *et al. Moving out of the Shadows: a report on mental health and wellbeing in later life.* 2005. Available from: http://www.changeagentteam.org.uk/_library/mootsreport.pdf

9 Department of Health. *The Journey to Recovery.* London: HMSO; 2001.

10 Roberts G, Wolfson P. The rediscovery of recovery: open to all. *Adv Psychiatr Treat.* 2004; **10**: 37–49.

11 Buchanan-Barker P, Barker PJ. *The Tidal Model: a guide for mental health professionals.* London: Brunner-Routledge; 2004.

12 Petch A. *Intermediate Care: what do we know about older people's experiences?* York: Joseph Rowntree Foundation; 2003.

13 Quinn A, Snowling A, Denicolo P. *Older People's Perspectives: devising information, advice and advocacy services.* York: Joseph Rowntree Foundation; 2003.

14 Oishi S, Unutzer J. Overcoming barriers to effective depression care in older adults. *Understanding Mental Health.* 2001. Available from: http://www.depression.org.uk

15 Collins E, Katona C, Orrell MW. Management of depression in the elderly by general practitioners: referral for psychological treatments. *Br J Clin Psychol.* 1997; **36**: 445–8.

16 Gallo JJ, Ryan SD, Ford DE. Attitudes, knowledge and behaviour of family physicians regarding depression in later life. *Arch Fam Med.* 1999; **8**: 249–56.

17 Department of Health. *The National Service Framework for Older People.* London: HMSO; 2001.

18 Office of the Deputy Prime Minister. *A Sure Start to Later Life: ending inequalities for older people.* London: Social Exclusion Unit; 2006.

19 Joseph Rowntree Foundation. *Older People Shaping Policy and Practice.* York: Joseph Rowntree Foundation; 2004.

20 Department of Health. *A New Ambition for Older People.* London: HMSO; 2006.

21 National Statistics and Government Actuary's Department. *Social Trends 2006, 36.* London: National Statistics.

22 Humphries C, Thiara RK. Mental health and domestic violence: 'I call it symptoms of abuse'. *Br J Soc Work.* 2003; **33**: 209–26.

23 House of Commons Health Committee. *Elder Abuse: second report of session 2003–04.* 2004.

24 Care Services Improvement Partnership. *Everybody's Business: integrated mental health services for older adults: a service development guide.* London: HMSO; 2005.

25 Department of Health. *Better Information, Better Choices, Better Health: putting information at the centre of health.* London: HMSO; 2004.

26 Sainsbury Centre for Mental Health. *Choice in Mental Health Care.* Briefing 31. Sainsbury Centre for Mental Health; 2006.

27 Hyde P, Davies HTO. Service design, culture and performance in health services: consumers as co-producers. *Hum Relat.* 2004; **11**: 1407–26.

28 Boyle D, Burns S, Conisbee M. *Towards an Asset-based NHS.* London: New Economics Foundation; 2004.

29 Batson CD, Ahmad N, Tsang J. Four motives for community involvement. *J Soc Issues.* 2002; **58**(3): 429–45.

30 Tait L, Lester H. Encouraging user involvement in mental health services. *Adv Psychiatr Treat.* 2005; **11**: 168–75.

31 Rethink. *Just One Per Cent: the experiences of people using mental health services.* Kingston Upon Thames, Surrey: Rethink; 2003.

32 Department of Health. *In the Public Interest: developing a strategy for public participation in the NHS.* London: HMSO; 1998.

33 Department of Health. *Patient and Public Involvement in the New NHS.* London: HMSO; 1999.

34 Department of Health. *Research and Development for a First Class Service.* London: HMSO; 2000.

35 Department of Health. *Research Governance Framework for Health and Social Care.* London: HMSO; 2005.

36 Beresford P. Theory and practice in user involvement in research: making the connection with public policy and practice. In: Lowes L, Hullat I editors. *Involving Service Users in Health and Social Care Research.* London: Routledge; 2005.

37 Fadden G, Shooter S, Holsgrove G. Involving carers and service users in the training of psychiatrists. *Psychiatr Bull.* 2005; **29**: 270–4.

38 Heslop P. *Direct Payment for Mental Health Users/Survivors: a guide to some key issues.* London: National Centre for Independent Living; 2005.

39 Arnstein SR. A ladder of citizen participation. *J Am Plan Assoc.* 1969; **35**(4): 216–24.

40 Department for Communities and Local Government. 2006. http://www.communities.gov. uk/index.asp?id

41 Warren L, Cooke J. Working with older women in research: benefits and challenges of involvement. In: Lowes L, Hullat I editors. *Involving Service Users in Health and Social Care Research.* London: Routledge; 2005.

42 Rose A. Having a diagnosis is a qualification for the job. *BMJ.* 2003; **326**: 1331.

43 Minogue V, Boness J, Brown A, *et al.* The impact of service user involvement in research. *Int J Health Care Qual Assur.* 2005; **1892**(3).

44 Telford R, Boote J, Cooper CL. What does it mean to involve consumers successfully in NHS research? A consensus study. *Health Expect.* 2004; **7**: 1–12.

45 Faulkner A. *The Ethics of Survivor Research: guidelines for the ethical conduct of survivor research.* Bristol: Policy Press; 2004.

46 Department of Trade and Industry. *The Employment Equality (Age) Regulations 2006.* SI No. 2006/1031; 2006. Available from: http:/www.opsi.gov.uk/si/si2006/20061031.htm

47 Barnes M, Blom A, Cox K, *et al. The Social Exclusion of Older People: evidence from the first wave of the English Longitudinal Study of Ageing.* London: Social Exclusion Unit; 2006.

CHAPTER 15

Cultural aspects of affective disorders in older people

ANILKUMAR PILLAI

Introduction

We live in a society which is rapidly embracing and amalgamating different cultures and races. This trend is becoming universal and is increasingly seen in rapidly developing countries such as China and India. This could be attributed to the migration of population between countries. Migration can also happen within a nation, across states and counties. People migrate for various reasons, chiefly political and socioeconomic. This migration results in dynamic changes to the structure of a society. It can lead to positive exchanges of values between cultures. Migration has gained momentum in the past few years due to the effect of globalisation.[1]

One of the main themes in the issue of migration is its impact on the economy. Economic activity depends on age, educational status, skill and proficiency in the local language. For example, in the United Kingdom the current first generation migrants generally do well and make a net fiscal contribution.[2] Older migrants may not be seen engaging in visible economic activities, but they may contribute significantly to childcare and other domestic duties. They also provide advice and support to family members in crisis and often take up the role of an informal 'psychotherapist'.

The presence of ethnic minority groups in a community is not always the result of continuing migration. Some groups will have been living in a country for generations. Among them, some will have absorbed the cultural values and norms of the host nation. They will consider themselves as belonging to the host nation, at the same time keeping their cultural identity. We may also find migrant communities locked in cultural ghettoes without integration or assimilation. This can lead to suspicion and feelings of insecurity both in the migrant population and local people.

Race, ethnicity and culture

These terms are controversial and difficult to define, and they are often used to convey the same meaning.

Culture has been defined as

> shared learned behaviour that is transmitted from one generation to another for purposes of human adjustments, adaptation and growth. Culture has both external and internal referents. External referents include artefacts, roles and institutions. Internal referents include attitudes, values, beliefs, expectations, epistemologies and consciousness.[3]

The US Department of Health and Human Services defines culture as a common heritage or set of beliefs, norms and values.[4] It refers to the shared attributes of one group. The dominant culture for much of United States history focused on the beliefs, norms and values of European Americans, but America is now essentially a multicultural nation.[5] Anthropologists often describe culture as a system of shared meanings. Many people consider themselves to have multiple cultural identities as cultural groups can be defined by ethnicity, religion, geographic region, age group, sexual orientation or profession. Culture is dynamic and ever changing. It helps people to adapt to their external and internal environments.[6]

Race is perceived by appearances and is attributed to biological and genetic traits. The UK Race Relations Act distinguished race as referring to physical differences and ethnicity to cultural differences. It is possible for people to be culturally similar but racially different.

A working definition for ethnic minorities is 'individuals with a cultural heritage distinct from the majority population'.[7] An ethnic group is a group of people who identify with each other, on the basis of a presumed common ancestry. Ethnic groups are sometimes united by common cultural, behavioural, linguistic or religious practices. Ethnic minority groups may comprise migrants who are first generation, second generation or those who migrated to the host country many generations ago.

On looking at these definitions it is easy to see the complexity of these concepts and the controversies these could evoke. Discussions on these definitions are beyond the scope of this chapter.

Attitudes towards elderly people vary across cultures. Many elders of Afro-Caribbean origin live alone whereas many of those from Asian cultures live with their families, possibly reflecting what happens in their country of origin or other unknown factors.

Migration

The 2001 census showed that one in 12 people in the United Kingdom are born overseas. The minority ethnic population constituted about 4.6 million, 7.9% of the total population of the UK.[8] Indians (1.8%) formed the largest minority group. This was followed by Pakistanis (1.3%), those of mixed ethnic backgrounds (1.2%), Black Caribbeans (1%), Black Africans (0.8%) and Bangladeshis (0.5%). The remaining minority ethnic groups together accounted for a further 1.4% of the population. This includes people who were foreign born and those who were born and brought up in the UK. Just over three-quarters of the UK population reported having a religion. More than seven out of 10 people said that their religion was Christian (72%). After Christianity, Islam was the most common faith with nearly 3% describing their religion as Muslim (1.6 million). The next largest religious groups were Hindus, followed by Sikhs, Jews, Buddhists and people from other religions. Fifteen per cent of people from non-white ethnic minority groups were aged 50 and over (around 672,000 people). The White Irish group had the oldest age structure in 2001, with one in four aged 65 and over. Among the non-White group, Black Caribbeans had the largest proportion aged 65 and above.

Figures from the US Department of Health and Human Services show that 13% of the population were Black in 2002.[9] They were the second largest minority population, following the Hispanic/Latino population. Only 8% of the Blacks were 65 and above compared with 14% of non-Hispanic whites.

Acculturation and mental health

Acculturation is defined as a culture change that is initiated by the conjunction of two or more autonomous cultural systems.[10] It is a dynamic process, which helps in the adaptation of the value systems resulting in the integration of an individual to the host community. On the other hand when this does not occur individuals may become alienated and feel unwelcome. This sense of not belonging may make them feel powerless, isolated and estranged. The process of acculturation is affected by age, socioeconomic status, language and belief systems.

The migrant population may take any of the following paths in the process of adapting or integrating to the host culture. First is a process by which they fully accept the host culture and reject or even disown their parent culture, leading to lack of cultural identity.

Second is a process of integrating well with the host culture by embracing its richness and at the same time creating an environment for enabling the next generations to understand and perpetuate the positive aspects of the parent culture.

Third is a situation where the migrant population fails to integrate with the new culture. They may have an isolationist attitude towards the new culture. They look at culture around them with suspicion, and their insecurity makes them close the doors to the host culture. This leads on to development of 'cultural ghettoes'.

The second process described above is the ideal situation, but in reality all three situations may occur in varying degrees among migrant populations depending on their age, value systems, education and other factors.

Extreme cultural transition can cause severe distress, which is sometimes called 'culture shock'. The stress is less when the move is planned, there are other persons involved and there is overlap in cultures. A Swedish study found that immigrants had 1.5 times greater risk of suicides than natives.[11] This may be explained by lack of ethnic community integration, as social support has consistently been found to be a protective factor against psychological distress associated with migration.[12,13] It is thought that the possible protective effect of traditional culture on mental disorders is reduced when the migrant population face adverse socioeconomic conditions leading to disruption of extended family structure, inability to follow social obligations and failure to keep religious affiliations.[14] All these may occur as part of acculturation. Studies suggest that social support and cultural integration, rather than acculturation, are protective factors for immigrants.[15]

Migration, culture and mental health

Migration is a social process by which an individual or group of individuals move from one cultural setting to another for economic, political or family reasons. This may be a permanent or transient activity. As discussed earlier this could occur within a country or across nations. People who emigrate are known to be vulnerable to mental heath problems. Migration can be a very stressful experience, but not all migrants go through the same process. Coping strategies as well as resilience among migrants can affect this.[16] The preparation for migration, the receptiveness of the host society and the acceptance the individual receives all affect the risk of psychological problems in the migrant community. At an individual level, factors such as personality, social support, psychological strength and inherent flexibility and adaptability may act as significant factors determining future psychological well-being. The association of mental illness with migration has been attributed to a variety of reasons. One theory is that people who are mentally ill are the most likely to emigrate.[17] Another is that the stress of migration can also lead to mental illness.[17] People migrate for various reasons, but it is rare for older people to migrate for economic reasons. They usually move to join their families. However, migration can occur for other reasons as well. For example, there has been increased migration activity from the UK to other parts of the world, particularly for retired individuals who seek better weather and improved quality of life. The loss of social networks, inflexibility due to ageing and poor physical health, rigid value systems and language difficulties may make the process of migration and settling down difficult for the elderly. Hence older migrants may be more vulnerable to mental health problems.

The elderly from minority ethnic communities have unique and complex mental health needs. There is difficulty in accurately assessing the prevalence of mental health problems among this population. One important factor contributing to this is that they are less likely to seek help for psychological problems. There are a number of other reasons including the following.

⟩ Diagnostic difficulties due to language barriers, lack of culturally appropriate diagnostic and screening instruments, etc.
⟩ Difference in presentation of mental health problems among this population compared to the native population.
⟩ Stigma attached to mental illness.
⟩ Lack of knowledge of mental illness and symptoms of mental illness among the family members.
⟩ Professionals' lack of understanding of their mental health problems and needs.

Epidemiology

Though studies on the prevalence of mental health problems in elderly immigrants are sparse, current available information suggests that migrants have higher rates of mental illness than the population in the country of origin and the host country.[18] There are no studies to support this in the elderly. A community study on the prevalence of psychiatric disorders among elderly South Asian immigrants from the Indian subcontinent living in Bradford (UK) showed depression to be around 20% and anxiety neurosis about 4%.[19] The Islington study[20] showed a total of 18.3% of migrant elders had depression. The prevalence studies on bipolar disorder among elderly ethnic minority group are scarce. In contrast to the reported increased likelihood to self-harm in young Asian women the risk of self-harm is less in the older Asian population.[21] Assessing the prevalence of substance misuse, alcohol abuse and forensic issues in older ethnic communities is difficult as it may be under-reported. One study[22] showed that African Americans were more likely to report hopelessness, poor appetite, poor concentration and lack of energy but when controlled for certain confounders the racial differences were found to be insignificant.

The AESOP study (2005) determined the incidence of bipolar disorder in three cities in the UK.[23] The study found a significantly higher incidence of bipolar affective disorder in black and minority ethnic groups compared with white groups. The study excluded the elderly population.

Mental health issues in asylum seekers pose particular challenges. Many may have experienced torture in their homeland. When they migrate to a new country they might face detention, enforced dispersal and discrimination.[24] Although issues related to asylum seekers are commonly talked about, information on mental health issues in this population is limited, in particular elderly asylum seekers.

Globalisation

Globalisation is a term used to describe a complex series of socioeconomic, technological and political changes that accelerated in the latter half of the 20th century. Advances in transport, communication and information technologies have assisted the process of crossing of borders. Globalisation has led to a great increase in migration. This process has been enhanced in the recent years by fast and efficient means of travel, deregulation of commerce and widened access to technology.[1] This has led to increasing interdependence and interaction between people and communities in distant locations. This is breaking down natural boundaries and has had an impact on economies. Migration of younger generations from developing countries in search of economic security has resulted in older people relocating to join their family (or being left behind).

Culture and mental health of elderly migrants with affective disorders

Elderly people living in a country may belong to different ethnic groups and cultures. The cultural aspects of mental health problems of the majority ethnic group are usually better identified and managed. This may be due to a better understanding of their culture by mental health professionals.

Identifying and managing mental health problems in older people from minority ethnic groups are complicated issues. The ethnic elders may be first, second or third generation immigrants. The first among these are likely to present complex cultural issues that affect their mental health. Even third generation migrants are likely to be affected if the integration with the host society has not occurred. We shall look at some of these issues in relation to affective disorders.

Aetiology

The migrant elder may bring with them to the new country a predisposition to some of the illnesses pertaining to his or her ethnicity. A combination of genetic, social or psychological factors may be contributory. For example, people from the Asian subcontinent may have a higher predisposition for somatisation.

Loss of home country and loved ones, multiple deprivations leading to learned helplessness, alienation, isolation and powerlessness leading to low self-esteem[7] have been identified as factors leading to depression. Other causes postulated include reasons for migration (torture, political and economic) and stress associated with migration.[18] Racism, difficulty of accepting the reality of not being able to return home,[25] concerns about the social values of the younger generations, social isolation due to bereavement, retirement and rejection from the family[25,26] have all been put forward as possible contributory factors for depression in ethnic elderly.

Symptomatology and presentation

The stigma of mental health problems may lead to expressing distress in a culturally acceptable way. Many cultures accept physical illness but mental distress is often considered a sign of weakness. In such situations the distress may be expressed as unexplained physical symptoms. This is very common in the elderly population with depression. Failure to recognise underlying depression can lead to needless investigations, prolonging the symptoms and reinforcing beliefs in their physical nature.[17] Individuals from certain cultures attribute external forces (fate or astrology) as driving factors in their behaviour or actions, which may also contribute to under-reporting of symptoms.[6]

The presentation of the illness may itself take varied forms depending on culture, belief and attitudes. Hence some of the delusional beliefs may be related to cultural beliefs. Depression may manifest with different patterns of symptoms depending on cultures. Some may present with psychological symptoms of sadness and low mood and others may present with pain and somatic symptoms.[27] Bhugra and Cochrane,[28] quoting various studies, point out that depression may be characterised by somatic symptoms rather than by guilt, self-blame or suicidal ideations in some ethnic groups. This can lead to diagnostic difficulties. Some religious rituals may be misinterpreted as obsessions. Magical cures may just be part of the culture and often culturally appropriate reactions may be misdiagnosed as mental illness.

Diagnosis

The migrant population may have different views on how they should address and manage psychological distress. They may believe that modern medicines cause side-effects and may prefer alternative remedies, magical cures or get help from faith healers, which may not be easily available in their new country. Many of them may not know the existing service provisions in the country they have migrated to. In many of the developing countries doctors are highly revered and patients are reluctant to approach doctors for reasons they may consider trivial. There could also be economic reasons which prevent them from seeking help if the healthcare is not state funded. Some may not seek help for fear of being ostracised, owing to the stigma attached to mental illness. It may be more pronounced if the female member of the family is affected. However, a recent study in the United Kingdom found that immigrant elders, in general, accessed primary and secondary care services at least at the same level as an older UK born.[29]

Where mental health services are sought, however, if the professionals involved are unaware of the cultural beliefs and value systems, they may often fail to recognise the underlying mental health problem, which can lead to delay or misdiagnosis.

Various scales and tools often complement psychiatric assessments and management. There is a dearth of reliable and valid assessment tools for the ethnic population, which can complicate these issues further. The languages of distress may be different from that in structured diagnostic tools, which can underestimate distress levels. One study found that a lower cut-off point is more appropriate for older black people living in the UK for screening depression.[30] The elderly person may not speak the local language and even if they do there may be difficulties arising due to accents and expressions. These language barriers and the person's inability to express distress in their mother tongue can make diagnosis difficult.

Management

The most important aspect of managing affective disorders involves engaging the service user and family in the process. Knowledge of their culture will be invaluable in understanding how it influences illness presentation, management and outcome. Dein[17] identifies the following common issues:

» The assessing doctor should try to know the views of patient's family and close friends to find out their assumptions about the symptoms.

» It may be better to involve independent interpreters if there are language barriers hindering the assessment process as family members may be biased for various social and cultural reasons.

» It may be decided that a mental health problem does not exist and the behaviour is culturally appropriate. In such situations utilising traditional healers (Hakims, Vaids, etc.) may be more relevant.

» Even in situations where Western treatments, including ECT, are appropriate, it is still important to attempt to understand the patient's illness concept and explain the treatment based on this. This will enhance the therapeutic relationship.

» Ethnic minority patients may have a different response to psychotropic drugs. South Asian patients show higher plasma concentration of some antidepressants than white patients on similar doses. Hence they may be more sensitive to side-effects and respond to lower doses.

In clinical practice many ethnic elders prefer an authoritarian (paternalistic) approach from healthcare providers. They would prefer a prescriptive solution for their problems. In spite of this, psychotherapeutic approaches are found to be very useful in managing affective disorders. Almost half of the participants in a study, however, expressed a strong desire to seek psychological treatments, which was positively associated with degree of assimilation, age, female gender and English fluency.[31] Most of the psychotherapies available are based on Western values. In many situations translating this across cultures for therapeutic purposes may not be appropriate or effective. Hence culturally appropriate psychotherapeutic approaches need to be developed. There may be informal traditional 'psychotherapists' within the extended families and the community. This may be a religious leader or a respected elder. Professionals and service providers should be their help. Their wisdom may be utilised appropriately in situations which demand their involvement.

There may be occasions when compulsory detention is necessary. This could place the professionals involved in a difficult situation. Involving the family and understanding their concerns can play a pivotal role. Family resources available in supporting the individual in the community may avoid the need for a compulsory admission and it is worthwhile exploring this.

Assessment of capacity forms an important part of mental health assessments and management. Professionals are called on to assess the individual's capacity to refuse treatment, decide on their care, make enduring power of attorney and make a valid will. Although capacity is a universal concept some of the issues assessed may have Western values attached to them. An older person belonging to an ethnic minority may not be able to grasp concepts such as enduring power of attorney or 24-hour care. Their understanding may depend on fluency of the native language and socioeconomic status. Hence time should be spent to explain these concepts in detail.

Prognosis

Non-compliance with medication is an important factor affecting prognosis. This can affect the ongoing management of affective disorders, especially in patients who need maintenance medications such as lithium. Minority ethnicity was found to be a factor affecting adherence to antipsychotic medications in bipolar disorders.[32] Compliance could be improved if the concerns of patients were addressed and reasons for medications were appropriately explained. Some patients may be using traditional medicines from their country of origin, when they visit their family and some of these may interact with drugs. An awareness of this is important as these medications may interact with prescribed medication or cause unwanted side-effects. Unfortunately, there are a number of traditional medicines which are used in treating 'nerves'. The side-effects of many of them are not known.

There is growing evidence that religious activity may be a significant protective factor against depression. Active religious practice is likely to provide considerable social support as well as a sense of a meaningful role.[33]

Specific syndromes

While considering the aetiology of mental health problems in migrant populations a factor that may come into prominence is the vulnerability for certain illnesses they carry with them to the new country. As previously mentioned somatisation is common in the South Asian population. There are certain patterns of behaviour which are seen only in specific cultures or countries and are known as culture bound syndromes. These include Amok, Koro and Dhat syndrome, etc. An awareness of the existence of these is important when addressing mental health problems in ethnic minorities.

Service provision

A substantial body of research indicates that the black and Asian ethnic minority population differ from white people in accessing and utilising mental health services.[34] This may be due to attitude towards services, previous experiences or cultural appropriateness. Provision of psychogeriatric services for ethnic minorities is important in any multi-ethnic society. There are considerable debates about integrating or segregating services. It is suggested that segregated services may further marginalise ethnic minority communities. Funding for such services may also be an issue. Hence in the current situation psychogeriatric services for this population may be delivered as part of the existing mental health service. This service should be sensitive to cultural needs, values and beliefs. The tools used in assessment should be culturally sensitive. Various tools, such as the geriatric depression scale and mini mental state examination, are available in different languages, and could be utilised.

The Royal College of Psychiatrists council report[35] on psychiatric services for black and minority ethnic elders recommends setting up acute psychiatric services for this population within mainstream psychiatric services. Staff should be trained to be culturally sensitive. Services providing continuing care should be developed for the appropriate user group. The College report also suggests recruiting a racial mix of multidisciplinary staff, reflecting the population served and involving general practitioners and other key players in establishing good practice for this group. Many have spiritual needs which may not be met within the current available mental health services. Psychotherapy services are also limited. In Britain there are psychotherapy centres providing care for ethnic minorities, the best known being the Nafsiyat Inter-Cultural Therapy Centre.[17]

Good partnerships between primary care team and other pathway agency teams is essential in providing care for this group.[36] Specialised teams (e.g. liaison) in general hospital and other settings (e.g. nursing homes) providing mental health assessments should be aware of cultural issues which may contribute in precipitating and maintaining affective symptoms in ethnic elders. There should be provision for culturally sensitive day care, respite and residential care to encourage ethnic minority elders to utilise such services.

Dewsbury experience

Dewsbury is a small town in Yorkshire (England) with a significant ethnic minority population, the majority from the Asian subcontinent. As part of psychogeriatric services, a specialised team provided assessment and support for this population. The team included a specialist nurse and link support workers with experience in transcultural issues. The team also provided translation services and had access to culturally appropriate day care and respite care. The project gained recognition in its attempts to break the barriers against taking the mental health service to the user – by raising awareness among the ethnic minority population of mental health issues and the services available to them.

KEY POINTS

- Over the next few years the number of elderly people from ethnic minority groups will increase. This is not only as a result of increased migration but also due to an increase in life expectancy.
- Attention needs to be focused on their health, social and economic needs.

Catering for the mental health needs of this population is complex and needs careful planning. The stigma attached to age, ethnicity and mental illness can all contribute to a 'triple whammy'.[37] This seems to be having an impact on mental healthcare delivery to this group.

> There should be conscious effort and policies in place to tackle the problems and provide appropriate care to this group.

> There is limited research in this area. There needs to be a concerted effort to improve this.

REFERENCES

1 Kelly BD, Globalisation and psychiatry. *Adv Psychiatr Treat.* 2003; **9**: 464–74.
2 Gott C, Johnston K. *The Migrant Population in the UK: fiscal effects.* London: Home Office Report; 2002.
3 Marcella AJ, Kameoka VA. Ethnocultural issues in the assessments of psychopathology. In: Wexler S, editor. *Measuring Mental Illness.* Washington, DC: American Psychiatric Association; 1989.
4 US Department of Health and Human Services. *Mental Health: a report of the Surgeon General.* Rockville, MD: US Department of Health and Human Services; 1999.
5 Office of the Surgeon-General. *Mental Health: culture, race, and ethnicity. A supplement to Mental Health: a report of the Surgeon General.* United States Public Health Service, Office of the Surgeon General; 2001.
6 Bhugra D, Ayonrinde O. Depression in migrants and ethnic minorities. *Adv Psychiatr Treat.* 2004; **10**: 13–17.
7 Manthorpe J, Hettiaratchy P. Ethnic minority elders in the UK. *Int Rev Psychiatr.* 1993; **5**: 171–8.
8 *UK population: by ethnic group: Census update.* Census 2001.
9 McKinnon J. *The Black Population in the United States: March 2002.* Washington, DC: US Census Bureau, Current Population Reports, Series P20–541; 2002.
10 Social Science Research Council. Acculturation: an exploratory formulation. *Am Anthropol.* 1954; **56**: 973–1002.
11 Ferrada-Noli M. A cross-cultural breakdown of Swedish suicide. *Acta Psychiatr Scand.* 1997; **96**: 108–16.
12 Chung RC, Bemak F, Kagawa-Singer M. Gender differences in psychological distress among Southeast Asian refugees. *J Nerv Ment Dis.* 1998; **186**: 112–19.
13 Ritsner M, Ponizovsky A, Ginath Y. Changing patterns of distress during the adjustment of recent immigrants: a 1-year follow-up study. *Acta Psychiatr Scand.* 1997; **95**: 494–9.
14 Foliaki S. Migration and mental health: the Tongan experience. *Int J Ment Health.* 1997; **26**: 36–54.
15 Tai-Ann Cheng AA, Chang J-CB. Mental health aspects of culture and migration. *Curr Opin Psychiatry.* 1999; **12**(2): 217–22.
16 Bhugra D. Migration and mental health. *Acta Psychiatr Scand.* 2004; **109**(4): 243–58.
17 Dein S. ABC of mental health: mental health in a multiethnic society. *BMJ.* 1997; **315**: 473–6.
18 Lipsedge M. Transcultural aspects of psychiatry. *Pract Rev Psychiatr.* 1986. **8**: 1–2.
19 Bhatnagar KS, Frank J. Psychiatric disorders in the elderly from the Indian subcontinent living in Bradford. *Int J Geriatr Psychiatr.* 1997; **1212**(9): 907–12.
20 Livingston G, Leavey G, Kitchen G. Mental health of migrant elders: the Islington Study. *Br J Psychiatr.* 2001; **179**: 361–6.

21 Bhugra D, Desai M, Baldwin DS. Attempted suicide in west London. I. Rates across ethnic communities. *Psychol Med.* 1999; **5**: 1125–30.

22 Blazer DG, Landerman LR, Hays JC, *et al.* Symptoms of depression among community dwelling elderly African-American and white older adults. *Psychol Med.* 1998; **28**: 1311–20.

23 Lloyd T, Kennedy N, Fearon P, *et al.* Incidence of bipolar affective disorder in three UK cities: results from the AESOP study. *Br J Psychiatr.* 2005; **186**: 126–31.

24 Silove D, Franz CP, Steel Z, *et al.* Policies of deterrence and the mental health of asylum seekers. *JAMA.* 2000; **284**: 604–11.

25 Boneham M. Ageing and ethnicity in Britain: the case of elderly sick women in a Midlands town. *New Community.* 1989; **15**: 447–59.

26 Blackemore K. The state, the voluntary sector and new developments in provision for the old of minority racial groups. *Ageing Society.* 1985; **5**: 175–90.

27 Livingston G, Sembhi S. Mental health of the ageing immigrant population. *Adv Psychiatr Treat.* 2003; **9**: 31–7.

28 Bhugra D, Cochrane R, editors. *Psychiatry in Multicultural Britain.* London: Gaskell; 2001.

29 Livingston G, Leavey G, Kitchen G. Accessibility of health and social services to immigrant elders: the Islington Study. *Br J Psychiatr.* 2002; **180**: 369–73.

30 Abas MA, Phillips C, Carter J, *et al.* Culturally sensitive validation of screening questionnaires for depression in older African-Caribbean people living in south London. *Br J Psychiatr.* 1998; **173**: 249–54.

31 Barry DT, Grilo CM. Cultural, psychological and demographic correlates of willingness to use psychological services among East Asian immigrants. *J Nerv Mental Dis.* 2002; **190**: 32–9.

32 Sajatovic M, Valenstein M, Blow FC, *et al.* Treatment adherence with antipsychotic medications in bipolar disorder. *Bipolar Disord.* 2006; **8**(3): 232–41.

33 Butler R, Orrell M. Late-life depression. *Curr Opin Psychiatry.* 1998; **11**(4): 435–9.

34 Bhui K. Service provision for London's ethnic minorities. In: Johnson, Ramsay R, Thornocroft G, *et al.*; editors. *London's Mental Health.* London: King's Fund; 1997.

35 Council Report CR103. *Psychiatric Services for Black and Minority Ethnic Elders.* London: Royal College of Psychiatrists; 2001.

36 Bhui K, Bhugra D. Mental illness in Black and Asian ethnic minorities: pathways to care and outcomes. *Adv Psychiatr Treat.* 2002; **8**: 26–33.

37 Rait G, Burns A, Chew C. Age, ethnicity and mental illness: a triple whammy. *BMJ.* 1996; **313**: 1347–8.

CHAPTER 16

Religion/spirituality and depression in old age

RACHEL DEW AND HAROLD KOENIG

Introduction

Over the past three decades, medical science has begun to pay greater attention to the spiritual needs of many types of patients. This movement has been spurred on, in large measure, by research demonstrating psychological and physical benefits of religious involvement.[1] Among the more well-researched groups in the religion/health literature are the elderly and the depressed.[2] This chapter will review the religion/health literature as it pertains to the depressed elderly and offer practical advice to the clinician interested in addressing or learning more about the spiritual or religious needs of older depressed patients.

Ageing population

The international population is ageing. Global demographic changes over the next 25 years will result in the proportion of the population aged 65 or older increasing from 6.9% to 12%. In developed countries, the number of persons aged 65 or greater is expected to nearly triple.[3] This change in demography, contributed to by increasing life expectancy and decreasing fertility, will inflate the proportion of people coping with chronic disease and disability, as well as decrease the proportion of the population available to care for them.

The strain this situation will place on healthcare delivery is tremendous. It is therefore imperative that research address chronic diseases such as depression, a condition that the World Health Organization (WHO) projects to be the world's second leading cause of disability by 2020 (behind only heart disease).[4]

Estimates of the prevalence of geriatric depression have varied from 1% to 15%.[5-7] The presence of other chronic diseases increases the incidence by up to 10%.[8] Older adults with depression also suffer an increased rate of disability as compared with their non-depressed peers.[9] Thus, there is reason to believe that as the elderly population increases, depression and its associated disability will become an even more important burden both on individuals and society.

Religion/spirituality and older adults

Key considerations in understanding the lives of older adults are religion and the related concept of spirituality. These are complex terms and likely mean different things to different people. As such, we will offer the operative definitions to be used for this chapter. Religion here will refer to a collection of beliefs and behaviours, embraced by a group, which regard the transcendent.[1] Spirituality, although having at least a handful of popular definitions, will here refer to a more personal search for a relationship with the transcendent, not necessarily institutionally related.[1]

These concepts are important for the clinician interested in understanding patients because they are central to the lives of most older adults. Recent US polls indicate that 89% of adults over 65 report they are certain or have little doubt in the existence of God,[10] and a mere 4% of those over 65 report no religious preference.[11] Nearly 90% of Americans over 65 and 60% of Britons over 65 say religion is important in their lives.[12]

Religion and spirituality are also important to older adults facing illness. Koenig and colleagues found that 34% of nursing home residents called religion the most important factor in enabling them to cope with their problems, and nearly 60% said they used religious coping to a large extent.[13] Almost 60% of a sample of depressed psychiatric inpatients in Canada endorsed theistic beliefs and 51% endorsed belief in the Bible as literal truth.[14] Religious beliefs are common and important in the lives of medical and psychiatric patients. Thus, medical providers who do not consider the religious and spiritual needs of depressed elderly patients may be missing an important part of the clinical picture.

Religion and health connections

Not only are religion and spirituality identified as personally important to the elderly, but there is accumulating evidence that they relate to health outcomes.[1] Two interrelated lines of investigation have developed, one linking religious variables with mental health outcomes, and another linking such measures to physical health outcomes. Examples of religious and spiritual variables used in religion/health research are church attendance, private religious activities such as prayer or scripture reading, self-identification as religious or spiritual, intrinsic religiosity, and using religion to cope with adversity. These and others variables have been compared with such outcomes as general mortality, cardiac disease, blood pressure, cancer, substance abuse, depression, sociopathy and health services use.[1,15,16] This religion/health literature has revealed complex relationships, but for the most part has found consistent small to moderate health benefits for those who embrace religion in their lives. This has held true in cross-sectional and longitudinal studies.[1]

Measurement

A vital issue in the religion/health field is measurement. As touched on at the beginning of this chapter, even experts struggle to agree on definitions of religion and spirituality. How then can such constructs be assessed reliably and validly in widely varying research populations? This difficulty, combined with the newness of the field, has led to a relative lack of standardisation of measurement among studies that makes comparison and meta-analysis challenging.

Probably the most frequently assessed variable is attendance at religious services. Attendance could be construed by some as a superficial measure that may fail to capture a person's true level of faith or spirituality; yet, as a concrete concept, it is perhaps more easily ascertained. Some researchers have opted to leave definitions of religion and spirituality to the research subject to determine; these investigators have merely asked subjects whether they consider themselves to be religious or spiritual without regard to what that might mean to the individual.

Often religious preference or denomination is measured in religion/health research. This enterprise is made somewhat difficult by the large variety of Protestant denominations, which may leave some groups with too small a number of subjects to be meaningfully analysed. Another approach is to attempt to quantify the intentions behind someone's religiousness; a well-known construct is 'religious orientation', first described by Allport and Ross.[17] In this scheme, a person with an 'intrinsic' religious orientation is thought to participate in religion primarily because of a deep commitment to the divine or transcendent, whereas someone with an 'extrinsic' religious orientation is thought to primarily participate in religion for another reason, e.g. to make social contacts.

Another important category of measurement seen in the religion/health literature is religious coping.[18] The literature on religious coping seeks not only to determine whether subjects use religion to cope with life's adversities, but precisely how they use it. Types of religious coping include giving up control of a situation to God, seeking support from one's religious congregation, or looking to religion for guidance in decision making.[18]

Measurement is a complex issue that is largely beyond the scope of this chapter. However, in evaluating a study of religion and health, it is important to consider how religion or spirituality was assessed. Each of the above modalities has its own strengths, weaknesses and contradictions. For the most part, public religious activities such as church attendance have most often been correlated with health outcomes. This may be due to ease in measurement, which may minimise variance (variance due to measurement error makes it more difficult to discover statistical relationships between variables). As the field grows, multidimensional measurement may allow for more comprehensive assessments of the role of religion and spirituality in the research subject's life (see Multidimensional Measurement of Religiousness/Spirituality for Use in Health Research: http://www.fetzer.org/PDF/Total_Fetzer_Book.pdf).

Religion/spirituality and mental health

Mental health, particularly depression, has been examined in relation to religion. A large portion of these studies focused on older adult populations.[1,19] For the most part, this line of research has found religious involvement to be associated with lower levels of depression, anxiety and suicidality, and with higher levels of well-being. The evidence also points to a protective effect against problematic behaviours such as substance abuse and criminal activity.[1,20]

The study of well-being focuses on human flourishing and positive adaptation rather than pathology. Specific outcome variables used in this field include such concepts as life satisfaction, happiness, psychological well-being, existential well-being and quality of life. Koenig and colleagues found that 79% of 100 studies examining well-being found at least one correlation linking greater levels of religious involvement with greater levels of well-being.[1] Ten of these were prospective cohort studies; of these 10, nine found correlations between baseline religious variables and later well-being.[20] Many of these studies specifically investigated populations of older adults, including four of the longitudinal studies finding greater religiousness correlated with greater well-being.[1]

In their systematic review, Koenig and colleagues located 93 observational studies examining the relationship between religion and depression. Fifty-nine of these found lower rates of depression associated with greater levels of religious involvement measured by at least one variable. Sixteen more found mixed positive and negative associations between religious variables and depression. Fifteen of the 22 longitudinal studies found baseline religiousness to predict lower levels of depression later on.[20] Two of these studied recovery from depression (both in older adults) and found that religious patients recovered more quickly than non-religious patients.[21,22] Earlier and more recent longitudinal studies in Dutch older adults supported these findings.[2,23]

There have also been a few clinical trials in which religious content was used to augment usual treatment for depression. An example of this would be cognitive behavioural therapy that also addresses religious issues.[24] Koenig and colleagues found that in five of eight of such trials, religious subjects receiving religiously augmented therapy recovered more quickly than those in the usual care or control groups.[20]

Anxiety disorders frequently accompany and complicate depression. Koenig and colleagues' systematic review located 69 observational studies of religion and anxiety, 35 of which found at least one significant relationship in which those with greater religiousness were less anxious. Seven of the remainder found mixed results.

Six of 7 clinical trials using religious or spiritual interventions showed success in treating anxiety.[20] More research in this area has been recommended.[25]

Koenig and colleagues' systematic review also uncovered 68 studies of attitudes towards suicide or rates of suicidal behaviour. Fifty-seven of these found that greater religiousness was associated with lower incidence of suicidal behaviour or more negative attitudes towards suicide.[20]

Other important areas of research in religion and mental health are psychotic disorders, substance abuse and crime. Research on schizophrenia and other psychotic disorders in relation to religion and spirituality is a new and growing field. Conclusions about such a relationship are premature at this point.[1,26] However, there is evidence that a substantial proportion of those suffering major psychoses employ religious and/or spiritual coping techniques.[26]

A large literature examines the relationship between religious involvement and substance abuse. Consistently inverse correlations between religious involvement and substance abuse have been noted in both adolescent and adult samples; several studies feature very large samples, and several include longitudinal data.[1,20] This area has been so well studied that avoidance of substance abuse has been hypothesised as a mechanism by which religion affects general health (see below).[19]

Criminal behaviour for decades has been thought to be inhibited by religious involvement.[1] This tenet has not been uncontroversial, as a seminal 1969 study found no correlation.[27] Subsequent studies, however, support the idea that crime and religion are inversely related. Koenig and colleagues found 36 studies addressing this issue, 28 of which found an inverse correlation between religion and delinquency.[20] One problem with this literature is the infrequent separation of substance abuse from other types of delinquency. Substance abuse, which, as seen above, has been found to strongly relate to religion, also relates to non-substance-related crime, and thus may serve as a confounder.

Although most studies of religiousness and mental health in older adults point to salutary effects, an emerging literature describes the phenomenon of 'religious struggle'.[28] Religious or spiritual struggle is sometimes called 'negative religious coping' and involves themes such as abandonment by God or church, anger with God, feeling one's circumstances are a form of divine punishment, and coming to believe that God is powerless to help.[18,28] Religious struggle has been found to be relatively common and to frequently coexist with the more positive forms of religious coping, such as turning to God or church for help, or helping others.[28] Negative religious coping has been associated with higher levels of psychological distress.[18,28]

Religion/spirituality and physical health

Physical illness, chronic pain, disability and impending death are germane to the practice of geriatrics, and frequently complicate or exacerbate late-life depression. The study of religion and/or spirituality in relation to physical health outcomes has been somewhat more controversial,[15] but has nonetheless provided evidence of salutary effects, especially in the elderly.[1,16,19] Some of the most striking findings in this field have been in regard to all-cause mortality. Koenig and colleagues found that 39 of 52 studies discovered enhanced longevity in more religious subjects.[29] A recent review by Powell and colleagues concluded that there is compelling evidence that church attendance delays death. Their conclusions were based on critical review of 11 longitudinal studies that used religious attendance to predict mortality.[15] Another recent review by Hummer and colleagues concurred.[30]

There is also evidence that religiousness protects against morbidity and mortality from major diseases such as coronary artery disease, hypertension and cancer. Powell and colleagues examined four prospective studies and concluded that there is some evidence that religiousness protects against cardiovascular disease.[15] In Koenig and colleagues' literature review, 12 of 16 studies of cardiovascular disease found lower levels of morbidity and mortality in more religious subjects.[29] Furthermore, review of 16 observational studies, including two prospective cohorts, found strong evidence for lower blood pressures among more religious subjects. Five of seven studies found that subjects with greater levels of religiousness had lower rates of cancer mortality.

Several studies have examined possible correlations between religiousness and immune or neuroendocrine function. Higher levels of IgA,[1] and lower levels of interleukin-6,[31] a marker of inflammation, have been shown to relate to religious experience or involvement. One study found that CD4 counts were higher in religiously active HIV patients.[32] Religious variables have been associated with immune markers in cancer patients.[29] Some research has also linked religiousness with risk of contracting sexually transmitted diseases and tuberculosis.[29]

With ageing and illness often come chronic pain and physical disability. Relationships between these phenomena and religious variables appear to be complex. Several cross-sectional studies have found that private religious activities such as prayer are related to greater levels of pain. This could be because prayer increases levels of pain. More likely, in light of all of the above research findings, severe pain probably leads victims to pray more in an attempt to gain relief.[29] One prospective study found that over time prayer was associated with decreased pain, even though it was initially related to greater pain.[33] Longitudinal studies have examined the relationship between religion and physical disabilities, which may result from late-life depression.[9] Idler and colleagues have discovered links between greater religiousness and lower emergence of disability, and between greater religiousness and less self-reported disability.[34]

Possible mechanisms

How can the religion-health connection be explained scientifically? This is a growing field of interest. Several social, psychological and biological mechanisms have been proposed, which may be independent, synchronous, or interrelated.

Enhanced social support has been hypothesised to mediate some of the observed benefit of religious involvement. Proponents have theorised that those who participate in religious activities widen their social network and secure instrumental social support, such as transportation, etc., which may contribute to improved health outcomes.[19] The largest source of support for older adults outside of immediate family comes from members of their church.[35]

Lifestyle patterns associated with religiousness or spirituality may also convey health benefits, especially over a lifetime. As noted above, religious involvement has been found to correlate with lower levels of substance use. Substance abuse, of course, carries wide-ranging risks for physical and emotional health that may be avoided by religious persons.[19]

Meaning and coherence of worldview may also mediate health benefits of religiousness, especially for older adults who may be wrestling with the purpose and meaning of their lives. Feeling that the world is predictable and makes sense, or feeling that one's time on earth serves a purpose, may convey psychological benefits; this may also ultimately lead to physical health enhancement.[19]

The emerging discipline of positive psychology studies the relationship between positive emotions such as joy, calm, contentment, etc. on health and well-being.[36] It has been proposed that positive feelings may be a mechanism by which religion alters health outcomes.[1]

How psychological well-being relates to or leads to physical well-being is a wider area of research. Depression and psychological stress, for example, have been found to increase risk of myocardial infarction, while social support may be protective against coronary artery disease.[37] Another burgeoning area of investigation is psychoneuroimmunology.[38]

Psychoneuroimmunology is concerned with how the brain, as a result of psychological experiences/perceptions, may undergo changes, and can in turn alter physiological systems outside of the brain.[38] An example of such a brain-body connection is alteration of immune cell function, precipitated by cortisol secretion, brought on by a frightening experience, such as fleeing from a wild animal.

Such psychoneuroimmunological phenomena may turn out to be an underlying mechanism related to all the previously proposed mechanisms. For example, social support from a faith community may create a psychological experience of comfort and relaxation that, via neurohumoral pathways, optimises immune function. Lack of social support, on the other hand, may lead to increased psychological stress, which may, through brain-body connections, depress immune function. Beyond the direct toxic effects of drugs and alcohol on the human body, the kind of social and psychological experiences that come along with substance abuse, i.e. interpersonal conflict, lack of intimacy, legal problems, poor self-esteem, etc., may affect physical health through psychoneuroimmunological pathways. Cognitions related to a sense of meaning and purpose in life may lead to feelings of comfort, joy, relaxation and fulfilment that may enhance immune function, whereas feeling that life is meaningless or that one is not fulfilling one's destiny may cause anxious feelings that ultimately suppress immune functioning. That may be particularly true for older adults whose immune systems may already be weakened due to ageing.

How does immune function relate to health outcomes that have been studied in relation to religiousness? Research in immunology continues to elucidate the importance of immune function for the health of a wide range of physiological systems. Although obviously related to HIV/AIDS, which has now claimed the lives of 25 million people worldwide,[39] immunity also relates to heart disease[40] and cancer,[38] two of the most important killers in the Western world. Research continues into possible connections between suboptimal immune function and such issues as wound healing and autoimmune diseases.[38]

Clinical applications

What clinical use can be made of these findings in the care of older patients with depression? Possible applications are many and varied.[29] Firstly, given the aforementioned importance of religion/spirituality for the majority of older adults, as well as the connection between religiousness and depressive disorders, the clinician treating the depressed elderly may wish to know more about this aspect of patients' lives. Spontaneous or systematised enquiry into the religious and/or spiritual lives of patients has been called a religious or spiritual history. A standard format for initiating such a conversation with patients has been proposed.[41]

Should a spiritual history reveal that religion and/or spirituality serve as important coping resources for a patient, a clinician may want to make that patient feel supported in this facet of his/her life, and enquire about whether the patient has any spiritual needs or questions that a chaplain might help in answering.

Although religion and spirituality have been shown to be important to the majority of older patients, conversations on these topics between patients and doctors rarely happen.[42] There are many reasons for this. Clinical encounters may be too short to allow for such conversations. Physicians may feel this part of patients' lives is unrelated to healthcare. Alternatively, patients may feel that clinicians don't want to hear about their religion, and that, as scientists, physicians would view religiousness with disdain. After all, in previous clinical encounters, the physician may have given the patient explanations for their state of health that, often filled with scientific jargon, contrasted starkly with their own views of their lot in life within the framework of religious beliefs. A patient who feels depression is a special challenge sent to them by God may have been told instead that depression is a state of low serotonin. Such a patient may not expect a physician to be interested in his/her religious life.

A patient for whom religion/spirituality holds import may profit from being told that research indicates it may have health benefits. If nothing else, the accepting attitude that leads the physician to have such a conversation has been shown to strengthen the clinician-patient bond.[43]

Sometimes a spiritual history will reveal that the patient is struggling with religious or spiritual issues. A patient, particularly if depressed, may contemplate the meaning of their illness. Is God punishing her? Has she been abandoned? In such a situation, merely stating research findings concerning the probable salutary effects of religiousness on depression could leave the patient feeling worse. Does this mean the illness came because she wasn't sufficiently devout? Furthermore, arguments presented to the patient concerning feelings of divine punishment or abandonment will likely ring hollow. After all, very few clinicians are also trained religious authorities.

In extreme cases, such situations could become coercive. In most cases they may be unproductive; clinicians are not trained to challenge and possibly alter patients' religious beliefs, even if well-versed in or a member of the patient's religious tradition. Therefore, in cases of spiritual struggle, clinicians may explore the matter with clients but should then consider referral to chaplains or pastoral counsellors. Clinicians should not attempt on their own to alter patients' religious beliefs, however dysfunctional they may appear to the clinician.

Many patients want their doctors to pray with them.[42] Should a physician do this? This is a controversial area.[29] We recommend that such activity always remain 'patient-centred'. The patient should initiate. If the physician feels comfortable, he/she may silently pray as the patient takes the lead in this activity. Care must be taken if the physician initiates this religious activity that this does not serve the needs of the physician rather than the patient.[29]

As life expectancy increases and chronic disease becomes more and more prevalent, clinicians need to pay heed to the lives of those who care for the elderly. Spouses, children and others who assist the depressed elderly are themselves at risk for depression and may suffer spiritual struggles such as those described above.

Finally, religious/spiritual needs of patients may never be more salient than at the end of life. Even when the physician can offer no more life-saving or even life-enhancing therapy, it is his/her job to be with the patient through suffering and anguish. As death nears, issues of ultimate meaning, moral regret and the afterlife may loom large for the dying. Despite whatever personal discomfort the clinician may feel with these topics, becoming a compassionate listener will make that clinician more helpful for his/her dying patients.

KEY POINTS

▶ Worldwide demographic changes will increase the proportion of elderly patients suffering chronic diseases, such as depression, throughout the 21st century.

▶ Religion and spirituality are not only important to older adults, including those with chronic diseases, but also related to both their mental health outcomes, and, possibly through psychosocial and neuroimmunological mediators, to their physical health outcomes as well.

▶ Clinicians who care for the elderly should be aware of this connection and consider patient-centred discussions of religious and/or spiritual needs with their patients.

▶ Issues of spiritual struggle should precipitate consideration of referral to chaplains or other pastoral care resources.

Funding/correspondence

Funding provided by a grant from the John Templeton Foundation. Correspondence: Harold G Koenig, MD, Box 3400, Duke University Medical Center, Durham, NC 27705, USA.

REFERENCES

 1 Koenig HG, McCullough ME, Larson DB. *Handbook of Religion and Health.* New York: Oxford University Press, 2001.

 2 Braam AW, Hein E, Dorly JHD, *et al.* Religious involvement and 6-year course of depressive symptoms in older Dutch citizens: results from the Longitudinal Aging Study Amsterdam. *J Aging Health.* 2004; **16**(4): 467–89.

 3 Goulding MR, Rogers ME, Smith SM. Public health and aging: trends in aging – United States and worldwide. *MMWR Morb Mortal Wkly Rep.* 2003; **52**(6): 101–06. Available from: http://www.cdc.gov/mmwr/preview/mmwrhtml/mm5206a2.htm (accessed 23 June 2006).

 4 World Health Organization. *The World Health Report 2001: Mental Health: new understanding, new hope.* Geneva: World Health Organization; 2001.

 5 Regier DA, Boyd JH, Burke JD, *et al.* One month prevalence of mental disorders in the United States: based on five Epidemiologic Catchment Area sites. *Arch Gen Psychiatr.* 1988; **45**: 977–86.

 6 Cullum S, Tucker S, Todd C, *et al.* Screening for depression in older medical inpatients. *Int J Geriatr Psychiatr.* 2006; **21**: 469–76.

 7 Beekman ATF, Deeg DJH, Geerlings SW, *et al.* Emergence and persistence of late life depression: a 3-year follow-up of the Longitudinal Aging Study Amsterdam. *J Affect Disord.* 2001; **65**: 131–8.

 8 Koenig HG, Blazer DG. Epidemiology of geriatric affective disorders. *Clinics in Geriatr Med.* 1992; **8**(2): 235–51.

 9 Callahan CM, Kroenke K, Counsell SR, *et al.* Treatment of depression improves physical functioning in older adults. *J Am Geriatr Soc.* 2005; **53**: 367–73.

10 Newport F. Who believes in God and who doesn't? *The Gallup Poll.* 2006. Available from: http://poll.gallup.com/content/?ci=23470 (accessed 24 June 2006).

11 Winseman AL. Religion in America: who has none? *The Gallup Poll.* 2005. Available from: http://poll.gallup.com/content/default.aspx?ci=20329 (accessed 24 June 2006).

12 Ray J. Worlds apart: religion in Canada, Britain, US. *The Gallup Poll.* 2003. Available from: http://poll.gallup.com/content/default.aspx?ci=9016 (accessed 24 June 2006).

13 Koenig HG, Weiner DK, Peterson BL, *et al.* Religious coping in a nursing home: a biopsychosocial model. *Int J Psychiatry in Med.* 1997; **27**(4): 365–76.

14 Baetz M, Larson DB, Marcoux G, *et al.* Canadian psychiatric inpatient religious commitment: an association with mental health. *Can J Psychiatr.* 2002; **47**: 159–66.

15 Powell LH, Shahabi L, Thoresen CE. Religion and spirituality: linkages to physical health. *Am Psychol.* 2003; **58**(1): 36–52.

16 Levin J, Chatters LM, Taylor RJ. Religion, health, and medicine in African Americans: implications for physicians. *J Nat Med Ass.* 2005; **97**(2): 237–49.

17 Allport GW, Ross JM. Personal religious orientation and prejudice. *J Pers Soc Psychol.* 1967; **5**(4): 432–43.

18 Pargament KI, Koenig HG, Perez LM. The many methods of religious coping: development and initial validation of the RCOPE. *J Clin Psychol.* 2000; **56**: 519–43.

19 George LK, Ellison CG, Larson DB. Explaining the relationships between religious involvement and health. *Psychol Inquiry.* 2002; **13**(3): 190–200.

20 Koenig HG. Religion and medicine. II. Religion, mental health, and related behaviors. *Int J Psychiatry Med.* 2001; **31**(1): 97–109.

21 Koenig HG, Cohen HJ, Blazer DG, *et al.* Religious coping and depression in elderly hospitalized medically ill men. *Am J Psychiatr.* 1992; **149**: 1693–1700.

22 Koenig HG, George LK, Peterson BL. Religiosity and remission from depression in medically ill older patients. *Am J Psychiatr.* 1998; **155**: 536–42.

23 Braam AW, Beekman ATF, Deeg DJH, *et al.* Religiosity as a protective or prognostic factor of depression in later life: results from the community survey in the Netherlands. *Acta Psychiatr Scand.* 1997; **96**: 199–205.

24 Propst RL, Ostrom R, Watkins P, *et al.* Comparative efficacy of religious and nonreligious cognitive-behavioral therapy for the treatment of clinical depression in religious individuals. *J Consult Clin Psychol.* 1992; **60**(1): 94–103.

25 Shreve-Neiger AK, Edelstein BA. Religion and anxiety: a critical review of the literature. *Clin Psychol Rev.* 2004; **24**: 379–97.

26 Mohr S, Huguelet P. The relationship between schizophrenia and religion and its implications for care. *Swiss Med Wkly.* 2004; **134**: 369–76.

27 Hirschi R, Stark R. Hellfire and delinquency. *Soc Probl.* 1969; **17**(2): 202–13.

28 Fitchett G, Murphy PE, Kim J, *et al.* Religious struggle: prevalence, correlates and mental health risks in diabetic, congestive heart failure, and oncology patients. *Int J Psychiatry Med.* 2004; **34**(2): 179–96.

29 Koenig HG. Religion and medicine. IV. Religion, physical health, and clinical implications. *Int J Psychiatr in Med.* 2001; **31**(3): 321–36.

30 Hummer RA, Ellison CG, Rogers RG, *et al.* Religious involvement and adult mortality in the United States: review and perspective. *Southern Med J.* 2004; **97**(12): 1223–30.

31 Lutgendorf SK, Russell D, Ullrich P, *et al.* Religious participation, interleukin-6, and mortality in older adults. *Health Psychol.* 2004; **23**(5): 465–75.

32 Woods TE, Antoni MH, Inronson GH, *et al.* Religiosity is associated with affective and immune status in symptomatic HIV-infected gay men. *J Psychosom Res.* 1999; **46**(2): 165–76.

33 Turner JA, Clancy S. Strategies for coping with chronic low back pain: relationship to pain and disability. *Pain.* 1986; **24**(3): 355–64.

34 Idler EL, Kasl SV. Religion among disabled and nondisabled elderly persons. II. Attendance at religious services as a predictor of the course of disability. *J Gerontol.* 1997; **52B**: 306–16.

35 Cutler SJ. Membership in different types of voluntary associations and psychological well-being. *Gerontologist.* 1976; **16**: 335–39.

36 Seligman MEP, Steen TA, Park N, *et al.* Positive psychology progress: empirical validation of interventions. *Am Psychol.* 2005; **60**(5): 410–21.

37 Koenig HG. Religion and medicine. III. Developing a theoretical model. *Int J Psychiatry Med.* 2001; **31**(2): 199–216.

38 Koenig HG, Cohen HJ, editors. *The Link Between Religion and Health: psychoneuroimmunology and the faith factor.* New York: Oxford University Press; 2002.

39 AIDS' relentless march leaves legacy of misery. *Newsweek.* 5 June 2006.

40 Pepys MB, Hirschfield GM, Tennent GA, *et al.* Targeting C-reactive protein for the treatment of cardiovascular disease. *Nature.* 2006; **440**: 1217–21.

41 Lo B, Quill T, Tulsky J. Discussing palliative care with patients. *Ann Int Med.* 1999; **130**: 744–49.

42 King DE, Bushwick B. Beliefs and attitudes of hospital inpatients about faith healing and prayer. *J Fam Pract.* 1994; **39**(4): 349–52.

43 Kristeller JL, Rhodes M, Cripe ID, *et al.* Oncologist assisted spiritual intervention study (OASIS). *Int J Psychiatry Med.* 2005; **35**: 329–48.

CHAPTER 17

An overview of human drug development

CHRIS BUSHE

Introduction

Drug development rarely gets attention until something goes wrong.[1] In March 2006 six healthy male volunteers participating in what to all extents and purposes was a routine phase 1 clinical study in an independent research clinic at Northwick Hospital had an unexpected and in many respects unprecedented reaction to an experimental compound, TGN1412.[1,2] Within minutes of receiving small doses of this anti-inflammatory compound each of the volunteers began complaining of severe symptoms that within a few hours would lead to them suffering multiple organ failure. The newspaper coverage was extensive and suggested that the future of clinical trials might appear to be in jeopardy.[1]

An investigation by the Medicines and Healthcare Products Regulatory Agency (MHRA) found that there were no errors in the manufacture, formulation, dilution or administration of TGN1412. They concluded that the most likely cause of the adverse reaction was an 'unpredicted biological action of the drug in humans'.[2]

Many compounds enter clinical testing in humans and few ever find their way successfully to market. The route to develop any pharmaceutical is complicated and expensive. There is consensus that in the future development of drugs for affective disorders attention needs to be given to faster regulatory process, discovering biomarkers of response and inclusion of the increasing elderly populations in clinical trials.

Clinical studies phases 1–3

In broad terms pre-clinical testing of compounds is done predominantly in the laboratory and in animals prior to them being administered to human subjects. Animal testing is the ongoing subject of much debate over its necessity with a plethora of views in existence. The role of animal testing is two-fold. Firstly, to establish that in using an animal model to simulate the illness there is evidence of likely effect in humans. There is the clear difficulty that there are no exact animal models of psychosis or mental disorders. Secondly, to provide critical safety data prior to the compound being administered to humans. To date many animal species have been used but mostly rodents. European guidance dictates that at least two species are tested, one of which has to be non-rodent. The dosing frequency and duration of animal studies is dependent on the intended dosing frequency and duration in humans. Toxicological testing in animals over an extended period of time, for example to assess the possibility of any carcinogenic potential, has been routine in past years and is usually done in parallel with Phases 1–3 studies. The exact timing of these studies is dependent on the perceived risk and duration of treatment patients are subject to in clinical trials. After such testing a critical decision is made whether to progress into human subjects. Although the decision is taken by the pharmaceutical company they must then get formal ratification from MHRA (or applicable competent authority when trials run outside of the UK), which authorises around 350 Phase 1 trials annually.[3] These initial subjects are usually medically well human volunteers who will be paid for their time to take part in the study, although in the development of oncology drugs patients are used due to the nature of the illnesses being treated.

These initial studies are called Phase 1. It can be estimated that between 20 and 100 subjects will receive the compound in Phase 1. The case of TGN1412 is not exceptional in that the doses reportedly administered to the six unfortunate males was around 500 times less than that given to monkeys in pre-clinical testing.[1,2] The general principles of Phase 1 studies are clear. Generally, pharmaceutical companies will start with 'single-dose toxicity studies', where each patient gets one dose only with incremental doses as the study proceeds. These lead on to 'repeat dose toxicity studies' where the same patient gets multiple doses, and sometimes dose increases over a period of time as the trial subjects are extensively investigated as to the effects, predominantly safety, in an inpatient setting. Many Phase 1 studies are administered in their entirety by contract research companies as opposed to the pharmaceutical company. They may build a specific research unit on or near a hospital site. The volunteers are given stringent medical examinations to ensure that they are appropriate to participate in such studies. The nature of these volunteers has changed over the last 20 years. In the 1980s it was not uncommon for all healthy volunteers to be staff members of the pharmaceutical company. More commonly nowadays adverts are placed in newspapers and at other locations to attract potential subjects, often students, who might welcome the financial rewards of taking part in these studies. What has not changed is that predominantly these volunteers are males and young. The outcome following the MHRA investigation is that they are reported to be seeking expert advice before authorising any more Phase 1 studies of compounds such as TGN1412.[2]

In Phase 2 studies small doses of the compound will be given to ill patients. In general terms the dose given initially will be a fraction of the expected eventual dose and represents the dose that has been established in Phase 1 as being 'safe' and possibly efficacious. Often a number of different doses are trialled in so-called 'dose finding' studies. The effectiveness and safety of the compound are evaluated by performing a battery of tests that include biochemical, haematological, urinary screening and cardiovascular monitoring, in addition to the relevant efficacy measurements. Around 100–1000 patients may participate for a single compound. A critical decision will then be made as whether to put the compound into Phase 3 clinical trials. These are the trials that predominantly will allow the compound to become licensed and hence are large trials. Around 1000–5000 patients may participate. These are also often the trials that provide data that will form the mainstay of the promotion of the compound to clinicians when licensed. In order to appropriately assess the compound, Phase 3 trials will include placebo and/or an active comparator. This is in order to assess the efficacy in comparison to existing therapies or, if none, to allow for the placebo effect.

There is variation dependent upon the illness but in general terms these Phase 3 trials may fail to include specific trials in elderly subjects. The resulting effects are that in some cases compounds are licensed for usage with certain caveats, despite not having had extensive testing in the elderly. The case of duloxetine is an example. The data generated in the Phase 3 trials allowed a post-hoc analysis of the elderly cohort which has been subsequently published.[4] A specific study in the elderly population was, however, not part of the original registration dossier but has recently been completed.[5] Thus the original marketing authorisation from the European Agency for the Evaluation of Medicinal Products (EMEA) included a warning regarding usage in the elderly. The manufacturers of duloxetine have now submitted data to the EMEA on safety and efficacy in an elderly population, and the warning has been removed from the summary of product characteristics.[6]

In general terms if data is not available to support use of a medication in a specific population (e.g. severe renal impairment or severe spinal injury or elderly), the summary of product characteristics will state there is no data available. The EMEA or licensing body are then likely to ask for caution when using the drug in this population or even to state it is contraindicated.

Generalisation might be unfair but the proportion of total prescriptions received by older people in the UK increased from 39% in 1985 to 50% by 1998. One can estimate that by 2020 this figure will have increased to around 65%.[7] There is little evidence in the global pharmaceutical industry of specific expertise or research strategy that addresses the broader issue of drug development and use in an elderly population.

Exclusion of the elderly from treatment trials (mostly Phase 3) may be for many reasons. The challenge in bipolar disorder is to determine best treatment strategies to reduce relapse. A recent review concluded that such trials should essentially exclude females and the elderly.[8,9] The rationale was that this would enhance the likelihood of all patients having identical chances of relapse. In the majority of cases there is no such rationale for not having a decent sized cohort of elderly subjects, specifically in affective disorder and psychosis trials where treatments can often be lifelong. The other issue is the reporting of data specifically in elderly cohorts. Clearly, some patients up to 65 years do enter depression trials and post-hoc analyses of the database can be undertaken to specifically report the efficacy and safety data. There are good examples of publications that report this type of data.[4,10] In many published studies, however, data are generally reported only as mean values and not in an additional categorical manner. This does not make it easy for clinicians to compare drug response in the various age cohorts. This is evidenced in recent trials of exemplary standard in bipolar disorder that report mean ages of the participants receiving olanzapine 39.2 (SD 11.9),[11] 42.9 (SD 13),[12] 39.99 (SD 12.8).[13] In contrast, the inclusion criteria for these trials were up to 18 years, over 18 years, 18–75 years. There is no data reported on the numbers of subjects up to 60 years or their response to treatment and it can be surmised from the standard deviations that the numbers of elderly subjects included in the trial are not so large. In contrast, the EMEA specifically requests in drug submissions that data from differing age cohorts is presented and comparisons made.[14–16] These regulatory submission requirements are discussed in more detail later in the chapter. For psychiatrists who look after older people with mental health problems it may be beneficial for them to have data that is specific to this age group.

EMEA approval and submission

At the Phase 3 stage drug development becomes not only more expensive but more complex. Since 1995 with the arrival of the EMEA and the centralised evaluation system the majority of compounds will now be submitted to the EMEA for assessment of their application for a licence.[17,18] The assessment period is in many ways surprisingly quick. Following the submission the scientific committee that is responsible for the review of these applications, the Committee for Medicinal Products for Human Use (CHMP), formulates a scientific opinion on the granting of a marketing authorisation in seven months. At around the four-month point the CHMP identifies any major and minor objections that may exist (typically 100 questions will be received). At this time the review timeline is stopped, and is restarted once the company responds. This 'clock-stop' occurs at least twice in the seven-month period. During the procedure the company has a number of options that include withdrawal of the application, addressing the objections or altering the scope of the application. The EMEA has recently reported that from September 1997 until May 2001 in the 111 successive applications 29% failed to reach a positive decision.[18] To put this into perspective, 66% were new chemical entities and 34% biopharmaceuticals. Somewhat surprisingly, in 42.3% of all applications a major objection was raised on the lack of adequate randomised controlled trials. Indeed the average number of major objections per application was 6.8. In only 6% of applications was there no major objection. This might seem surprising in that during the development phase of the compound companies can liaise with CHMP to request scientific advice, although there is no obligation. Positive partnerships with regulators including EMEA have been shown to be productive in terms of complex regulatory submissions.[17] This has been recently evidenced by the global registration of olanzapine where Lilly achieved regulatory submissions in 21 countries within days of one another. The numbers of drugs that fail to receive a licence from the EMEA has remained remarkably constant, being 28% between 1995 and 1999.[18] Companies can appeal a CHMP decision. At the end of the review process, if successful, the European Commission grants a marketing authorisation valid throughout the EU.

EMEA requirements for drug licensing in affective disorders and elderly

The EMEA and the USA Food and Drug Administration (FDA) both set out their individual and often different requirements for clinical trials that are needed to achieve a successful marketing authorisation. As an example, for an antipsychotic agent to receive marketing approval as a mood stabiliser in bipolar disorder there are stringent requirements from EMEA for substantial studies that assess both proportions of patients relapsing and time taken to relapse, for both manic and depressive phases. Patients must be stable at entry and there should be a placebo cohort.[19]

In many regards the advice given by the EMEA is clear and is set out in the many notes for guidance on the clinical investigation of medicinal products.[15,18,19] In addition pharmaceutical companies remain free to discuss and liaise with EMEA regarding their proposed package of clinical trials for submission. There is, however, an awareness that the current US system with the FDA is perhaps more open for discussion than the EMEA. The CHMP publishes the various sets of 'notes for guidance' on the EMEA website. The main guidance notes relevant to depression and the elderly are contained within 'Note for guidance on clinical investigation of medicinal products in the treatment of depression', issued in April 2002, and the more specific International Conference on Harmonisation (ICH) Topic E7, 'Note for guidance on studies in support of special populations: Geriatrics', which provides generic advice for clinical trials in the elderly.[15,16]

The EMEA will consider granting a marketing authorisation only for major depressive disorder as defined by DSM-IV or ICD-10. The expectation is that moderate major depressive disorder (MDD) will be the diagnosis in the majority of the patients included in the trials. The expectation for a submission for an antidepressant agent is that clinical trials are included to show efficacy and safety within an acute depressive illness and maintenance of that response (continuation of treatment). There is no obligation, however, to submit data on recurrence prevention.

An acute antidepressant response requires trial duration of six weeks with an essential requirement to have a placebo arm and in practice three-arm trials including both placebo and an active control are recommended.[15] The EMEA demands unambiguous evidence of efficacy which translates into showing clear efficacy versus placebo or the active comparator. This is one situation in which a non-inferiority trial versus an active comparator would not be deemed acceptable. This arises due to the fact that a non-inferiority margin cannot be determined, as in over a third of trials in which an active control is used as a third arm, the effect of the third arm could not be separated from placebo, thus giving an uncertain effect size. Conversely, including placebo also has ethical considerations and any short-term trials over six weeks need to be fully justified. The next challenge is to show that a short-term response can be maintained throughout the duration of the depressive illness, estimated to be around six months but possibly longer in older patients. Such a relapse prevention study randomises responders to the antidepressant following 8–12 weeks of open treatment to either placebo or antidepressant for around six months. Both of these trial designs involve placebo subjects and there has been much debate over the ethical issues involved. The EMEA is, however, clear over its views that without use of placebo it is simply not possible to show undoubted evidence of antidepressant activity and hence they argue it would be detrimental to public health and ethically unacceptable to grant a product licence to such a medicinal product. The ethical trade-offs are that the short-term trials do not exceed six weeks and in the six-month relapse prevention trials the protocol needs to allow rescue medication and/or switches. These latter events sometimes make interpretation of data complicated.

The use of placebo-controlled studies in depression has been rigorously debated by clinicians and featured in the fifth revision of the Declaration of Helsinki.[20] The broad consensus among psychiatrists is in agreement with EMEA in that placebo studies are 'necessary, ethical and feasible'. A major reason behind this consensus derives from a recent review of 75 placebo-controlled trials of antidepressants published between 1981 and 2000. Not only is there a striking variability of placebo response (10–50%) but crucially the number of placebo responders has increased by 7% per decade, reflecting variable patient recruitment criteria.[21] There also appear to be no negative long-term sequelae for the placebo subjects with no reported increase in suicidal behaviours.[20]

Recurrence prevention is not an obligatory part of a registration package and where included they need to be one to two-year placebo-controlled studies. The specific trial length might reflect the recurrence rate in the trial population.

In a similar manner any additional claims need to be supported by specific trials; for example, in psychotic depression.

There is an encouraging consistency throughout the various guidance notes in that EMEA often refers to the need to include categorical data (responder or remission rates) in addition to mean change data. There is little doubt that such categorical data is clinically more meaningful for healthcare professionals and patients alike. Hence although no current treatments are indeed licensed for therapy-resistant patients there is unambiguous advice that remission rates in this population are more relevant than mean changes on a rating scale.

The assessment of what constitutes efficacy is no less important than the choice of trial types. Results need to be presented and discussed in terms of both clinical and statistical relevance. Thus in short-term trials both baseline to post-treatment scores and responder rates (protocol pre-specified) must be reported and a 50% improvement in a rating scale is widely accepted as a clinically relevant response. For longer term trials both the relapse rates and time to this event should be reported with one chosen as a clear primary end-point. The general principle prevails that within the protocol there are clear definitions of primary and secondary end-points, with the statistical power of the trials being calculated in respect of the primary end-point. There remain a curiously large number of trials published in peer-reviewed publications for various therapeutic modalities that fail to state either the primary study end-point or provide standard deviations/errors around efficacy data. The commonest rating scales used in depression are the Hamilton Rating Scale of Depression (17-item scale) and the Montgomery Asberg Depression Rating Scale for primary end-points. Investigators must also be fully trained and conversant with all rating tools with inter-rater reliability scores being documented for all investigators. Investigators need not necessarily be medically qualified clinicians and often are other healthcare professionals (nurses, etc.) but will be carefully supervised by the primary investigator, a physician who is held responsible for the conduct of the trial at that site.

The design features for the trials also warrant some discussion. There remains little doubt that clinical trial populations within a given therapeutic area can be highly heterogeneous and this in part is the reason why a non-inferiority comparison with an active comparator cannot be acceptable proof of efficacy. The majority of patients should be outpatients and the patients evaluated in these large Phase 3 studies should preferably be homogeneous with those used in the dose-finding and pivotal proof of concept studies that constituted Phases 1 and 2 studies.

The numbers of studies needed may vary between compounds evaluated for various reasons. Clearly, new chemical entities need more testing and trials than new molecular versions of existing types. One of the major challenges is to establish not only the optimal dose but also the lower end of the clinical effective dose. Thus the EMEA demands that controlled parallel fixed-dose short-term studies using at least three dosages and preferably placebo and an active comparator are performed, additional to the three-arm studies previously discussed.[15] Many other studies may be performed; pharmacodynamic, pharmacokinetics and interaction studies are usually essential. For antidepressants there is clear need based on precedent to determine whether rebound or withdrawal phenomena may occur and trials will be designed to evaluate this possibility.

The specific evaluation of antidepressants in the elderly is of much debate. The generic ICH 7 document available from the EMEA website that gives guidance on studies in the elderly indicates that the efficacy and safety for a compound can be determined for the elderly population from the total database.[16] This is feasible for an antidepressant in clinical trials with a few provisos. Firstly, that the agent derives from a known pharmacological class and, secondly, that sufficient elderly patients are included in the database to allow a prospective subgroup analysis. For many antidepressants it may be preferable to conduct specific trials in an elderly population. ICH 7 defines the elderly as over 65 years but states the importance of including patients over 75 years and furthermore suggests there should be no arbitrary upper age cut-offs in clinical trials.

The elderly are a very different population to their younger counterparts in relation often to pharmacodynamic, pharmacokinetic, hepatic and renal functions. There has also sometimes been the tacit assumption that the depressive illness is also identical to that seen in younger patients. Recently, placebo-controlled studies of the same design and dose have failed to show evidence for efficacy in the elderly when similar trials in adults had already done so.[15,16] There are also clear issues with determining the correct dosage and the EMEA recommends that this is a matter addressed prior to licensing. The optimal study proposal in the elderly would thus be a placebo-controlled dose response study or series.

If a licence to treat the elderly is desired, the overall dossier should evaluate age-related differences in adverse events rates, effectiveness and dose-response.

Drug development and depression: any clues for the future?

There are no immediate signs that the regulatory framework will change for anti-depressants requiring efficacy to be determined on the basis of clinical symptoms. Yet it is not unreasonable to presume that assessment of efficacy will one day be complemented by neuroimaging. Positron emission tomography (PET) has shown that patients with major depression have altered patterns of activity in limbic and cortical regions.[22] Neuroimaging may also provide predictive biomarkers of depression. PET studies have indicated that there is increased activity in a specific region of the limbic system, the amygdala of the left hemisphere, which may represent an indicator of potentially increased vulnerability to future depressive episodes. Such biomarkers may potentially lead to the need for reduced numbers of patients in efficacy trials of relapse prevention. Magnetic resonance imaging (MRI) may also have a role to play in determining biomarkers of depression or its response to treatments. MRI studies demonstrate that hippocampal volume is reduced in long-term depression patients. MRI, PET and other functional imaging tools are currently in their early days in terms of providing regulatory relevant data for putative antidepressants.[22]

While there are clear challenges in relation to developing the next successful antidepressant class there are many compounds in development. The Internet has provided a useful tool to track the development of potentially new compounds. Many pharmaceutical companies now voluntarily provide a list of ongoing trials and when appropriate place the results of such trials on their websites.[23,24] At time of writing in mid-2007 at least nine compounds are in Phase 3 trials, 17 in

Phase 2 and 11 in Phase 1, giving a total of at least 37 new antidepressant drugs in development.[25] A variety of differing chemical entities are represented that range from DVS-233 SR desvenlafaxine (a metabolite of venlafaxine) through to 5-HT1A partial agonists, beta-3 adrenoceptor agonists, melatonin receptor agonists M1/M2, NK2antagonists (all new types of chemical entity in development currently) – and many other putative antidepressant agents that include purified omega-3. Many of these new compounds are very different from the current antidepressant agents that essentially target the monoamine system. For example, aside from tolerability issues a major problem with the SSRI class is their delayed onset of action resulting from long-term changes in neurotransmitter systems. One of the novel approaches is to target 5-HT1A receptors, which are involved in augmenting serotonergic transmission, directly. However, these compounds have not been without development problems. For example, Gepirone ER (a new chemical entity in development) was not approved by FDA in 2004, although a new amended New Drug Application (NDA) may be submitted in the near future, and Vilazodone failed to demonstrate efficacy versus placebo while demonstrating comparable efficacy with a currently marketed antidepressant.[25–27]

Drug development and affective disorders in the elderly: any clues for the future?

There will always be problems with recruitment of elderly patients into Phase 3 clinical trials. Aside from the increased practical difficulties of including the elderly in clinical trials, only 4.2% of elderly patients with major depression meet the increasingly rigorous inclusion and exclusion criteria of Phase 3 studies.[28] The situation in bipolar disorder may be even more difficult notwithstanding recommendations for such studies that if applied would effectively outlaw the inclusion of elderly patients.[29] However, despite such nihilism randomised double-blind placebo-controlled trials of antidepressants (including the recently licensed duloxetine) which included decent-sized cohorts of patients have been undertaken in elderly patients with major depression.[5] Such data generated in specific trials in the elderly can add to the efficacy and safety data that have been already derived from post-hoc analyses of patients aged over 55 years (and thus technically not elderly patients) who participated in registration studies.[4]

The future for drug development in general

In 2004 only 24 new active substances were first marketed, which is the lowest figure for well over a decade and there is no sign of this trend reversing.[30] The total number of new drugs approved by the FDA and EMEA in 2005 actually dropped from 151 in 2004 to 121.[31] Furthermore, despite development times for successful compounds remaining around 10–12 years on average during the last decade, over the last three to four years development time has begun to increase.[31] The consensus seems that regulatory agencies are becoming more risk averse and are requesting more safety data. Despite this climate or possibly because of it pharmaceutical research and development (R&D) expenditure increased during 1995–2004 at an average annual rate of 6.5% to $US56 billion (£27 billion) in 2004. Fortuitously, sales during this period grew at a faster rate of 7.7% per annum and 17% of such pharmaceutical sales were reinvested in R&D.[30]

As a result of regulatory requirements and the perceived deficiencies in the dossiers submitted by pharmaceutical companies (mean 6.8 major objections per dossier) the current cost of bringing a new medicine to market is estimated at $US802 million (£387 million).[18,30] Part of this high expenditure relates to the high attrition rates of Phase 3 compounds with only 55% estimated to make it to the marketplace. Attention is thus falling on the single most costly component of drug development, the clinical trials. Many companies now perform trials in lower cost countries such as Eastern Europe and South East Asia but this by itself will not be enough to reduce costs significantly. What may pay greater dividends is the possibility that the regulatory model, Phases 1–3, might change to shorten development times. The development and validation of biomarkers might allow smaller or shorter trials that have been enriched for potential responders. PET scanning, for example in Alzheimer's disease, may reduce patient numbers needed. A provisional approval phase with controlled early market access that subsequently leads to a full approval with updated clinical and safety data has been another possible option to consider.[30] This model essentially would include observational studies in the regulatory dossier as this late-stage development would take place in a real world population. Drastic as it may seem, this suggestion has some merit. Dropout rates in RCTs are often around 75% over even a six-month study, rising to 84% at 12 months in contrast to dropout rates in naturalistic forms of research which may be as low as 20% over two years.[13,32,33] Drugs are used very differently in a real world population and many side-effects, although qualitatively the same, are quantitatively very different in naturalistic studies. For example, weight gain associated with antipsychotic treatment is consistently lower in naturalistic studies than in RCTs.[34]

There is little doubt that a challenging era lies ahead for drug development, with the increasing advent of effective generic compounds in many therapeutic areas. The elderly populations are increasing worldwide and they mostly retain their illnesses into old age. A real challenge exists to determine the most effective treatments for their disabling mental illnesses while not compromising their physical health. An effective partnership needs to be created between the pharmaceutical industry and the regulatory agencies to maximise the development and potential of significant new chemical entities.

KEY POINTS

▶ Drug registration is a well-defined process by the drug regulatory agencies, often specifying trial types and allowing discussion with pharmaceutical companies.

▶ Speed of registering new compounds is surprisingly quick with final decision in most cases under 12 months.

▶ Around 30% of drug registration applications to EMEA do not reach a positive opinion.

▶ At least 37 new antidepressant compounds are currently in development in 2007.

▶ Future drug registration may look to utilise biomarkers and complex neuroimaging in addition to clinical symptoms and biochemical measurements.

REFERENCES

1   Moss L. Guinea pigs drug ordeal remains a mystery as no errors found. *The Scotsman*. 6 April 2006.

2   MHRA. Clinical trial final report; 25 May 2006. Available from: www.mhra.gov.uk

3   http://www.mhra.gov.uk

4   Nelson JC, Wohlreich MM, Mallinckrodt CH, *et al*. Duloxetine for the treatment of major depressive disorder in mature and elderly patients. *Am J Geriatr Psychiatr*. In press.

5   Raskin J, Wiltse C, Dinkel J, *et al*. Duloxetine versus placebo in the treatment of elderly patients with major depressive disorder. Poster presented San Diego: American Association for Geriatric Psychiatry; 3–6 March 2005.

6   Summary of Product Characteristics Duloxetine 2006.

7   Ford G. *Drug Development in an Ageing World*. 2002. Available from: http://www.ncl. ac.uk/peals/ageing/

8   Angst J, Baastrup P, Grof P, *et al*. The course of monopolar depression and bipolar psychoses. *Psychiatr Neurol Neurochir*. 1973; **76**(6): 489–500.

9   Tyrer S. What does history teach us about factors associated with relapse in bipolar affective disorder? *J Psychopharmacol*. 2006; **20**(Suppl.2): S4–11.

10   Wohlreich M, Mallinckrodt CH, Watkin J, *et al*. Duloxetine for the long-term treatment of major depressive disorder in patients aged 65 years and older: an open-label study. *BMC Geriatrics*. 2004; **4**: 11.

11   Tohen M, Calabrese J, Sachs G, *et al*. Randomised placebo controlled trial of olanzapine as maintenance therapy in patients with bipolar I disorder responding to acute treatment with olanzapine. *Am J Psychiatr*. 2006; **163**: 247–56.

12   Tohen M, Greil W, Calabrese JR, *et al*. Olanzapine versus lithium in the maintenance treatment of bipolar disorder: a 12-month, randomized, double-blind, controlled clinical trial. *Am J Psychiatr*. 2005; **162**(7): 1281–90.

13   Tohen M, Ketter TA, Zarate CA, *et al*. Olanzapine versus divalproex sodium for the treatment of acute mania and maintenance of remission: a 47-week study. *Am J Psychiatr*. 2003; **160**(7): 1263–71.

14   European Medicines Agency. http://www.emea.eu.int/

15   European Agency for the Evaluation of Medicinal Products. *Note for Guidance on Clinical Investigation of Medicinal Products in the Treatment of Depression*. London: European Agency for the Evaluation of Medicinal Products; 2002. Available from: http://www.emea. europa.eu/pdfs/ewp/051897.pdf

16   European Agency for the Evaluation of Medicinal Products. *Note for Guidance on Studies in Support of Special Populations: geriatrics*. London: European Agency for the Evaluation of Medicinal Products; 1994. Available from: http://www.emea.europa.eu/pdfs/human/ ich/03799Sen.pdf

17   Worthen S, Kasher J, Saunders J, *et al*. The global registration of Zyprexa (olanzapine). *Drug Inf J*. 1997; **31**: 49–55.

18 Pignatti F, Aronsson B, Gate N, *et al.* The review of drug applications submitted to the European Medicines Evaluation Agency: frequently raised objections, and outcome. *Eur J Clin Pharmacol.* 2002; **58**(9): 573–80.

19 European Agency for the Evaluation of Medicinal Products. *Note for Guidance on Clinical Investigation of Medicinal Products for the Treatment and Prevention of Bipolar Disorder.* London: European Agency for the Evaluation of Medicinal Products; 2001. Available from: http://www.emea.europa.eu/pdfs/human/ewp/056798en.pdf

20 Baldwin DS, Broich K, Fritze J, *et al.* Placebo-controlled studies in depression: necessary, ethical and feasible. *Eur Arch Psychiatr Clin Neurosci.* 2003; **253**: 22–8.

21 Walsh BT, Seidman SN, Sysko R, *et al.* Placebo response in studies of major depression. *JAMA.* 2002; **287**: 1840–47.

22 Nemeroff CB. Contributions from imaging. *Scientific American.* 1998; June [journal online]. Available from: http://www.sciam.com/1998/0698issue/0698nemeroffbox2.html

23 http://www.lillytrials.com

24 http://www.clinicaltrials.org

25 http://www.neurotransmitter.net/newdrugs.html Accessed 14 September 2006.

26 http://www.fda.gov/cder/regulatory/applications/default.htm

27 *Depression: a bleak future?* Available from: http://www.imshealth.com

28 Yastrubetskaya O, Chiu EO, Connell S. Is good clinical research practice for clinical trials good for clinical practice? *Int J Geriatr Psychiatr.* 1997; **12**: 227–31.

29 Rush AJ, Post MR, Nolen WA, *et al.* Methodological issues in developing new acute treatments for patients with bipolar disorder. *Biol Psychiatr.* 2000; **48**: 615–24.

30 McAuslane N. The future of the pharmaceutical industry: need for a fundamental change? *J Br Assoc Pharm Physicians.* 2006; **16**: 4–9.

31 Pharmaceutical Regulatory Industry. http://www.bccresearch.com/editors/RB–215.html

32 McQuade RD, Stock E, Marcus R, *et al.* A comparison of weight change during treatment with olanzapine or aripiprazole: results from a randomized, double-blind study. *J Clin Psychiatr.* 2004; **65**(Suppl.18): S47–56.

33 Bushe C, Yeomans D, Smith S, *et al.* A well being programme (WSP) in severe mental illness: reducing risk for physical ill-health: a post programme re-audit at 2 years. Poster presented Chicago, IL: 25th Biennial Congress of the Collegium Internationale Neuro-Psychopharmacologicum; 2006.

34 Haddad P. Weight change with atypical antipsychotics in the treatment of schizophrenia. *J Psychopharmacol.* 2005; **19**(Suppl.6): S16–27.

Index

Abbreviated Mental Test Score 146
ABC approaches 186
acculturation 232–3
ACE inhibitors 36
aetiology
    for bipolar disorder 26–7
    for depression 27, 55
        altered brain structure 31–5
        limbic and fronto-subcortical circuitry
            30–1
        medication-induced 18, 35–7
        organic conditions 27–30
affective disorders
    classification systems 3–4
    current trends 1–2
    see also individual disorders
ageing
    and depressive symptoms 18–19
    models and social expectations 195–6, 218–19
    neurobiology 25, 30–5
    and occupation 194–6
    and spirituality 243
alcohol misuse 182
Alzheimer's disease (AD)
    and depression 21, 130
    pathology 33
amitriptyline 56–7, 65, 134
Amok syndrome 238
amygdala enlargement 27

analgesics 36, 154–5
anhedonia 196
anti-cholinergic effects 134, 148
anticonvulsants 36
antidepressants 56–71, 134–7
    choice considerations 65–9, 130, 167–8
        acute stage 67
        continuation treatments 67–8
        maintenance 68
        physically ill patients 69, 134–7, 148, 149
        treatment-resistant conditions 70–1
    classes 56–62
        MAOIs (monoamine oxidase inhibitors)
            60–1
        NaSSAs (noradrenaline and serotonin
            synaptic antagonists) 61–2
        RIMA (reversible inhibitors of
            monoamine oxidase) 61
        SNRIs (serotonin and noradrenaline
            reuptake inhibitors) 59–60
        SSRIs (selective serotonin reuptake
            inhibitors) 57–9
        TCAs (tricyclic antidepressants) 56–7
    combination therapies 72
    compliance issues 68–9
    mechanisms of action 56
    prescribing practices 62–3, 139
        and Parkinson's disease (PD) 148
        role of nurses 181–2

antihypertensives 36
antipsychotics
    and bipolar disease 87–9
    and depression 71
anxiety 179–80
    and depression 20
apathy, and Parkinson's disease (PD) 130,
    147
apolipoprotein E genotype 28
aripiprazole 71, 89
aspirin 71
assessment instruments 176, 185
    see also diagnostic instruments; screening
        measures
attention, and pain management 152

back pain 18, 151
basal ganglia 31
BASDEC see Brief Assessment Schedule for
    Depression in the Elderly
benefits and allowances, care entitlement 208,
    209–12
benzodiazepines 89
bereavement
    and depression 9, 18, 38, 177–8
    and dysthymia 69
β-blockers 36, 133
bipolar disorders 80
    aetiology 26–7
    classification and definitions 80–1
    course and outcome 81
    and dementia 22
    and depression 11–12, 22
    epidemiology 234
    guidelines 82
    management principles 82
        acute episodes 89
        maintenance and prevention 90–1
        rapid cycling 91
    pharmacological management 82–91
        drug types 82–9
        indications and choice 89–91
    suicide risk 91
blindness 130–1
bone disorders 130
brain imaging 35
brain structure changes 31–5
    see also neurobiology
Brief Assessment Schedule for Depression in
    the Elderly (BASDEC) 4, 11

calcium channel blockers 36
cancer and depression 7, 129–30
carbamazepine 86
    dosages 87
cardiac conditions and depression 6–7, 145

cardiovascular disease and depression 6–7, 21,
    28–9, 128
    brain structure changes 33–5
    see also stroke and depression
care approaches 217–18, 226
    collaborative primary care 168
    nurse roles 173–89
    occupational therapy roles 194–204
    policy guidance 221–2
    see also primary care issues; social services
care entitlement 208
    case studies 209–12
care managers 208
Care Programme Approach 188–9
Care Services Improvement Partnership
    (2005) 203, 223
carers 179, 217–27
    establishing needs and wants 220–1
choice issues 220–1, 221–3
cholinesterase inhibitors 148
chronic obstructive airways disease (COPD)
    128
chronic pain and depression 18, 150–4
    cognitive-behavioural models 153–4
    Gate Control Theory 151–2
citalopram 57–9, 66, 135
classification systems
    for bipolar disorder 80–1
    for depression 3–4, 17–18, 178
clomipramine 65
clonidine 36
clothiepin 56–7
cognitive assessments 146
cognitive behavioural therapy (CBT) 63, 111,
    112
    case study 116–17, 118
    guidelines 64
    indications 112, 154–5
    mode of action 112
    training 112
cognitive impairment and depression 8, 20–2,
    27–30, 146
    assessment 146
cognitive-behavioural models of chronic pain
    153–4
communication difficulties 129
community involvement initiatives 221
community psychiatric nurse (CPN) 168
compliance issues 68–9
COPD see chronic obstructive airways disease
Cornell Scale 21–2
corticotropin-releasing factor antagonists 73
cortisol 30
cultural aspects 6, 230–40
    epidemiological studies 234
    globalisation 234–5

migration issues 232–4
  acculturation and mental health 232–3
  with elderly mental health patients 235–40
Cushing's disease 130

deafness 130–1
delusions 22
dementia
  aetiologies 27–30
  and bipolar disorders 22
  and depression 8, 27
    diagnosis 146
    reversible conditions 21
demographic changes 1–2
'demoralisation syndrome' 165–6
dependency issues 7
depot medications 90–1
depression
  aetiologies 25–39, 55
  classification and definitions 3–4, 17–18,
    178
  diagnosis
    clinical features 2–3, 17–19, 146
    investigations and tests 4, 10–11, 19–20,
      133, 146
    under-recognition 127, 131–3, 165–6
  differential diagnosis 133, 146
  epidemiology 5–11, 54–5, 126–7
  impact on health 145
  medication-induced 18, 35–7, 133
  pharmacological management 54–74
    acute stages 67
    continuation and maintenance stages
      67–8
    in physically ill patients 69, 133–40
  physical conditions 6–7, 18, 55–6, 127–40,
    144–56
  risk factors 20
  screening 10–11, 19–20
  treatment-resistant conditions 69–73
  use of ECT 63, 72–3, 89, 94–102
'depression-executive dysfunction syndrome'
  21
'depressive pseudodementia' 21
Dewsbury psychogeriatric services 239
Dhat syndrome 238
DHEA (dehydroepiandrosterone) 29
diabetes mellitus 130
diagnosis
  clinical features 2–3, 17–19
  differential 133, 146
  under-recognition problems 127, 131–3,
    165–6
diagnostic instruments 4, 7, 133, 146
  see also screening measures
differential diagnoses 133, 146

Direct Payments 211
disability, and depression 8–9
distractional coping strategies 152
dopamine reuptake inhibitors 73
dopaminergic agents 71
dosulepin 65, 134
doxepin 56–7
drug-induced conditions see medication-
  induced depression
DSM-IV-TR classification 17–18
duloxetine 67
DWML (deep white matter lesions) 33–5
dys-executive symptoms 109
dysphoria 165–6
dysthymia 69, 164

EBAS-DEP scale 11
ECT (electroconvulsive therapy) 63, 72–3, 89,
  94–102
  administration protocols 98–9
  adverse effects 99–101
  efficacy 101–2
  future developments and other treatments
    103
  indications for use 95–7
    age-related 96–7
    continuing treatments 102
    diagnostic 95–6
    physical illnesses and risk 97–8, 138–9,
      148
  long-term prognosis 101–2
  with Parkinson's disease 148
ELSA (English Longitudinal Study of Ageing)
  162
emotionalism 129, 150
endocrine disorders 130
engagement processes 184–5
epidemiological studies
  for bipolar disorder 234
  for depression 5–11, 54–5
    and culture/ethnicity 6, 234
    and dementia 8
    and disability 8–9
    and exercise 9
    and gender 9–10
    and mortality 6
    and physical illness 6–7
    and settings 5
epilepsy 134
escitalopram 57–9, 66, 135
ethnicity 231
  and depression 6
  see also cultural aspects
Everybody's Business (CSIP 2005) 203, 223
evidence-based approaches 1
exercise therapies 9, 138

FACS (Fair Access to Care Criteria) 208
  case studies 209–12
falls and fractures, medication-induced 135
familial affective conditions 28
family issues, recognising depression 131
fluoxetine 57–9, 66, 135
flupenthixol 67
fluvoxamine 57–9
folate deficiency 133
frontal lobe changes 33, 109
fronto-subcortical circuits 30–1, 32
functional brain imaging 35

GABA 32
Gate Control Theory of pain 151–2
GDS *see* Geriatric Depression Scale
gender, and depression 9–10
genetic markers 28
genito-urinary disorders 131
geographical prevalence studies 126
Geriatric Depression Scale (GDS) 4, 10–11,
  19–20, 133
Geriatric Mental State (GMS) Examination 4
globalisation 234–5
Glucocorticoid Cascade Hypothesis 29
glutamatergic modulators 73
GMS *see* Geriatric Mental State (GMS)
  Examination
'Gospel Oak' studies (London) 8–9
government policies 221–2
GP consultations
  and depression 19
    frequent attenders 132
    investigations and tests 4, 7, 133
    under recognition 131–3
  and psychiatric referrals 139
  see also primary care issues
'Grandma Moses' 196
grief, cf. depression 177–8
guided self-help 64, 113
guidelines for management
  bipolar disorder 82
  depression 9, 63–4

habits and routines 197–8
HAD *see* Hospital Anxiety and Depression
  (HAD) Scale
Hamilton Depressive Rating Scale 7
health promotion, and nursing practices 175–7
health services
  partnership and integrated working 168,
    207–8, 214–15
  see also nursing practices; occupational
    therapy interventions; primary care issues
herbal remedies 62, 137–8
hereditary conditions 28

hippocampus 29–30, 33
Hospital Anxiety and Depression (HAD)
  Scale 4, 7, 11, 146
hospital settings, and depression 5, 127–8
HPA (hypothalamo-pituitary-adrenal) axis 25,
  29–30
5-HT 25, 30
5-HT receptor antagonists 73
hypnotics 36
hypochondriasis and depression 150–4
hypomania 11–12
hyponatraemia, and SSRIs 135
hypothyroidism 133

ICD-10 systems, for mood disorders 3–4
imipramine 56–7, 65
immune responses, and spirituality 248–9
incidence of depression 126
Individual Budgets 212
insomnia 2–3, 18–19
international perspectives 126
interpersonal therapy (IPT) 111, 112
  case study 116–17, 118–21
  indications 112
  mechanisms of change 112
IPT *see* interpersonal therapy
isoniazid 60–1

joint diseases and depression 130
Joint Inquiry into Mental Health and
  Wellbeing in Later Life 203
Joseph Rowntree Foundation 218, 222

Koro syndrome 238

lamotrigine 86–7, 90
life review therapy 111, 114
limbic system 30–1
Link-Age Plus 223
lipid lowering agents 36
lithium 71, 83–4, 87, 90–1, 136
  adverse effects 84
  dosages 87
  efficacy 83–4, 90–1
  mode of action 83
Local Area Agreements (LAAs) 214–15
lofepramine 56–7, 65, 134
loneliness, and depression 9
LUNSERS medication scale 185

magnetic seizure therapy (MST) 73, 103
management approaches
  cultural considerations 237–8
  current trends 2
  see also care approaches; pharmacological
    management; psychotherapies

mania
  acute episodes 89
  bipolar depressive episodes 90–1
  secondary episodes 89
manic-depressive illness *see* bipolar disorder
MAOIs *see* monoamine oxidase inhibitors
Matisse, Henri 196
measuring outcome *see* outcome measurement
  studies
medical conditions *see* physical illnesses
medication management *see* pharmacological
  management
medication-induced depression 18, 35–7, 133
melatonergic agonists 73
mental capacity 181
mental health promotion
  role of nurses 175–7
  see also prevention initiatives
mental health services 211
  collaborative care approaches 168
  see also social services
mianserin 61–2, 66
migration issues 232–4
  see also cultural aspects
Mini Mental Test Score 146
mirtazapine 61–2, 67, 136
  combination therapies 72
moclobemide 61
Model of Human Occupation 194–5
monoamine oxidase inhibitors (MAOIs) 60–1,
  66–7, 136
  combination therapies 72
  dietary restrictions 136
Montgomery Asberg Scale 10
mood stabilisers
  definitions 82
  drug types 83–9
  see also individual agents
MOOTS *see* Moving Out of the Shadows
  (MOOTS) report (2005)
mortality rates, and depression 6
motivation issues 195, 196–7
Moving Out of the Shadows (MOOTS) report
  (2005) 217–18, 219, 223

NARIs *see* noradrenaline reuptake inhibitors
NaSSAs *see* noradrenergic and specific
  serotoninergic antidepressants
National Service Frameworks for Older
  People 166, 176, 207, 218
neck pain 18
neurobiology
  brain structure alterations 31–5
  neural pathway changes 30–1
  neurotransmitter changes 25
neurodegenerative diseases 130

neurokinin receptor antagonists 73
neurotransmitters 25
'A New Ambition for Older People' (DoH
  2006) 219
NHS
  partnership and integrated working 168,
    207–8, 214–15
  see also nursing practices; occupational
    therapy interventions; primary care issues
NICE guidelines
  for anxiety 180
  for bipolar disorder 82
  for depression 9, 63–4, 178
  on ECT (electroconvulsive therapy) 95–6
nifedipine 133
noradrenaline reuptake inhibitors (NARIs) 62
noradrenergic and specific serotoninergic
  antidepressants (NaSSAs) 61–2, 136
nortriptyline 56–7, 65
NSAIDs 36
nursing practices
  assessment and diagnosis 173–5
  health promotion 175–7
  pharmacological management 181–2
  for psychosis and psychosocial conditions
    183–9
  working with alcohol misuse 182

occupational performance assessments 198–200
  history interview 199–200
occupational therapy interventions 194–204
  assessment 198–200
  in early stages 200–2
  in later stages 202–3
oestrogen receptor modulators 36
olanzapine 71, 88, 90
older people, demographic changes 1–2
omega-3 fatty acids 71, 138
opioids 155
organic conditions 27–30
  dementias 8, 21–2, 27
  familial conditions 28
  see also physical illnesses
Our Health, Our Care, Our Say (DoH 2006) 214
outcome measurement studies, for depression
  10–11

pain and depression 18, 150–4
  cognitive-behavioural models 153–4
  Gate Control Theory 151–2
panic disorder 20
Parkinson's disease (PD) and depression 7, 30,
  69, 130, 147–9
  psychological and social factors 148–9
  use of ECT 148
  use of psychotropic drugs 148

paroxetine 57–9, 66, 135, 148
partnership working 214–15
patient choice 220–1, 221–3
patient education 63
person-centred care 217, 226
personality factors 37
pharmacological management
  of bipolar disorder 82–91
    drug classes 82–9
    guidelines 82
    indications and drug choices 89–91
    long-acting drugs 90–1
    treatment principles 82
  of depression 54–74
    choice considerations 65–9, 130, 148,
      167–8
    combination therapies 72
    compliance issues 68–9
    discontinuing treatments 73
    drug classes 56–62
    future developments 73–4
    guidelines 63–4
    maintenance treatments 68
    mechanisms of action 56
    in physically ill patients 69, 133–40,
      147–8, 149
    prescribing practices 62–3, 139
    role of nurses 181–2
    treating acute stages 67
    treatment-resistant conditions 69–73
phenelzine 60–1, 66
phobic disorder 20
physical activities *see* exercise therapies
physical health and depression 145
physical illnesses 6–7, 18, 55–6, 127–40, 144–56
  assessment and identification 127, 131–3,
    146
  conditions
    bone and joint disease 130
    cancer 7, 129–30
    cardiovascular disease 6–7, 21, 28–9,
      128
    chronic obstructive airways disease
      (COPD) 128
    genito-urinary disorders 131
    neurodegenerative diseases 7, 30, 69,
      130
    stroke 7, 21, 28–9, 129, 149–50
  investigations and tests 4, 10–11, 19–20, 133
  management approaches 154–5
  pharmacological management issues 69,
    133–40, 148, 149
  use of ECT 97–8, 138–9, 148
platelet activation 145
policy guidance 221–2
prescribing practices 62–3, 139

prevalence studies
  for depression 5, 54–5, 126–7
  see also epidemiological studies
prevention initiatives 213–15
  see also health promotion
primary care issues 161–9
  challenges 165–6
  contexts 161–3
  depression course and outcomes 163–5
    management approaches 167
  good practice components 166–7
  use of collaborative approaches 168
  see also GP consultations
psychiatric referrals 139
psychoanalysis 111, 113–14
psychological treatments, *see also*
  psychotherapies
psychoneuroimmunology 248–9
psychosis
  assessment tools 185
  nurse interventions 183–9
  prevalence 183
psychosocial factors 37–8
  bereavement 9, 18, 38
  role of nurses 183–9
  social isolation 37–8
  social withdrawal 18
psychotherapies 108–22
  guidelines 64
  models and approaches 110–15
    cognitive behavioural therapy 111, 112,
      117, 118
    culturally specific 237–8
    interpersonal therapy 111, 112, 117–21
    life review therapy 111, 114
    psychoanalysis 111, 113–14
  use with older people 115–16, 217–18
    case studies 116–21

quality of life 218–19
Quality and Outcomes Framework (QOF) 162
quetiapine 88

race relations 231
raloxifene 71
rating scales *see* diagnostic instruments;
  screening measures
reboxetine 62
Recovery Model 217
relapse prevention 189
religious beliefs 37–8, 243–51
  coping mechanisms 244
  faith-based support groups 221
  impact on mental health 245–6
  impact on physical health 246–7
  measurement and assessment 244–5

mechanisms 247–9
  possible clinical applications 249–50
religious struggle 246
repetitive transcranial magnetic stimulation
  (rTMS) 73, 103
reserpine 36
residential care homes 213
  and depression 5, 127–8
reversible inhibitors of monoamine oxidase
  (RIMA) 61, 66
rheumatoid arthritis 130
RIMA see reversible inhibitors of monoamine
  oxidase
risk factors for depression 20
risperidone 71, 88
roles and expectations
  motivation issues 195, 196–7
  routines and habits 197–8
  skills 198
  social environments 195–6, 218–19
routines and habits 197–8

St John's Wort 62, 137–8
SAP see Single Assessment Process
schizoaffective disorder 183
schizophrenia 183–4
  see also psychosis
screening measures
  for depression 10–11, 19–20
    guidelines 64
selective serotonin reuptake inhibitors (SSRIs)
  57–9, 66, 71, 90, 134–5
  combination therapies 72–3
  side-effects 135–6
self-assessment measures 4
self-harming 10
self-help programmes 111, 113
  guidelines 64
self-identity, and roles 197–8
sensory impairments 130–1
serotonin and noradrenaline reuptake
  inhibitors (SNRIs) 59–60, 66–7, 136
  contraindications 136
sertraline 57–9, 66, 135
service users 218–20
  establishing needs and wants 220–1
  involvement and choice 221–3
Short-CARE schedule 4
SIADH 135
Single Assessment Process (SAP) 176–7, 188,
  213
skills and roles 198
sleep disturbances 2–3, 18–19
SNRIs see serotonin and noradrenaline
  reuptake inhibitors
social environment, and ageing 195–6

Social Functioning Scale 185
social isolation 37–8
social services 205–15
  background and context 205–7
  entitlement to support 208–12
  joint working 207–8
  partnership working 214–15
  preventative measures 213–15
  residential care homes 213
  user engagement initiatives 223–5
social withdrawal
  and depression 18
  disengagement mechanisms 197–8
somatoform disorders and depression 150–4
spirituality 243–51
  impact on mental health 245–6
  impact on physical health 246–7
  measurement and assessment 244–5
  mechanisms 247–9
  possible clinical applications 249–50
SSRIs see selective serotonin reuptake
  inhibitors
statins 36
steroids 36
stroke and depression 7, 21, 28–9, 129, 149–50
  treatments 149–50
substance-induced depression 18, 35–7
subsyndromal depression 19
suicide risk
  bipolar disorder 91
  depression 3, 10, 20
Sure Start programmes 219, 223
syncope 134

tachycardia 135
tamoxifen 36
temporal lobe atrophy 33
Tidal model 21
tranylcypromine 60–1, 66
trazodone 66
treatment-resistant depression 69–73
tricyclic antidepressants (TCAs) 56–7, 65–6,
  134–5
  combination therapies 72–3
  with Parkinson's disease 148
trimipramine 134
tryptophan 137

ulcer healing drugs 36
unipolar disorder 22
  aetiology 27
user involvement initiatives 223–5

vagal nerve stimulation 73, 103
valproate 37, 85
  adverse effects 85

valproate (*continued*)
   dosages 87
   efficacy 85
   mode of action 85
vascular dementia 130
'vascular depression' 21, 35
vascular disease 28–9
   brain structure changes 33–5
venlafaxine 59–60, 67, 71, 136
   combination therapies 72
   contraindications 136

ventricular volume changes 31–3
vigabatrin 37
violence and abuse issues 219
vitamin B_{12} 133

'watchful waiting', guidelines 64
weight loss 2, 18
Wesley, Mary 196
white matter hypertensities 33–5
Who Cares Wins (RCP 2005) 145